Skin Cancer

2nd edition

An illustrated guide to the aetiology, clinical features, pathology and management of benign and malignant cutaneous tumours

Skin Cancer

2nd edition

An illustrated guide to the aetiology, clinical features, pathology and management of benign and malignant cutaneous tumours

Rona M MacKie

MD, DSC, FRCP London and Glasgow, FRCPath, FRSE

Professor of Dermatology, University of Glasgow
Honorary Consultant Dermatologist, Greater Glasgow
Health Board
Western Infirmary, Glasgow, and Royal Hospital for
Sick Children, Glasgow
Honorary member of French, German, Dutch,
Italian, Polish and Swedish Dermatological Societies
President, British Association of Dermatologists

MARTIN DUNITZ

© **Rona M MacKie 1989, 1996**

First published in the United Kingdom in 1989
by Martin Dunitz Ltd, 7–9 Pratt Street, London NW1 0AE

Second edition 1996

A CIP record for this book is available from the British Library

ISBN 1-85317-203-0

Composition by Scribe Design, Gillingham, Kent
Originated, Printed and Bound in Singapore by Toppan Printing Company (S) Pte Ltd

Contents

Introduction

Since the first edition of *Skin Cancer* was published in 1989 there has been a continuous increase in the incidence of skin cancers annually. The problem of skin cancer is being increasingly recognized at national and intenational level; in the UK, the government's *Health of the Nation* document sets out a target of halting the year-on-year rise in the incidence of skin cancers by the year 2005.

For these reasons and others, the second edition of *Skin Cancer* has been revised and updated in the hope that it will be of value to a wider audience. In particular I hope that those involved in primary care, including general practitioners, will find it useful. Chapter 15 has been rewritten and expanded in the hope that those concerned with achieving a reduction in the incidence of skin cancers will consider the value of early detection and primary prevention in their everyday practice in many parts of the world.

R.M.M. 1995

1
Skin biology

Within the epidermis, dermis and skin appendages, there is a very wide range of cell types. On basic biological principles, any cell that is capable of entering mitosis and dividing is potentially capable of malignant change due to faulty programming during cell division. The range of cutaneous malignancies is thus very extensive, ranging from the common so-called basal cell carcinoma to the much rarer skin appendage tumours and soft tissue tumours found in the dermis.

Benign proliferation of one of the many cell types found in the epidermis and dermis is an even commoner event. The range here includes congenital naevoid or hamartomatous lesions, acquired naevoid lesions and proliferations commonly associated with aging skin. Epidermal proliferation stimulated by the human papilloma virus – warts – is possibly the commonest benign skin tumour, and many studies are in progress investigating the role of the human papilloma virus as a possible carcinogen or co-carcinogen in various types of cutaneous and mucosal malignancy.

Both benign and malignant skin tumours are logically classified according to their cell of origin, and these cell types in turn may be grouped according to their location in the epidermis, the dermis, or one of the skin appendages. The main types of skin appendage are the apocrine and eccrine sweat glands, and the pilosebaceous apparatus, which comprises the hair follicle, sebaceous gland and arrector pili muscle.

The epidermis

The keratinocyte

Within the epidermis (Figures 1.1 and 1.2) the predominant cell is the keratinocyte. This is a terminally differentiated cell of ectodermal origin. Differentiation is seen commencing with the basal cells situated in the deepest parts of the epidermis. The basal cells are the only keratinocytes seen to divide in normal epidermis, and there is continuing controversy as to whether or not all basal cells are capable of division, or if there is within the basal cell population a subset of stem cells that are specifically committed to epidermal renewal.[1] Stem cells are defined as a subpopulation of cells capable of division almost indefinitely, and mathematical models of cell division suggest that not all basal cells are in this category. Recently, attention has switched from the basal layer to the bulge area of the hair follicle adjacent to the insertion of the arrector pili muscle. There is in this area a slowly cycling morphologically primitive label-retaining population that has many of the characteristics of stem cells.[2] Further studies are in progress to try to establish whether or not these cells are stem cells either for the hair follicle area or for a larger population. Within the basal layer, dividing basal cells leave one daughter cell in the basal layer, and the other cell resulting from division is then committed to terminal differentiation. The middle zone of the epidermis, best seen in the thicker epidermis of the palms of the hand and soles of the feet, is composed of polygonal keratinocytes adhering one to the other as a result of a specialized type of intercellular adhesion, the desmosome (Figure 1.3). Desmosomes form junctions between the epithelial cells and help to explain the resilience and plasticity of normal epidermis.

The granular layer in the upper epidermal area marks the critical transition zone between living keratinocytes and the anuclear cornified layer or stratum corneum. The granular layer is so named

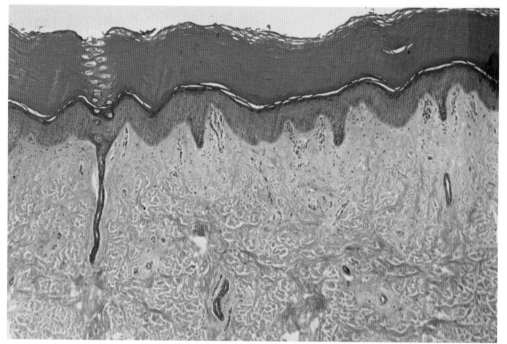

Figure 1.1 Normal epidermis, sole of foot, showing outer cornified layer, granular layer, prickle cell layer and underlying dermis.

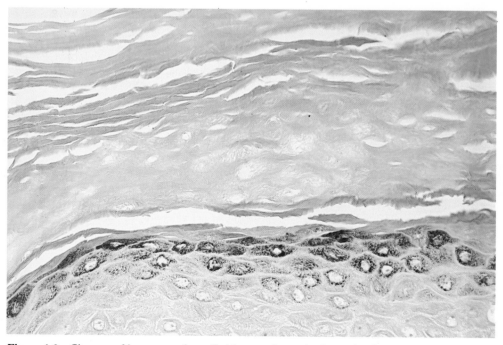

Figure 1.2 Close-up of lower part of cornified layer and granular layer, showing granules composed of disintegrating nuclei.

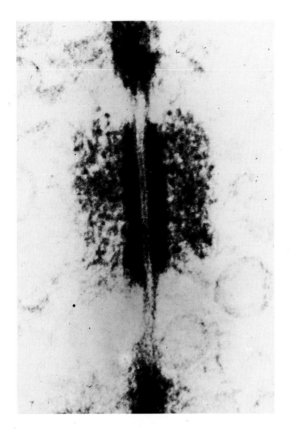

because of the presence of keratohyaline granules seen in the cytoplasm. These granules are the remnants of keratinocyte nuclei, and above this layer the stratum corneum is composed of anucleated dead cells. These non-nucleated cell 'ghosts' form orthokeratotic epidermis (see Figure 1.2). In some pathological situations parakeratotic epidermis is formed (Figure 1.4). This consists of an outer layer of stratum corneum which has retained nuclei, and may be seen in an interesting regular alternating pattern in actinic keratoses (see page 82). In certain body sites, such as on some mucosal surfaces inside the mouth, parakeratotic epithelium is the normal physiological appearance.

The thickness of the cornified layer varies greatly with body site and, clearly, specific site adaptation is important in epidermal differentiation. Areas such as the inner surface of the upper arm have a very thin stratum corneum, while areas such as the palms of the hands and soles of the feet have a very much thicker

Figure 1.3 Ultrastructural view of desmosome, showing the complex structure by which adjacent keratinocytes adhere one to the other.

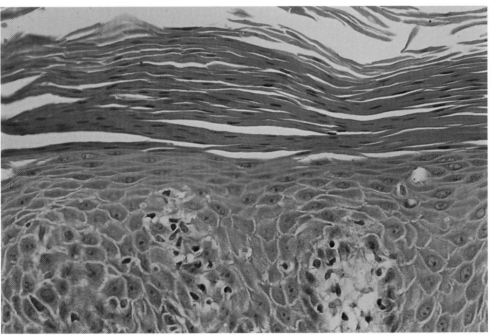

Figure 1.4 Pathological parakeratosis. Note the presence of nuclei in the outer layers. The granular layer is absent.

outer epidermal layer. This pattern of anatomical site adaptation breaks down in many benign, premalignant and malignant keratinocyte-derived epidermal skin tumours. An example of this is the striking hyperkeratosis frequently seen in the premalignant actinic keratosis (see Chapter 6).

Another important feature giving rise to variation in thickness of the entire epidermis, not just the stratum corneum, is the age of the subject from which the epidermis is taken. There is a decrease in epidermal thickness with age,[3] and some evidence to suggest that this change in epidermal thickness also varies according to the quantity of previous exposure to the sun of the site in question.[4,5]

The keratins synthesized within the epidermal keratinocytes are members of the intermediate filament family, and are the structural proteins which provide the protective cytoskeleton within keratinocytes. Keratins coexist in pairs, each being a member of the type I or type II keratin class. In the normal basal layer, there is strong expression of keratins 5 and 14, while in the suprabasal layers there is expression of keratins 1 and 10. Expression of keratin is associated with rapidly dividing cells, but as yet there is no pattern of expression of keratins which is exclusively and specifically associated with any form of cutaneous malignancy.

Non-keratinocyte epidermal cells

There are three other cell types currently recognized in the epidermis. These are the melanocyte, the Langerhans cell and the Merkel cell.

The melanocytes are mainly situated within the basal and suprabasal layers of the epidermis. They are dendritic cells of neuroectodermal derivation, and have the ability to synthesize melanin pigment, which is subsequently distributed to surrounding keratinocytes as melanosomes or melanin granules. These melanin granules tend to cluster above the nucleus of keratinocytes, particularly in skin that has been exposed to sun. This pattern of pigment distribution, together with the fact that melanin synthesis is stimulated by ultraviolet (UV) exposure, gives rise to the theory that the function of melanin pigment is to protect dividing cells from UV radiation. This theory does not explain all the known facts about melanin and recently some interesting additional theories have been advanced.[6] A recent observation of clinically normal skin and vitiliginous skin from the same individual suggests that the protective effect of melanin against UV radiation may not be its only function.[7] (Vitiligo

is the condition in which there is a localized absence of melanocytes in the epidermis, causing a lack of ability to tan.) If melanocytes and melanin pigment were the only photoprotective mechanisms in the epidermis, then one might anticipate that on areas of skin on which vitiligo had been present for many years the incidence of skin malignancy would be high. In fact the incidence of skin malignancy is no different in areas of vilitigo in comparison with adjacent areas of normally pigmented skin. This observation does not apply to albino skin, in which the incidence of non-melanoma skin cancer is greatly increased.[8]

The ratio of melanocytes to basal-layer keratinocytes varies according to body site, age, and degree of exposure to the sun.[9] Traditionally, counting of numbers of melanocytes in histological sections has been carried out on the conventional vertical sections of epidermis. This method allows the ratio of melanocytes to basal-layer keratinocytes to be calculated. An alternative method of studying melanocytes is to use epidermal sheet preparations, which are obtained by separating the epidermis from the underlying dermis by a variety of methods, such as incubation of whole skin in sodium bromide. The horizontal spread of epidermis thus obtained allows calculations to be made on the number of melanocytes per unit of horizontal surface area of the skin under study.

The presence in the melanocyte of the enzyme tyrosinase and its capacity to catalyse synthesis of melanin protein from tyrosine is utilized in the specific dopa staining techniques used to identify melanocytes. It must be emphasized that it is the demonstration of the capacity to produce melanin pigment that proves that a cell is a melanocyte, not merely the presence of melanin pigment, which can be taken up by a variety of cell types.

The Langerhans cell is the second major dendritic cell type recognized within human epidermis.[10] It is derived from the bone marrow,[11] and is found mainly at a higher level within the epidermis than is the melanocyte. Until recently, Langerhans cells could be positively identified only at the ultrastructural level by recognition of the specific Langerhans cell or Birbeck granule within the cytoplasm of the cell (Figure 1.5). This granule has a distinctive tennis-racquet-like shape. The function of the granule is unknown. More recently the availability of monoclonal antibodies of the CD 1 group, which recognize Langerhans cell surface membrane determinants, has made it possible to use the immunofluorescence and immunoperoxidase techniques to identify Langerhans cells (Figure 1.6). These antibodies have stimulated a flood of papers on Langerhans cells in a wide variety of benign and

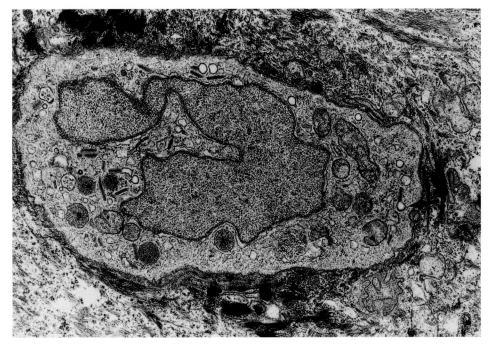

Figure 1.5 Ultrastructure of Langerhans cell showing classic Birbeck granules (tennis-racquet-shaped structures in the cytoplasm, arrow).

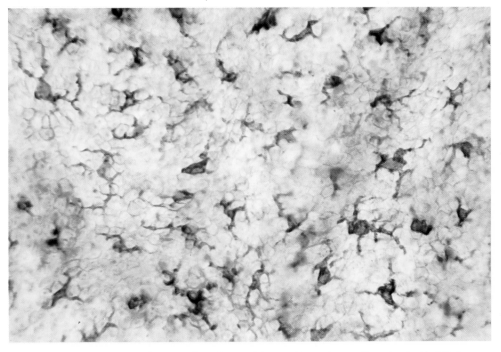

Figure 1.6 Horizontal-spread preparation of normal human Langerhans cells stained with CD 1 monoclonal antibody.

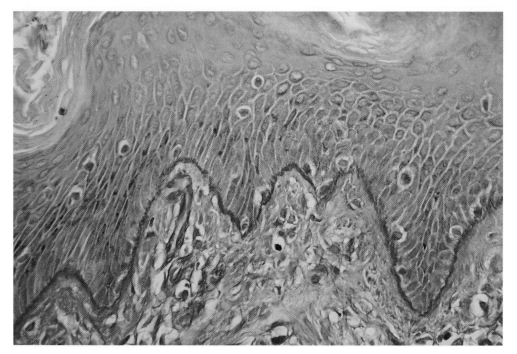

Figure 1.7   Periodic acid–Schiff stained basement membrane.

malignant skin tumours. As with the melanocyte, both vertical and horizontal epidermal section methods have been used to quantitate Langerhans cells.

The function of the Langerhans cell is still a matter of some discussion. In 1973, Silberberg[12] reported that, on ultrastructural study, patients with contact dermatitis showed lymphocytes in the epidermis in contact with apparently damaged Langerhans cells. This observation was the start of a period of intense study of the Langerhans cell and its possible role in contact dermatitis. The Langerhans cell carries surface antigens of the HLA-Dr series, is an immunologically competent cell, and is capable of antigen presentation. Thus, a physiological role in the immune function of the epidermis seems likely.

In the past it has been suggested that the Langerhans cell may also play an additional role in the control of keratinization, in view of the fact that in the mouse tail there are striking variations in the number of Langerhans cells between areas of epidermis that are orthokeratotic and areas of epidermis that are parakeratotic – areas in which there is no granular layer and the outer layer of the epidermis retains nuclei. At present there is little evidence of such a role in humans.

One of the problems of further functional studies of the Langerhans cell is the difficulty of isolating a pure preparation of Langerhans cells from a whole epidermal population, and of establishing and maintaining Langerhans cells in culture. Langerhans cells are also involved in histiocytosis X (see page 238).

The Merkel cell[13] was identified over a century ago, and in mammals is related to the hair disc.[14] In humans it is thought to be a mechanoreceptor, and a member of the APUD system (amine precursor uptake and decarboxylation). The putative Merkel cell tumour is discussed in Chapter 13.

The basement membrane

Dividing the epidermis and dermis is the basement membrane. This membrane is not rigid, and cells can move freely across this complex multilayered structure. It is not easily seen in preparations using the conventional haematoxylin and eosin stain, but is clearer if a stain such as periodic acid–Schiff is used (Figure 1.7). The importance of the basement membrane in the context of cutaneous malignancy is that it is not an absolute barrier, and the presence or absence of a basement membrane beneath an area of possible epidermal malignancy does not in itself prove the benign or invasive nature of the epidermal lesion.

The dermis

The dermis is composed of fibrous, filamentous and amorphous connective tissue, in which the three predominant cell types are the fibroblast, the macrophage and the mast cell.

The fibroblast is responsible for collagen synthesis and is found in large numbers in the dermis in all body sites. Type III collagen is the variety found in greatest quantity in the dermis and accounts for 75 per cent of the dry weight of the dermis. Type IV collagen is an important component of the basement membrane, which separates the dermis from the epidermis.

The second cell type, the macrophage, is derived from the circulating monocyte, and is a terminally differentiated cell.

The third cell type is the mast cell, which has long been recognized as an important cell in type I hypersensitivity reactions on account of its rich supply of intracytoplasmic heparin granules. In addition, however, there is currently considerable interest in a further role of the mast cell in fibrotic processes such as keloids and chronic graft versus host disease.[15,16]

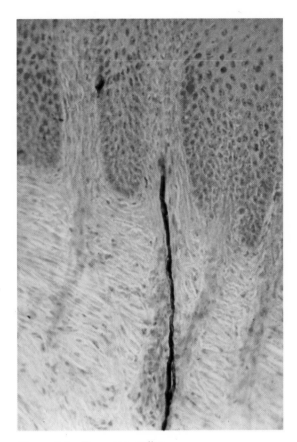

Figure 1.8 Free nerve ending.

The vasculature

The vascular supply to the dermis is from a rich capillary network forming the superficial and deep capillary plexus. The epidermis has no blood vessels actually within its substance, and draws nutrients from the capillaries in the papillary dermis. There are, therefore, large numbers of vascular endothelial cells in the dermis which can give rise to both benign and malignant proliferation. In the ascending arteriole there is a shunt mechanism called the glomus body, which can give rise to one of the spontaneously painful tumours of the dermis, the glomus tumour (Chapter 13).

In the deeper layers of the dermis there is a rich lymphatic system, which is responsible for draining tissue fluid. This lymphatic system is not easily identified on microscopy of clinically normal skin, and tends to be seen only in areas of chronic oedema. Benign lymphatic proliferation is seen in lymphangioma and, rarely, in a malignant situation such as the lymphangiosarcoma.

The dermal nerve supply

The skin is an important sensory organ and there are therefore large numbers of sensory nerves within the dermis. The number of nerve endings varies according to body site, being maximal on face and fingertips and less numerous on areas such as the lower back. Nerve endings may be simple free nerve twigs (Figure 1.8), encapsulated endings (Figure 1.9), or complex structures such as the Vater–Pacini corpuscle (Figure 1.10).

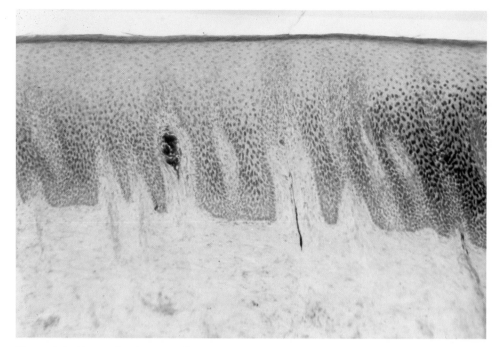

Figure 1.9   Encapsulated nerve ending.

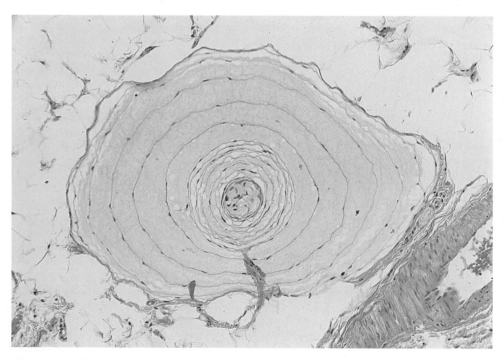

Figure 1.10   Vater–Pacini corpuscle.

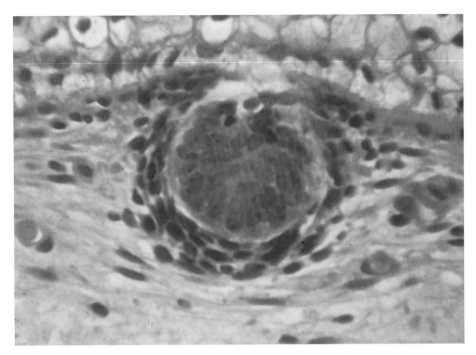

Figure 1.11 Fetal skin at 12 weeks' gestation showing hair germ developing from fetal ectoderm and starting to grow down into the dermis.

The dermis also has a smooth muscle population, both in the arrector pili muscles and in myoepithelial cells surrounding the skin appendages.

The dermis varies considerably in depth according to body site, being thinnest on areas such as the face and backs of the hand, and thickest in areas such as the lower back. The subcutaneous tissue deep in the dermis is composed mainly of fat, and participates in relatively few benign and malignant tumorous processes.

The skin appendages

The skin appendages can be divided logically into the structures associated with the pilosebaceous complex – the hair follicle, the sebaceous gland, the arrector pili muscle, and, in some body sites, the apocrine gland – and those associated with the eccrine sweat glands. It is important to be aware of the normal structure of these appendages, as an extensive array of biologically relatively benign tumours may develop from them. While these tumours are of great interest to the dermatopathologist, they are of relatively little epidemiological significance as their incidence in a large dermatopathology practice has been estimated at 1 in 50 000 specimens. They are, however, of great interest in trying to understand the potential for differentiation which is still present in adult cells in the dermis and epidermis.

The pilosebaceous complex

The hair follicle is an elegant example of interaction between epidermis and dermis. In early fetal life an invagination develops from the primitive ectoderm (developing epidermis) and grows downwards into the dermis to form the hair shaft (Figure 1.11). The dermal component of the hair follicle comprises the dermal papilla, which contains a rich blood supply and which is situated at the base of the epidermal component (Figure 1.12). In adult life the pilosebaceous complex comprises the hair shaft, the sebaceous gland, the arrector pili muscle, and, in some body sites, the apocrine gland (Figure 1.13).

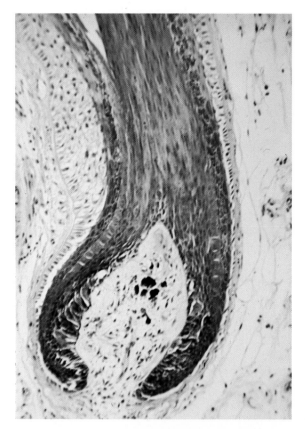

The control of growth of terminal scalp hair from the hair follicle is a poorly understood phenomenon. At any one point in time, approximately 80 per cent of scalp hair follicles are in the growth or anagen phase, and the remaining 20 per cent are either resting – in catagen – or are in the process of shedding the hair shaft – in telogen. Understanding the growth control mechanisms involved in hair follicle activity, and the possible role of growth factors, could well be of some significance in understanding other cellular growth control mechanisms and their abnormalities in both benign and malignant tumours in the skin and other tissues.

Benign and locally invasive tumours of the hair follicle are discussed in Chapter 13, and may arise from the intraepidermal component, the root sheath component, or the deeper area around the dermal papillae.

The sebaceous glands are found in association with hair follicles. On the scalp, the hair follicle is the morphologically predominant component of the complex, the sebaceous gland being present as a relatively small functional unit; on the face and upper back, however, particularly in adolescence, the sebaceous gland forms the larger part of the unit. It

Figure 1.12 Hair root showing hair bulb papilla, which is the dermal component of this structure.

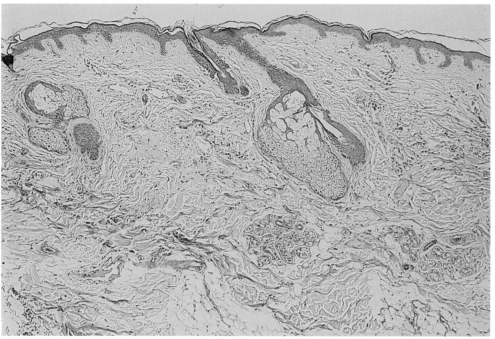

Figure 1.13 The pilosebaceous complex in adult life, showing sebaceous gland draining into hair follicles.

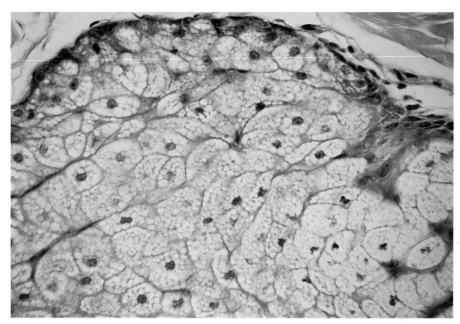

Figure 1.14 High-power view of sebaceous gland cells, showing characteristic foamy cytoplasm.

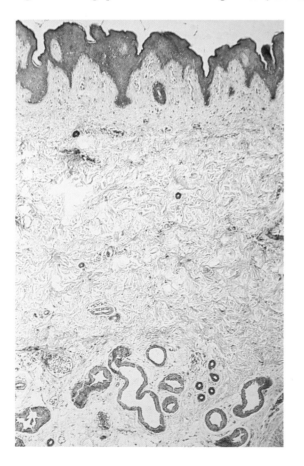

can be recognized as a lobulated structure composed of cells with abundant foamy cytoplasm and small nuclei (Figure 1.14). Sebaceous secretion is formed as a result of breakdown of these cells and is thus termed holocrine secretion. Around these sebaceous gland elements, a small number of myoepithelial cells may be seen. The sebaceous gland constituents discharge into the hair follicle and then pass to the epidermal surface along the hair shaft.

The arrector pili muscle is found in the root sheath at a level in the dermis similar to that of the opening of the sebaceous gland. It varies greatly in size and may be only vestigial in some body sites.

The apocrine glands

In the axilla and groin area apocrine sweat glands also discharge into the pilosebaceous complex. These glands are recognized by the fact that their secretory component is situated deep in the dermis and has an extremely large luminal area (Figure 1.15). The

Figure 1.15 Normal skin from axilla, showing deeply situated cells of the secretory component of the apocrine glands.

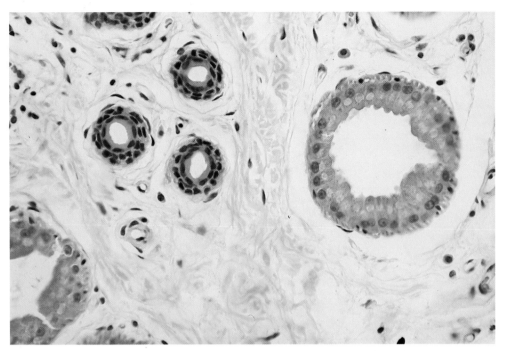

Figure 1.16 The secretory component of the apocrine gland is seen to the right, with the much smaller excretory ducts to the left. The secretory cells show the apocrine type of secretion particularly clearly.

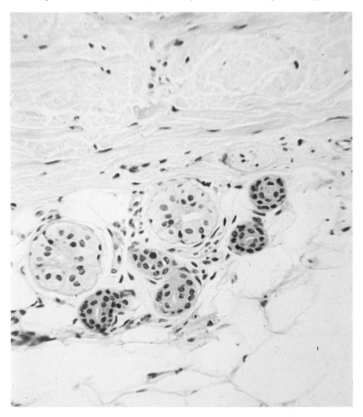

Figure 1.17 Secretory components of the eccrine sweat glands seen at the junction between the dermis and the subcutaneous fat. The larger, paler structures are the secretory elements and the smaller, darker structures just beneath them are the excretory ducts.

glands are lined with conical cells, giving rise in the past to the concept that secretion from these structures was by a nipping-off of cytoplasmic processes – so-called decapitation secretion (Figure 1.16).

The excretory portion of the apocrine glands comprises a series of double-layered tubules of darkly stained cells with a basophilic nucleus and darkly stained cytoplasm. Myoepithelial cells may be seen in small numbers around the secretory component of the apocrine glands.

The eccrine sweat glands (Figure 1.17)

Unlike the apocrine glands the eccrine glands are found in all body sites. Their secretory component is situated in the mid-dermis at a higher level than that at which the apocrine secretory components are found, and in these glands the lumen of the secretory component is very much narrower. Three cell types are found in the secretory element. These are the dark or mucoid cells, which stain positively with periodic acid–Schiff stain, the paler, clearer secretory cells, and the surrounding myoepithelial cells. The excretory component is composed of a bilayered tubular structure that connects directly with the outer epidermal surface.

Tumours of the eccrine sweat apparatus may arise from any of the cell types composing the secretory component, from the intradermal ductal component, or from the intraepidermal ductal component. These are described in Chapter 13.

2
Aetiological factors in cutaneous malignancy

Older laboratory studies on cutaneous carcinogenesis in animal models have relied heavily on chemical carcinogens. More recently, with the growing realization of the importance of natural sunlight as a cutaneous carcinogen in humans, the attention of laboratory workers has turned to UV radiation studies. There is currently great interest in the role of papilloma viruses as carcinogens or co-carcinogens on both skin and mucous membrane surfaces.

Chemical carcinogens
Ultraviolet radiation
Ionizing radiation
Topical cytotoxic drugs
The human papilloma viruses
Human immunodeficiency virus and malignancy
The significance of activated oncogene detection
Immunological aspects of cutaneous carcinogenesis

Chemical carcinogens

A traditional approach to the study of carcinogenesis in general is the use of animal models and the application of putative carcinogens to their epidermal surface. This has resulted in the identification of a very large number of chemical carcinogens.[1] The most common animal model is the mouse, and the usual pattern of observed changes is the development of multiple squamous papillomas and keratoacanthoma-like lesions after a relatively short period of time during which the carcinogen is applied topically at regular intervals. A proportion of these squamous

papillomas then regress spontaneously, and a smaller proportion go on to develop the cytological criteria of malignancy. It is, however, unusual for papillomas developed in this way to metastasize, although they may become locally invasive.

From models of this type have developed some of the current theories of carcinogenesis. Up to the present, three stages of progression have been identified. These are initiation, promotion, and frank carcinogenesis. A list of chemicals that are recognized as initiators is shown in Table 2.1, together with a list of recognized promoters. It should be noted that for a promoter to be effective it must act on previously initiated cells.

It is important to be aware that studies of chemical carcinogenesis have been carried out on relatively

Table 2.1 Recognized initiators and promoters of cutaneous carcinogenesis used in dermatological therapy.

Initiators	Promoters
Polycyclic aromatic hydrocarbons (tar)	Phenol
Quinolones	Phorbol esters
Nitrogen mustard	Anthralin
Psoralens	Benzoyl peroxide

UV radiation, mainly UVB, is considered to be both an initiator and a promoter.

small numbers of inbred strains of laboratory mice.[2] A particular strain commonly used in these studies is the sencar mouse. This is chosen because of its unusual sensitivity to carcinogens. These genetic factors, together with the facts that in humans there is no immediately obvious clinical equivalent of the regressing squamous papilloma and that much the commonest skin tumour is basal cell carcinoma, should be considered carefully when relating reports of chemical carcinogens in animal models to the human situation.

It is understood that in the course of initiation the cells in the tissue to which the initiating agent is applied undergo a basic change in DNA configuration which is thereafter permanent.[3] Subsequent progression to malignancy is not inevitable and the initiated cells may remain further unchanged throughout the lifetime of the tissue in question. In a number of initiated cells the presence of an activated *ras* oncogene has recently been recognized.

A functional and morphological correlate of the initiated cell is the fact that cells that are normally terminally differentiated lose this pattern of differentiation and retain their ability to divide. This pattern may be seen morphologically in actinic keratoses where suprabasal mitoses are present. The epidermis in psoriasis shares many features in common with initiated cells.

Promoters

Materials which act as promoters tend to cause inflammation and hyperplasia, although these two features are not invariably associated with promoting activity. Promotion is a reversible phenomenon, and the visible effects of a promoter may disappear when the stimulus is withdrawn. The phorbol esters, which are found in croton oil and include TPA,[4] are a group of promoters which have been used in the past in very large numbers of animal experiments. New developments in molecular biology in the past 5 years have recognized the existence of a receptor for phorbol ester on the cell membrane. This is protein kinase C, and the presence of phorbol ester activates this enzyme,[5] causing addition of phosphate groups to serine residues in specific protein substrate. The endogenous activator of protein kinase C is diacylglycerol, and protein kinase C participates in a second messenger system,[6] regulating the response to a number of hormones at the intracellular level. There is

currently great interest in the role of G proteins in this situation.[7] It can be seen in Table 2.1 that a number of substances recognized as initiators and/or promoters are found in regular therapeutic use in clinical dermatology. Tar, traditionally used in the treatment of psoriasis, contains polycyclic aromatic hydrocarbons, which are well-established initiating agents. Similarly, nitrogen mustard, which is used topically in the management of cutaneous T-cell lymphoma, is a recognized initiator. On the basis of animal studies UV light is thought to act as both an initiator and a promoter.

Promoters used therapeutically in dermatology include the anthralin group of preparations, used in the management of psoriasis, and benzoyl peroxide, used topically in the treatment of acne.[8] Recently there has been some concern about the effect of benzoyl peroxide and its use in patients, in view of the fact that one report suggests that benzoyl peroxide is a complete carcinogen,[9] that is, it can act as both initiator and promoter. It is important to recognize that this is an isolated report, and that the animal model studied was the sencar mouse. A recent epidemiological study looking at the incidence of melanoma in acne patients and appropriate controls has shown no increased incidence of this type of cutaneous malignancy in the acne group.[10] Obviously, this is reassuring. Nevertheless, the number of recognized partial or complete carcinogens used in therapeutic dermatology should give cause for thought, particularly with regard to the combinations and sequences in which they are used. For example, it could theoretically be argued that tar followed by anthralin treatment in psoriasis would be likely to lead to an increased incidence of malignancy, as in this example an initiator is followed by a promotor. However, as with acne, recent studies on the incidence of all types of cutaneous malignancy in patients with psoriasis who have been treated with these preparations over many years do not suggest that their long-term clinical use is associated with an increased incidence of malignancy.[11]

The study of chemical carcinogens has to date failed to identify chemicals that give rise to useful working models of either basal cell carcinoma or malignant melanoma. In the case of malignant melanoma, dimethyl benzanthracene does give rise to melanocytic lesions, particularly if applied to the skin of albino guinea pigs.[12] The majority of these lesions, however, appear to have the characteristics of blue naevi, and very few metastasize and kill the host.

Ultraviolet radiation

The classic experiments on the exposure of mouse skin to repeated doses of UV radiation and observation of the development of squamous cell cancer were carried out by Blum in the 1940s.[13] These experiments were the first to demonstrate the cumulative nature of UV damage, an observation which also holds good in clinical situations but is not widely appreciated by the general public.

In humans, epidemiological studies from all parts of the world strongly suggest that the most important aetiological factor for all types of cutaneous malignancy is UV radiation.[14] This evidence relates to the fact that in white-skinned populations the incidence of non-melanoma skin cancer and melanoma increases in a direct linear fashion with proximity to the Equator. In the case of non-melanoma skin cancer there is clear evidence that a quantitative relationship exists between lifetime sun exposure and risk of developing non-melanoma skin cancer. The most common sites of these lesions, on the head and neck and backs of the hands, also correlate well with the sites of maximum chronic sun exposure in outdoor workers. This pattern may change over the next few years as chronic sun exposure becomes less of an occupational and more of a recreational phenomenon.

For malignant melanoma, the evidence is rather more complex: there are epidemiological studies suggesting that episodes of short, intense sun exposure on skin that is normally protected from UV radiation constitute a significant risk factor. In addition, however, there is growing evidence, particularly from Australia and Western Canada, that there is a quantitative relationship between lifetime sun exposure and increased risk of developing malignant melanoma.[15,16]

All types of cutaneous malignancy are relatively rare in the dark skin of those of Afro-Caribbean ethnic descent. In large cities in the USA the incidence of malignant melanoma in the black-skinned population is approximately one-tenth that of the white-skinned population living in the same environment and having a similar lifestyle. Further evidence of the efficacy of melanin as a partial photoprotective agent comes from studies of albinos. In the African countries albinos have a very high incidence of cutaneous malignancy, mainly non-melanoma skin cancer, early in life. The malignancies on albino skin are actinic keratoses and squamous cell carcinoma, and occur almost exclusively on sun-exposed sites.[17] This high incidence of non-melanoma skin cancer in albinos contrasts with the lack of reports of non-melanoma skin cancer in those with vitiligo (see Chapter 1, page 4).

Depletion of the ozone layer[18]

There is considerable concern about the depletion of the ozone layer by a number of environmental chemicals (see Chapter 8). The ozone layer acts as a very powerful barrier in absorbing a proportion of UV radiation emanating from the sun and preventing it reaching the earth's surface. The chemicals responsible for the depletion of this ozone layer are chlorofluorocarbons (CFCs), which are found in the gases from refrigerators and in aerosol sprays. Reports indicate that the depletion of ozone over the southern hemisphere in the winter of 1993 was the most severe yet recorded.[19,20] It is, however, unlikely that the depletion of the ozone layer can be solely responsible for the rapid rise in both non-melanoma skin cancer and melanoma seen over the past 30 years, as it is estimated that before 1960 the amount of CFC escaping into the atmosphere was negligible. Since the mid-1970s, when the hazards of CFCs became apparent, a number of governments, including those of Scandinavia and parts of the USA, have taken action to reduce the amount of CFC escaping into the atmosphere. Current mathematical models suggest that it will take upwards of 50 years for the full effect of the depletion of the ozone layer to become apparent in the form of increased incidence of all types of cutaneous malignancy. Moan and Dahlbeck[21] have calculated on the basis of differing incidence figures for skin cancer in northern and southern Norway that 10 per cent ozone depletion will result in a 16–18 per cent rise in the incidence of squamous cell carcinoma in both sexes, a 19 per cent rise in melanoma in males and a 32 per cent rise in melanoma in females. Agreed international control of environmental pollution is required, but the combination of increased UV radiation striking the earth's surface because of a depleted ozone layer and changing habits of sun exposure will cause problems in terms of allotting responsibility for increased incidence of cutaneous malignancy in humans.

Therapeutic UVB radiation and skin cancer

Although UVB from artificial light sources has long been recognized as an important cutaneous carcinogen in the hairless mouse, and natural sunlight is recognized as an important carcinogen in humans, there are very few reports of therapeutic artificial UVB radiation causing malignancy. Thus there is a lack of reports of cutaneous malignancy in patients who have received UVB therapy in the past for both acne vulgaris and psoriasis. One clinical situation in which squamous cell cancer has been reported is in the scars of lupus vulgaris. It is, however, unclear whether the malignancy in this situation is associated with scar formation or is associated with past therapy with high but, in general, poorly quantified levels of UV radiation from a Kromeyer lamp.

Photochemotherapy with UVA[22]

Since the mid-1970s, the use of photochemotherapy in the form of oral psoralen and UVA (PUVA) has created a new iatrogenic potential carcinogen. PUVA is currently fairly widely used in the management of resistant plaque psoriasis, and also in the management of some patients with cutaneous T-cell lymphoma. Other less common indications for PUVA therapy include resistant atopic dermatitis and vitiligo. Since its introduction, the majority of patients receiving PUVA have been carefully monitored, as it was recognized from the beginning that this was a potentially carcinogenic form of therapy. Stern has published three important reports. The first, in 1979, suggested that in the USA, patients receiving PUVA did have a higher incidence of squamous cell carcinoma, and that the usual ratio of basal cell carcinoma to squamous cell carcinoma (normally 2 : 1) was reversed.[23] In this paper it was emphasized that those patients who developed squamous cell carcinoma had, without exception, received other carcinogens prior to starting PUVA therapy. These included X-ray and oral arsenic therapy. It was thus suggested that PUVA itself was not acting as a complete carcinogen but only as a co-carcinogen in association with other materials. However, in 1984 Stern published a second paper suggesting, on a longer follow-up of a larger number of patients, that PUVA itself could act as a complete carcinogen.[24] The risk of squamous cell carcinoma developing in this population 25 months after PUVA therapy was commenced was 13 times higher in those patients receiving high doses of UVA than in those receiving lower doses. No significant dose-related increase was noted for basal cell carcinoma. The disturbing factor in this report was that of squamous cell carcinoma developing in patients without a previous history of skin cancer or exposure to other cutaneous carcinogens. The most recent and worrying US report records metastatic spread of PUVA-induced squamous cell carcinoma in 7 of 1389 patients on long-term follow-up.[25]

Studies in Europe initially appeared to produce less disturbing results.[26] The European PUVA study reported first on 418 patients. In this group 9 patients who developed cutaneous malignancies were detected over a mean observation period of 8 years. These 9 patients developed 14 malignancies – 6 squamous cell carcinomas and 8 basal cell carcinomas. All the patients with malignancies had a history of previous X-ray or arsenic therapy. In a further, more extensive study,[27] 1643 patients have been followed, mainly in Germany and Austria, for an average observation period of 96 months. Thirty-six patients have been identified with 40 squamous cell carcinomas and 23 basal cell carcinomas. This European study failed to demonstrate a clinically-relevant increase in the risk of tumours induced by PUVA alone, with no history of previous use of other carcinogens, and has also failed to show a clear relationship between total PUVA dose and tumour development. All patients with tumours had been exposed to other carcinogens before the start of PUVA. The carcinogens associated with subsequent malignancy development after commencing PUVA were arsenic, methotrexate and X-ray therapy. In contrast, patients with a past history of UVB and/or tar therapy did not have a greater than expected incidence of malignancies.

These initially differing reports from the USA and Europe were explained by differences in approach to PUVA therapy. In the USA, the general policy has been to give frequent PUVA treatments with low doses of UVA treatment on each occasion. In other words, a given total dose of UVA is spread over a larger number of treatments. In contrast, in Europe the tendency has been to give higher doses at each individual treatment. There are theoretical reasons associated with DNA repair and reciprocity failure to suggest that a regime which gives higher doses of UVA at each individual treatment session but gives a smaller number of actual episodes of treatment may be associated with a greater potential for cells damaged by UV therapy to complete normal repair processes and thus be associated with a lower incidence of associated malignancy.[28] Unfortunately, however, a recent UK report on 69 patients who had received more than 2000 J/cm^2 records an 18 per cent incidence of squamous cell carcinoma[29] in this group, and there are now reports of metastases from PUVA-induced skin cancers. The current treatment implications of these findings are that PUVA should be given only where less aggressive methods of therapy have failed, and only as defined short courses, not as maintenance therapy; that careful records of cumulative total exposure should be kept; and that patients should be either on indefinite follow-up even after stopping PUVA or should be on an at-risk register.

The risk of developing primary cutaneous malignant melanoma in patients receiving long-term PUVA therapy is also at present under careful study. A large proportion of patients receiving PUVA develop striking large stellate freckles on light-exposed skin – so-called PUVA freckles. The pathology of these is that of a lentigo with some degree of melanocyte atypia.[30] Despite this common occurrence, there are at present only three reports of melanoma developing in patients on long-term PUVA therapy. In terms of the numbers of patient years of observation this figure is actually slightly lower than might have been expected in an untreated control population.

UVA as a carcinogen in the absence of psoralen

Both sencar and ordinary albino hairless mice have recently been reported to develop cutaneous malignancies when exposed only to long-wave UVA in the 310–60 nanometre range.[31,32] These are the predominant wavelengths in the UV tubes used in solaria and sunbeds. These data make it highly likely that UVA alone will also be shown to be a carcinogen in humans. Case–control studies carried out on patients with melanoma in Canada,[33] the UK[34] and Sweden[35] all show the use of sunbeds to be a weak but significant risk factor for developing melanoma.

Ionizing radiation

The studies of the risk of cutaneous malignancy associated with PUVA therapy have further stimulated more careful evaluation of the risk of malignancy in other situations. It has been established for many years that X-rays induce cutaneous malignancies in humans, commonly a mixture of basal cell carcinomas and spindle cell squamous cell carcinomas.[36]

Grenz ray therapy has in the past been a popular treatment for benign skin disorders. The Swedish cancer registry has been used to search for an increase of malignancy in 1440 patients who had received Grenz ray therapy between 1949 and 1975. No increase in either melanoma or non-melanoma skin cancer was reported, even in the 481 individuals in this study who had received a high cumulative dose of Grenz rays.[37]

Topical cytotoxic drugs and subsequent cutaneous malignancy

The use of agents that have proved their therapeutic value but also have carcinogenic potential has long been standard practice in cutaneous T-cell lymphoma. For many years topical nitrogen mustard has been recognized as a useful method of controlling this chronic lymphoma (Chapter 11). However, this therapy is also associated with an increased risk of non-melanoma skin cancer.[38] Skin tumours have been reported to develop two years or more after starting topical nitrogen mustard therapy. The range of tumours developing has included squamous cell carcinoma, basal cell carcinoma, keratoacanthoma and actinic keratoses. The striking feature of these tumours is that they have been reported to develop on habitually covered skin, such as the groin.

As such patients are regularly supervised, it would be anticipated that such tumours would be identified and excised at an early stage. There is, however, one report of a cutaneous squamous cell carcinoma metastasizing in such a patient.

The role of papilloma viruses in the aetiology of cutaneous malignancies

The papilloma viruses are a family of double-stranded DNA viruses. They are responsible for warts, and may play a role in some cutaneous malignancies, particularly in those who are immunosuppressed, and in mucosal malignancies. The genes required for replication of human papilloma virus (HPV) DNA are divided into early (E) and late (L) genes. E5, E6 and E7 are thought to be genes associated with malignant transformation, E1 and E2 are involved with simple replication, and L1 and L2 control formation of the capsid of the virion.[39,40] HPV has been difficult to study in vitro, but recent developments in molecular biology, in particular the use of the polymerase chain reaction to amplify minute quantities of HPV DNA (which is extremely stable in formalin-fixed tissue) have accelerated studies aimed at correlating the presence of differing types of HPV DNA with malignancy.

At present over 60 HPV types have been identified by hybridization techniques. They can be broadly divided into three main categories. These are those associated with cutaneous wart infection on the skin of otherwise healthy individuals, those found in oral and genital mucosal tissue (mainly HPV 6, 11, 16 and 18) and those associated with the rare genodermatosis, epidermodysplasia verruciformis (EV) (HPV 5 and 8). HPV 16 and 18 are found in genital malignancies, but not exclusively, whereas HPV 6 and 11 are not found in these malignancies.[41–43] Similarly, virtually all malignancies on the skin of EV patients carry HPV 5 and 8. There is at present great interest in possible interactions between HPV presence and expression of activated oncogenes such as *p53* in the development of cutaneous malignancy with regard to their role as carcinogens or co-carcinogens in a variety of situations,[44] but at present there is little, if any, evidence that in the immunocompetent host HPV acts as either a complete carcinogen or a co-carcinogen, although there have been sporadic case reports of the identification of one or other of the newly identified HPVs in keratoacanthoma, squamous cell carcinoma and actinic keratosis. It must, however, be stressed that these are individual case reports and there is no large series confirming these observations. In the case of the association of certain types of HPV with genital tract malignancy, it must also be noted that, although HPV 16 and 18 have been identified in the genital tracts of patients with both premalignant and malignant dysplasia, particularly of the cervix, control series of women with no such dysplasia have also shown the presence of these two types of HPV.[45]

Malignancy in patients receiving therapeutic immunosuppression

The situation with regard to the presence of various types of HPV and immunosuppression is very different. Careful studies of renal transplant patients in many parts of the world have shown that patients on long-term immunosuppression after receipt of a transplanted kidney are at increased risk of non-Hodgkin's lymphoma and cutaneous malignancy.[46] The cutaneous malignancy is most commonly squamous carcinoma. More recently, careful studies have further shown that patients undergoing therapeutic immunosuppression also have an increased incidence of warts, particularly on sun-exposed sites.[47] There is currently intense interest and speculation as to whether or not the normally more benign types of HPV can act as co-carcinogens in the immunosuppressed host. The identification of HPV 5 in cutaneous lesions of renal transplant patients confirms that the types of HPV present in transplant patients must be monitored with some care.[48]

Human immunodeficiency virus

There are many current studies on the clinical manifestations of infection with the human immunodeficiency virus (HIV) type 1 or human T lymphotropic virus (HTLV) type 3.[49] It is of interest to note that the acquired immunodeficiency syndrome (AIDS) was in fact first clinically recognized in homosexual individuals in New York who suffered from an epidemic type of Kaposi's sarcoma (KS).[50] At the present time the exact relationship between HIV and KS of the epidemic type is not entirely clear. By no means all patients who are HIV-positive develop KS, and KS would appear to be more common in homosexuals who develop AIDS than in individuals from other groups at risk, such as injecting drug users. The fact that as yet no subsection of the population that is not HIV-positive has developed the epidemic type of KS clearly suggests a strong aetiological relationship between the two conditions, but the current epidemiological evidence would suggest that a further co-factor in addition to the presence of HIV-1 is necessary for the development of KS. An excellent recent study suggests that this co-factor may be a newly identified member of the herpes family.[51] There is some evidence that patients with AIDS and concomitant KS have a better prognosis than AIDS patients who do not develop KS. Kaposi's sarcoma of all types is further discussed in Chapter 13.

HTLV-1 is strongly associated with acute T-cell leukaemia, a rare and rapidly progressive form of T-cell malignancy. A cluster of patients has been identified in a small area of Japan all of whom have antibodies to HTLV-1, and an aetiological association is suggested. Early reports suggested that a small proportion of European patients with cutaneous T-cell lymphoma had HTLV-1 antibodies, but more recent studies have found no evidence of HTLV-1 DNA in the skin of patients with cutaneous T-cell lymphoma using the sensitive polymerase chain reaction.[52]

Oncogenes, suppressor genes and cutaneous malignancy[53]

A reasonable working definition of an oncogene is a gene that encodes a protein that contributes to the malignant phenotype of the cell. The first reports of such a gene in a human solid tumour concerned bladder cancer, and involved a single point mutation. Currently, it is believed that oncogenes can act mainly by one of three mechanisms: point mutations, which may result in only one single amino acid substitution; amplification, which involves repetition of DNA sequences and causes over-amplification of the gene product; or chromosomal translocation. This is the transfer of the gene from its normal site to an alternative site, possibly on a different chromosome, and results in altered transcription. *Ras* oncogenes are almost always associated with point mutations, c- and N-*myc* oncogenes with amplification in leukaemias and neuroblastoma, and Burkitt's lymphoma with translocations between chromosomes 8 and 2, 14 or 22.

There are five main functional types of oncogene. These are protein kinases, natural growth factors such as platelet-derived growth factor, receptors such as the receptor for epidermal growth factor (*erbB* oncogene), guanine nucleotide precursors, and chromatin-binding proteins. A development from early work on oncogenes has been the recognition of the role of their normal precursors – proto-oncogenes – as important modulators of growth control in normal tissue. Thus the field of research into growth factor identification and function is closely related to oncogene research.

Suppressor genes which act as stabilizers of the cell are now also recognized, and it is accepted that the stepwise progression to malignancy may involve both activation of oncogenes and also loss of normal suppressor gene function. Two good examples of oncogenes and suppressor genes which appear to play some role in development or control of malignancy in humans are the *ras* family of oncogenes and the gene coding for p53 protein.

Ras oncogenes and cutaneous malignancy

The *ras* family of genes comprises the trio of Harvey, Kirsten and N-*ras*. All of these code for 21-kDa proteins which possess GTPase activity. Mutations in the *ras* family are usually point mutations, most commonly at codons 12 or 61. These point mutations have been identified in a relatively large proportion of human colonic cancers, usually at a late stage in tumour progression.

In cutaneous carcinogenesis, Balmain et al[54] used a mouse model and chemical carcinogens clearly to demonstrate point mutations in Harvey *ras* at an early stage in tumour induction; this work has been confirmed by others. However, in human non-melanoma skin cancer, the picture is less clear, with reports of *ras* mutations ranging from 46 per cent and 31 per cent, respectively, in a series of squamous cell and basal cell carcinomas reported from Texas,[55] to zero in a UK series of basal and squamous cell tumours and Bowen's disease. Two points which may explain these widely discrepant results are, firstly, the very different sun exposure history of patients in Texas and the north of England and, secondly, variations in methodology.

In human malignant melanoma, N-*ras* appears to be more commonly involved than either Harvey or Kirsten *ras*, but mutations are seen in less than 10 per cent of patients and then usually in patients with late-stage disease. Thus these mutations would appear to be a marker of tumour progression and do not appear to be involved in the early development of melanoma in humans.[56–58]

The p53 tumour suppressor gene and skin cancer

p53 is a gene whose normal function is to encode for nuclear phosphoproteins involved in control of the cell cycle. It is a very frequent target for mutations in human cancer, and is located on the short arm of chromosome 17 with 11 exons and 10 introns. *p53* interacts with the E6 protein of human papilloma virus, which may be of importance in some varieties of cutaneous or mucosal malignancy.[59]

The function of normal or wild type *p53* appears to be to allow damaged cells time to repair by delaying progression through the cell cycle and thus preventing expansion of DNA damage. This explains the term 'guardian of the genome' commonly applied to wild-type *p53*. Mutations seen in *p53* appear in some cases to be specific for the damaging agent, e.g. the aflatoxins associated with some types of liver cancer. In humans, Ziegler et al[60] have recorded the association between *p53* damage and C–T or CC–TT mutations. These mutations are associated with UV-induced damage. More recently, Ziegler and colleagues[61] have reported an association between sunburn-induced apoptosis, CC–TT mutations, actinic keratoses and human squamous cell carcinoma. UV exposure appears to induce *p53* mutations in previously normal skin. If wild-type *p53* is inactivated in mouse skin, apoptotic cells are reduced in number after sun exposure, and the assumption is that damaged cells are therefore allowed to replicate and perpetuate DNA damage. *p53* mutations of the same type as those found in squamous cell carcinoma are seen in precursor actinic keratoses, and in some cases loss of one normal allele is recorded in these actinic keratoses. Further UV exposure leads to further UV-induced damage, loss of the remaining normal *p53* allele, and progression to fully established squamous cell carcinoma.

Thus this study is the first to give molecular evidence for the role of UV as both an initiator and a promoter in the induction of squamous cell carcinoma.

The role of *p53* mutations in the initiation and progression of melanoma is not yet clear, and there are conflicting results in the literature concerning their frequency. This may in part be due to technical differences. Many studies have used only *p53* antibodies and immunocytochemical techniques. These are unreliable, and sequencing of *p53* after using the polymerase chain reaction to amplify the relevant areas is more likely to give relevant and accurate results.

Immunological aspects of cutaneous carcinogenesis

The concept that the immune system is of vital importance in the development of malignancy has a long history. There is a very large body of work relating to the detection of an immune response to tumours in experimental animals. The object of this work has been partly that of harnessing such responses in therapy. Both antibody- and cell-mediated cytotoxic antitumour responses have been detected in animal tumours, but in the clinical setting the frequency with which immunological reaction against tumour types is detected and the value to the host in destroying tumour cells is less well established. Macfarlane-Burnett[62] has in the past been a keen advocate of the importance of the immune response to tumours and introduced the concept of immune surveillance – the theory that large numbers of potentially fatal tumours are continually being detected and destroyed by the immune system before they are sufficiently large to permit clinical detection.

There are several areas in which the relevance to cutaneous malignancy of tumour immunology is currently under active investigation. The first is the utilization of large numbers of monoclonal antibodies raised against a wide variety of tumour types.[63] These antibodies can be used in pathological diagnosis or in tumour localization imaging studies.[64,65] Their value in both diagnosis and therapy is discussed in Chapter 3. The use of tumour vaccines in therapy is also a logical sequel to the concept that the human immune system can successfully protect against the development of malignancy. At present these are in active phase 1 trials in humans, mainly in the management of melanoma.

A further exciting area of activity in immunological aspects of malignancy is the investigation, stimulated mainly by the work of Kripke, into the effects of UV radiation on the immune system.[66] Kripke has shown that UV radiation, mainly UVB, has reproducible systemic effects on the murine immune system, giving rise to the proliferation of a subset of suppressor T-lymphocytes. A significant body of work has been carried out in this field since the mid-1970s, but at present its relevance to the human immune situation is not well established. Clearly, the interaction between UV radiation and the immune system is of considerable potential importance in the field of cutaneous malignancy, in which UV radiation is postulated as the main aetiological factor.

3
Diagnosis and management

This chapter covers general points on diagnosis and management in the following areas:

Diagnosis

Clinical diagnosis

Although in many cutaneous tumours the clinical diagnosis is obvious, there are a number of occasions when the differential diagnosis on clinical examination is extensive and includes problems ranging from the harmless basal cell papilloma or seborrhoeic keratosis to the life-threatening nodular melanoma. A good example of a situation in which clinical diagnosis may usually seem straightforward is that of the typical basal cell epithelioma or carcinoma situated adjacent to the inner canthus of the eye with a raised, rolled edge over which capillaries can be seen. Most dermatologists, and many doctors in other specialties, would feel reasonably confident that at least in this field their clinical diagnosis was likely to be correct. Unfortunately this confidence may be misplaced, as recent surveys of the pre-biopsy diagnostic accuracy of trained dermatologists with a special interest in cutaneous malignancy in both basal cell carcinoma[1] and malignant melanoma[2] indicate that even among a group of trained individuals there can be a disturbingly wide margin of error in clinical diagnosis. The problem is much greater in the field of the rare skin appendage tumours and in the dermal or soft tissue group of tumours. The former group tends to be diagnosed preoperatively as atypical clinical presentation of basal cell carcinoma, and for the latter no preoperative clinical diagnosis may be offered.

For these reasons, it is essential that pathological confirmation of a clinical impression be obtained in all skin tumours. Mistakes can be made in both directions, in that benign lesions, such as sclerosing angiomas, may be clinically confused with potentially fatal nodular melanoma and unnecessarily wide surgery carried out, or, in contrast, inadequate surgery may be performed on a malignant tumour. This point is particularly important now that an increasing proportion of minor skin surgery is carried out in the primary care sector. A biopsy or the entire specimen must be sent for pathological assessment, and the individual who performed the procedure must ensure that he or she sees and acts appropriately on the pathologist's report.

Clinical photography

Clinical photography is of value in the field of skin tumours. A useful teaching and learning collection can be generated, and if the photographs are reviewed when the pathological diagnosis is available, important lessons may be learned and future errors prevented. Wherever possible, clinical photographs with a centimetre scale adjacent to the lesion should be taken before any biopsy procedure. This should become routine in all minor surgery clinics as in this way a good collection of teaching slides will be built up. Unless photography becomes a routine procedure, it is difficult to gather a worthwhile collection of the rarer skin tumours.

Dermatoscopy or epiluminescence microscopy

These terms describe the technique of using bright light and moderate magnification in vivo to assist in the preoperative diagnosis of cutaneous lesions. The main area of activity has been in the field of pigmented lesions in the attempt to separate more accurately early melanoma from benign lesions such as naevi. The technique is not new, and early publications[3] suggested that preoperative diagnostic accuracy can be increased from around 60 per cent to over 80 per cent. In the past ten years there has been a resurgence of interest in this technique. Previously, the equipment used was cumbersome, expensive and non-portable, and was therefore only available in specialized centres. The development of small hand-held machines similar in size to an auriscope has brought the equipment within reach of a much wider potential user group. In addition to alterations to the actual equipment used,

there have been extensive efforts made to categorize accurately and reproducibly the surface appearance of the varying types of pigmented lesions. In summary, it is now relatively easy to separate pigmented lesions of the melanocytic series from non-melanocytic lesions, i.e. melanoma from pigmented basal cell carcinoma or histiocytoma, but differentiating benign from melanocytic lesions is not as yet so consistently achievable.[4,5] A vocabulary of dermatoscopy findings has developed, including terms such as 'milky veil' to describe the pattern of clusters of melanin pigment seen in the superficial dermis and 'pigment network' to describe the more superficial pattern of melanin distribution in both melanocytes and keratinocytes.[6] In the hands of those who see large numbers of melanomas, this technique can increase diagnostic accuracy to over 90 per cent,[7] but it is less useful at present for those who work in the primary care sector whose experience of seeing melanomas preoperatively is obviously much less. Current developments include linking dermatoscopy findings to computerized image analysis and this linkage may in the future greatly extend the applicability of dermatoscopy.

Biopsy techniques – excisional and incisional biopsies

In the majority of small skin tumours, the appropriate procedure is an excision biopsy with a narrow margin of 1–2 mm of clinically normal skin around the edge of the tumour. Even in the case of suspected melanoma this is an appropriate initial procedure, and if it is found that the tumour thickness is such that further tissue should be removed (Chapter 10) this can be carried out within a few days of obtaining a pathological diagnosis. There is no evidence whatever to suggest that this two-stage procedure alters the prognosis for melanoma patients.

In the case of larger tumours, an incisional biopsy is acceptable. In the case of large squamous cell carcinomas, basal cell carcinomas, and other tumours, there is no evidence that an incisional biopsy worsens the prognosis for the individual patient. In the case of malignant melanoma, there are conflicting reports as to whether or not an incisional biopsy could do so, but the larger series suggest that, provided such a procedure is followed in a few days by definitive surgery, the prognosis for the patient is unaltered. As public education campaigns result in patients presenting earlier with smaller, thinner melanomas, the number of occasions on which an incisional biopsy is necessary is falling.

For detailed guidance on cutaneous surgery techniques, the reader is referred to one of the standard texts.[8–10] In general, in biopsy procedures the choice lies between an elliptical biopsy using a scalpel blade and a punch biopsy using a disposable punch with a diameter of between 3 mm and 8 mm. Most pathologists prefer to report on an elliptical scalpel blade biopsy, although with the sharp disposable punches now available excellent material can be obtained for critical histological assessment, provided the volume of tissue submitted is adequate, and the tissue is taken from an appropriate and representative part of the lesion.

Incisional punch biopsies should not be carried out on possible melanomas, as published case reports have demonstrated that tumour cells had been driven deeper into the dermis following definitive excision of the specimen on which a punch biopsy had previously been performed. In the case of incisional biopsies, the choice of a representative area for biopsy is of utmost importance, and in the case of cutaneous lymphoma where multiple lesions are present, multiple biopsies may be an appropriate procedure.

Submitting the sample for histological assessment

Place the specimen in a pot containing appropriate fixative, usually 10 per cent neutral buffered formalin, label the pot and submit the sample with adequate clinical information. In the case of straightforward lesions, all that will be required will be processing and staining of the sample with standard procedures, usually only needing haematoxylin and eosin staining. If, however, the sample is more complex, additional tests and samples may be required.

Frozen sections

In a number of situations the important differential diagnosis lies between a benign and a malignant cutaneous lesion. In this situation a frozen section examination may yield useful information, as an instant diagnosis may be available while the patient is still on the operating table, but not all pathologists are prepared to give an opinion on only a small sample of the entire lesion in some of the more difficult situations. Examples of specific problems in differential diagnosis in which it might be wiser to wait an extra 24 hours for a conventionally processed slide to be examined include the situation where the clinical differential diagnosis lies between a Spitz naevus and early malignant melanoma. If, however, the broader question of whether or not the lesion is a malignant melanoma or a benign vascular lesion requires a rapid answer, frozen sections may be entirely acceptable. This will depend on the individual pathologist and it should be borne in mind that with modern tissue-processing techniques it is often possible to obtain a conventionally fixed and processed specimen for examination within 24 hours or less of surgery.

Electron microscopy[11]

If the lesion is clinically unusual and therefore it can be anticipated that there may be pathological problems, the reporting pathologist should be consulted before the biopsy is carried out so that tissue can be reserved for special techniques should these be required. In the case of electron microscopy, it should be borne in mind that there are no absolute ultrastructural criteria of malignancy, but that on occasion the ultrastructural pathologist can answer a specific question, such as whether or not melanosomes are present in the cytoplasm of the main cell type present. If the need for electron microscopy is agreed before biopsy, a tissue fragment not more than 1 mm in diameter should be dissected without any crushing or squeezing and fixed immediately in freshly prepared isotonic gluteraldehyde buffered to pH 7.4. If this procedure is carried out, the best possible ultrastructural preservation will be obtained. If, however, this has not been carried out, a small piece of tissue that has been retained in the routine pathological fixative will also yield useful information. The least satisfactory tissue for electron microscopy is tissue reprocessed from the paraffin block for ultrastructural examination.

The situation in which electron microscopy is most likely to be required and be of value is in the diagnosis of the undifferentiated and clinically non-diagnostic soft tissue tumour. This should be borne in mind when such a tumour requires biopsy. Prior liaison with the laboratory for provision of appropriate fixatives should be routine in such cases.

Immunocytochemistry[12]

In the past few years the use of monoclonal antibodies for accurate identification of cell types in cutaneous pathology has moved rapidly from being a research to a routine procedure. As with electron microscopy, it should be appreciated that there are at present virtually no monoclonal antibodies that will consistently differentiate between a benign and a malignant cell type. The value of the immunocytochemical technique lies in the use of monoclonal antibodies to identify accurately the cell type from which the tumour arises. It cannot yet answer the benign versus malignant question.

At present, monoclonal antibodies can be divided into those for which frozen tissue is necessary, and those that can be used on routinely processed material. This latter group is obviously extremely useful for retrospective analyses. If, however, it is recognized before biopsy that immunocytochemistry may be of value, a representative portion of tissue should be snap-frozen and stored at −70°C for use with monoclonal antibodies. Immunocytochemistry is most useful in the field of lymphoma pathology, in the accurate identification of Hodgkin's from non-Hodgkin's lymphoma, and in identifying T-cell and B-cell lymphomas in the skin. T-cell lymphomas can be further subdivided on the basis of the presence of T-helper and T-suppressor subsets. Although monoclonal antibodies are now available that can identify cells of the lymphoid series on routinely formalin-fixed and conventionally processed tissue, the more specific identification of T-cell subsets still requires frozen material. The antibodies currently available which can be used on routinely processed material include antibodies directed against the intermediate filaments (cytokeratins, vimentin and GFAP), antibodies that are associated with cells of the melanocyte series (S 100, NKI C3 and HMB 45), antibodies to factor V111, found in vascular tumours, and UCHT 1, which recognizes T-lymphocytes. This list is currently expanding rapidly.

Immunocytochemical techniques are well detailed in the standard texts and include variations on the immunoperoxidase and immunoalkaline phosphatase techniques.

DNA analysis

One of the newer techniques currently undergoing the transition from research to routine procedure is that of analysis of DNA, most commonly of the beta-chain of the T-cell receptor genes in patients with cutaneous lymphoma. Using this technique, clonal rearrangement of these genes has been demonstrated in patients with cutaneous T-cell lymphoma of the mycosis fungoides type.[13,14] Similar rearrangements have,

however, been identified in lymphomatoid papulosis and regressing atypical histiocytosis.[15] This technique is at the time of writing more a research tool than a routine investigative procedure, but the situation is changing rapidly. Approximately 1 000 000 tumour cells are at present necessary for DNA extraction, and it is important that the sample is as pure as possible, as DNA from adjacent normal or inflammatory cells may confuse the analysis. However, newer techniques using the polymerase chain reaction have made it possible to obtain useful information from ever smaller tissue samples. This tissue must be rapidly frozen and not re-thawed before DNA extraction takes place. Liaison with the laboratory before biopsy is essential if use of this technique is contemplated.

Management

Surgery

In the vast majority of both benign and malignant cutaneous tumours surgical excision is the routine preferred treatment. Total excision of small lesions has the obvious advantage that the entire specimen is available for pathological examination in a relatively non-traumatized state. Details of surgical procedures are beyond the scope of this volume, and will be found in standard texts.[8–10] In many countries there is a move to carry out an increased proportion of surgery in the primary care setting. While this may be very convenient geographically for the patient, it is obviously important that the same high standards are maintained whether the patient has the procedure carried out in an outpatient department or a doctor's surgery. In the UK, the British Association of Dermatologists and other associations run excellent courses devoted to skin surgery, and those interested in extending their skills in this area are encouraged to take advantage of these.

Cryotherapy, curettage and diathermy

Minor surgical destructive procedures that do not involve complete excision of the lesion include cryotherapy, curettage and diathermy.[16,17] All of these procedures may produce a cosmetically highly acceptable result for the patient, and are relatively easily carried out in situations where minimal surgical facilities are available. While they are quite acceptable in the management of such lesions as basal cell papillomas (seborrhoeic keratoses), they are of more questionable value in the management of locally malignant tumours, such as Bowen's disease, and are definitely not appropriate in the management of invasive malignant melanoma. It is important, therefore, that if such procedures are planned the operator should review carefully the grounds for the clinical diagnosis. It should be borne in mind that if any tissue is available for pathological examination after these procedures, it may well be so distorted that critical pathological assessment is not feasible.

Mohs' surgical technique and surgical techniques involving pathological control of excision margins[18]

In the 1930s, Frederick Mohs, while in Wisconsin and while still a medical student, evolved a technique of tissue fixation on the patient prior to examination of horizontally cut layers of tissue to assess completeness of excision of cutaneous tumours. The patients concerned were mainly farmers from the area, and a zinc chloride paste was applied to the face and acted as an in vivo fixative. This technique was revolutionary in its time, in that there was microscopic control of completeness of excision of tumour cells. Over the years the technique has been further refined and at the present time the usual approach is to use a fresh frozen tissue technique where the samples are taken, snap-frozen and cut parallel to the skin surface, in contrast to the usual vertical sections, and examined for residual tumour cells. Although it is self-evident, it must be stated that the basic premise behind this approach is that the tumour in question is invading by direct extension from the primary site rather than by satellite progression or by micrometastatic spread. The main value of the technique lies in assessing the completeness of excision of tumours such as a morphoeic basal cell carcinoma, particularly when it has recurred after initial excision. Those who are not acquainted with the technique should not assume that the pathological examination of the tissue obtained in this way is straightforward, as frequently it can be surprisingly difficult to differentiate between the lower part of a skin appendage and a small island of tumour tissue.[19,20]

From the above it will be seen that Mohs' technique, or a pathologically controlled and micrographically planned approach to surgical excision, is labour-intensive in terms of both surgical and pathological time. It should further be understood that this is not a technique that will guarantee 100 per cent excision of all tumour cells in all cases. It is, however, of great value in a limited number of situations, particularly that of recurrent tumour on the central panel of the face adjacent to vital structures such as the eyelid. It should further be borne in mind that modern plastic surgery techniques with elegant free-flap procedures, which give the ability to transpose relatively large areas of skin from one facial site to another, have provided an alternative approach to ensuring total clearance of tumour.

Radiotherapy[21]

The use of radiotherapy in the management of cutaneous tumours varies greatly according to local custom and available facilities. Although the use of radiotherapy is unusual in the case of benign tumours, in some parts of eastern Europe radiotherapy is regarded as the treatment of choice for many cutaneous malignancies. The choice of radiotherapy versus surgery will vary in many situations according to local availability of surgical and radiotherapy facilities, and also the relative lengths of waiting lists. In general, basal cell carcinoma, squamous cell carcinoma and vascular tumours such as Kaposi's sarcoma are radiosensitive tumours and respond well to radiotherapy, but malignant melanoma is relatively radio-resistant and surgery is preferred. From every tumour for which radiotherapy is planned as the main therapeutic procedure, a biopsy must first be taken to obtain a pathological diagnosis.

Types of ionizing radiation available in the management of skin malignancies include conventional tumour dose radiotherapy with X-rays, commonly used for squamous cell carcinoma, Grenz ray therapy, used in some centres for early cutaneous lymphoma, and also electron beam or beta-ray therapy, used for cutaneous lymphoma. Although in a number of centres in Europe and North America it has been the practice for dermatologists to operate their own X-ray machines, this is becoming less common and radiotherapy is now, in the great majority of cases, given by fully trained radiotherapists.

In situations in which there is some doubt as to whether radiotherapy or surgery is the treatment of choice, a combined clinic, at which patients are seen and subsequent management discussed by surgeons, radiotherapists, and dermatologists, is popular and forms an excellent teaching forum for trainees.

Chemotherapy

The value of chemotherapy in cutaneous malignancy is limited. There are few situations in which systemic chemotherapy is indicated, as neither basal cell nor squamous cell carcinoma commonly metastasize. Systemic chemotherapy has recently been advocated both in combination and as single-agent chemotherapy for the management of advanced cutaneous lymphoma (CTCL), although analysis of published trials does not suggest that current regimes confer a significant survival advantage. Similarly, both single-agent and multiple-drug regimes have been reported to be of some value in palliation of disseminated malignant melanoma but, once again, overall survival figures are disappointing and chemotherapy in melanoma is currently mainly used in the clinical trial situation.

Topical chemotherapy in the form of topical 5-fluorouracil (5-FU) and also topical nitrogen mustard is of proven value in a number of cutaneous malignancies. Topical 5-FU is of value in the management of actinic keratoses, and can be a most effective way of treating a large area, such as the entire cheek or forehead or the back of the hand. A preparation of 5-FU is applied topically to the site in question daily for 2–3 weeks. An intense erythematous reaction in areas of actinic dysplasia which are not yet clinically visible will develop, and the patient should be warned about this. In general, response to 5-FU is more impressive on facial skin than on the arms or legs, although on these sites the use of a combination topical preparation with both topical 5-FU and retinoic acid will increase efficacy. Both topical nitrogen mustard and hydroxyurea have been used to control plaque-stage cutaneous T-cell lymphoma.[22,23] Topical nitrogen mustard is better applied in an ointment base than in aqueous solution.[24]

Experimental therapy

There are a number of interesting and novel approaches to the therapy of cutaneous tumours that are currently undergoing clinical trials. The most encouraging preliminary results from these studies are in the field of cutaneous lymphoma and also, in some cases, melanoma. This may reflect the current very poor results of management of patients with both advanced melanoma and lymphoma.

Retinoids

Vitamin A itself has long been known to be essential for normal differentiation and maturation of epithelial tissues,[25] and vitamin A deficiency enhances the effect of a number of chemical carcinogens. Studies on animal models show that vitamin A supplementation can, at least in part, reverse the preneoplastic and neoplastic process.[26] The use of synthetic retinoids rather than vitamin A is because of their greater therapeutic ratio, in that greater clinical benefit and fewer side-effects are seen, particularly with regard to liver toxicity.

The current theory as to the mode of action of retinoids in preventing or reversing malignancy is that they act as anti-promoters (Chapter 2). Attention is at present mainly focused on their effect on the protein kinase C pathway. Retinoids do not block binding of phorbol esters to their protein kinase C receptor, but do appear to block subsequent activation of the cascade.

The current studies on the clinical value of retinoids in human tumours can logically be divided into studies on preneoplastic lesions and studies on established malignancy. In the former group, actinic keratoses have been studied most frequently, and have been treated by both oral and topical retinoid.[27] Regression of lesions has been reported with both treatment routes, although the lesions tend to recur when treatment is discontinued. This is a constant observation in the majority of clinical studies to date, but in the case of actinic keratoses it has been suggested that 2 months' treatment annually might be adequate to control the majority of lesions.

In the management of established malignant disease, oral and topical retinoids have been used in basal cell carcinoma,[28] squamous cell carcinoma,[29] melanoma,[30] and cutaneous lymphoma.[31] The most encouraging results to date are with cutaneous lymphoma. These are discussed in Chapter 11. The possibility of combining retinoids with the interferons (see below) is also at present under study. Over the next few years the exact place of retinoids, both those currently available and newer compounds, will be clarified. Current information suggests that they may find a specific role in the prevention of progression of premalignancy, or the reversal of premalignant changes.[32] The fact that premalignant changes are common on aging light-exposed skin and that these changes can be observed with the naked eye and biopsied for histological confirmation with minimal trauma makes the skin a most important organ for assessing these compounds.

Interferons

There are three varieties of interferon currently available: alpha, beta and gamma. To date most clinical studies have been carried out with recombinant alpha-interferon because of the availability of relatively large quantities of pure interferon due to recombinant DNA technology.

The most encouraging results are with hairy cell leukaemia, but in the field of cutaneous malignancy a response rate of around 15 per cent has been reported in melanoma patients treated to date.[33] Probable responders are those with subcutaneous lesions or pulmonary secondaries, and although the response rate is relatively low, reported responses are of long duration. Toxicity is generally dose-related, and includes fever and mild marrow toxicity. In clinical trials of new conventional cytotoxic drugs in cancer patients it is normal practice to use the drug first only on patients with relatively advanced disease and a large tumour burden. This situation may not be appropriate for the interferons and other biological response modifiers, as they may require to be used in a minimal residual disease situation to be maximally effective. Current trials in progress in the use of adjuvant interferon therapy in the management of melanoma after surgery suggest that subsets of patients may have an increased disease-free interval,[34] but there is not as yet any controlled randomized study showing a survival benefit. The use of interferons in cutaneous lymphoma in combination with photochemotherapy (PUVA) does appear to increase response rates compared with the use of either modality alone.[35] Several current studies suggest that intralesional interferon is of value in controlling individual lesions of Kaposi's sarcoma in AIDs-related Kaposi's sarcoma.[36-38]

Interleukin-2 and other cytokines

Interleukin-2 stimulates growth of T-cells in vitro, and in vivo also appears to activate killer cells. Early reports from the National Institutes of Health (NIH) of a 50 per cent response rate in advanced malignant melanoma[39] have not been confirmed, even by the original authors, and toxicity is significant, with three therapy-related deaths in the most recent report.

Gene therapy[40]

While the above results with administered interleukin-2 are disappointing, the principle of using cytokine activity to augment the body's ability to destroy tumour cells is sound. Current work in the field of gene therapy is concentrating in this area, and attempting to insert genes for appropriate cytokines into cells and return these to the patient. In vitro studies suggest that the granulocyte/macrophage colony-stimulating factor may be a promising candidate, and early studies in humans are in progress.

Monoclonal antibodies

Therapeutic use of monoclonal antibodies is still very much at the experimental stage in the management of cutaneous malignancies, mainly melanoma. They have been used as single agents, using the antiganglioside antibody GD 2 in melanoma, and encouraging early results have been reported.[41] One study gives details of responses of advanced melanoma treated with ricin A-chain conjugated to monoclonal melanoma antibody.[42] Anti-T-cell antibody has been used in the treatment of T-cell lymphoma with initially encouraging results, but a decline in response is seen with repeated therapy. The antibody used was mouse-derived, which is likely to explain this decline, but newer techniques of humanizing antibodies may overcome this problem.

Photopheresis[43,44]

Advanced cutaneous T-cell lymphoma is a disorder that responds poorly to conventional cytotoxic therapy. Edelson has introduced the concept and technique of photopheresis. The principle is to put a patient who has received oral psoralen on a leucapheresis machine and then to irradiate the white cells ex vivo with UVA, thus destroying only rapidly dividing white cells. These cells are then returned to the body. Early reports of this technique include encouraging long-term remissions in subsets of patients.[45] Ideally, a controlled clinical therapeutic trial should be carried out to establish exactly which patient groups will benefit most from this method of therapy.

Photodynamic therapy (PDT)[46]

This technique involves the combination of endogenous photosensitizers such as porphyrins and laser light to treat malignancies. The underlying basic principle is the use of photochemical reactions mediated by photosensitizing drugs and oxygen. Photosensitizers are selectively retained in tumours for reasons which are not yet understood,[47] and lasers have traditionally been used in this technique because of the high energy output, which reduces treatment times and also allows delivery of intense light down an appropriate bronchoscopy or endoscopy tube for treating internal malignancies such as carcinoma of the bronchus. Clearly this is not necessary in superficial cutaneous tumours, and the use of intense white light sources is equally acceptable. At present, clinical trials of the use of PDT in dermatological malignancies are mainly concentrated on basal and early squamous cell carcinomas. Response rates of 60–90 per cent are obtained, but local recurrence rates are higher than those obtained by conventional surgical excision.[48] Pigmented melanocytic tumours do not respond. The true value of PDT in cutaneous malignancies by comparison with simple surgical excision remains to be established, and at present the depth of some tumours is beyond the range of available light sources; however, PDT is likely to find a useful therapeutic niche in areas such as the management of widespread but superficial Bowen's disease on the lower legs of elderly patients.[49]

Tumour vaccines

The principle of tumour vaccines clearly depends on the presence of tumour-associated if not tumour-specific antigens against which the patient can be vaccinated and mount an immune response. At present experimental work in skin tumour vaccine therapy is virtually confined to melanoma. A number of vaccines have been developed directed against peptides and components of the melanin synthesis pathway, and some of these are in clinical use,[50] although evidence for their efficacy is slight and no randomized controlled trials have yet been carried out. In future they may well play a part in disease control after apparently successful surgery but may require to be combined with cytokines for maximum effect. Early reports of their use in the adjuvant setting are encouraging, with significant increases in disease-free survival time reported.[51]

Diet

A recent well-controlled study[52] suggests that a low-fat diet will reduce the rate of development of actinic keratoses, well-recognized precursors of squamous cell carcinoma. This study needs confirmation, and if this is forthcoming, dietary modification for older patients with sun-damaged skin might be an acceptable addition to current conventional treatment.

Preventive therapy

Actinic keratoses are well-recognized markers of sun-damaged skin, which is at increased risk of all types of skin cancer. The use of high sun protection factor (SPF) topical sunscreens over a 9-month period has been shown in a high solar intensity climate to reduce the rate of development of new actinic keratoses.[53] Longer-term studies are needed to assess the true value of this in relation to prevention of non-melanoma cutaneous malignancies. Similarly, reports of both clinical and histological improvement in photoaged skin after use of topical tretinoin[54,55] require longer-term assessment to establish whether in the longer term the incidence of skin cancer is reduced in tretinoin-treated skin.

4
Cancer-associated genodermatoses

These conditions divide naturally into two main groups (see below). Group 1 comprises those genodermatoses displaying cutaneous features that progress in a significant proportion to cutaneous malignancy. Group 2 comprises those cutaneous disorders associated with non-cutaneous malignancy. Thus, conditions in Group 1 show a logical and predictable progression of cutaneous lesions, whereas those in Group 2 appear to have multi-organ abnormalities.

At the present time, familial cancer and associated syndromes are an area of very active investigation in the elucidation of the role played by oncogenes and suppressor genes in these cancers, as this information may in turn give valuable clues to the roles of the same genetic factors in apparently sporadic cancers. One large informative family with three generations affected and available for investigation is a very valuable resource in this field.

While being of obvious interest to dermatologists, these groups of disorders are also of importance in the fields of paediatrics, clinical genetics, and oncology. Early recognition may allow delay or prevention of malignancy in the affected individual, and also allow genetic counselling and possibly prenatal diagnosis for the family.

GROUP 1. GENODERMATOSES ASSOCIATED WITH DERMATOLOGICAL MALIGNANCY

Xeroderma pigmentosum
Naevoid basal cell carcinoma
Familial atypical mole syndrome
Multiple self-healing epithelioma of Ferguson-Smith

GROUP 2. GENODERMATOSES ASSOCIATED WITH NON-CUTANEOUS MALIGNANCY

Torre's syndrome
Cowden's syndrome
Gardner's syndrome
Peutz–Jeghers syndrome
Dyskeratosis congenita
Carney's syndrome

Group 1

Xeroderma pigmentosum

Definition, epidemiology, and genetics

This rare skin disorder was first described in 1874 by Kaposi,[1] who classified it as a cutaneous atrophy. Xeroderma pigmentosum (XP) and the more recently recognized clinically related xeroderma pigmentosum variant (formally called pigmented xerodermoid) are rare diseases. Xeroderma pigmentosum is inherited by autosomal recessive transmission and its prevalence in the USA is estimated at 1 in 250 000.[2] The condition is relatively more common in Egypt and is also recorded more frequently in Japan.[3–5] There are no accurate incidence or prevalence figures available for the UK but the recent establishment of xeroderma pigmentosum registers in various countries should allow a more accurate assessment, both of the numbers of affected individuals and of the natural history of the disease. At present our knowledge of the latter is gleaned mainly from case reports. A recent excellent review of published details of 830 cases has been compiled by Kraemer.[6]

Clinical presentation (Figures 4.1–4.7)

Males and females are affected with equal frequency, and this disease is a rare example of a situation in which genetically pigmented skin shows damage on exposure to natural sunlight, even in childhood.[7] In true xeroderma pigmentosum the diagnosis should be apparent in the first summer of infancy. When the infant is exposed to sunlight he or she will be clearly uncomfortable and there is rapid development of unusually persistent erythema on all exposed sites. This is followed by freckling and other macular brown pigmentation on the face, hands and neck. If the condition is not recognized and sun protection introduced, the exposed skin will rapidly develop features suggestive of accelerated aging, even at the early age of 1–2 years. Atrophy and mottled pigmentary change, with areas of depigmentation and hyperpigmentation alternating, and extreme dryness with scaling are all seen on both skin and mucosal surfaces of the lips. The eyes are also affected, and the children have obvious photophobia and tend to shield their eyes from sunlight.

Five distinct complementation groups are now recognized, groups A–E, and the clinical features vary in these groups. Table 4.1 gives some of the distinguishing features seen in the groups.

Before the introduction of effective sunscreens, most children rapidly developed premalignant actinic keratoses followed by both melanoma and non-melanomatous malignancies. The average age in the

literature for development of non-melanoma malignancy in affected individuals is 8 years. Death in the second or third decade was the common pattern before the introduction of early and effective sunscreening regimes, and still applies in less developed and sunnier parts of the world. Forty-five per cent of published cases have non-melanoma malignancies, and 5 per cent have melanoma.

Many affected children have a rather bird-like facies with a rather pinched but protuberant nose in profile. The sun-exposed ocular tissue is rapidly affected, resulting in deterioration of vision associated with keratitis and corneal vascularization. Ocular melanomas are reported in addition to cutaneous malignant melanomas. Mucosal tumours are also reported and lesions on both the lower lip and the tip of the tongue occur with a fair degree of frequency (Figure 4.7).

In addition to the cutaneous ocular and mucosal changes, the central nervous system appears to be a major target site for degenerative damage. The extreme form of this was first recognized by Neisser in 1883, but reported by de Sanctis and Cacchione in 1932.[8] This is apparent in infancy with microcephaly, growth retardation and hypogonadism, progressing to cerebellar ataxia and spastic quadriplegia.

Now that affected individuals are living longer as a result of protecting their skin from UV radiation it is clear that as many as 50 per cent of patients suffering from xeroderma pigmentosum have a progressive decline in mental function. This is not associated with obvious initial mental retardation in infancy. A recent study of 32 patients in the UK emphasizes the growing importance of central nervous system complications now that UV-induced change can be partly prevented and delayed.[9] In the 32 patients there were three deaths but all were from non-malignant

Table 4.1 Current known complementation groups in xeroderma pigmentosum and their characteristics.

Group	Prevalence	DNA repair level	CNS involvement
A	Commonest	Very poor	Yes
B	2 families only	Very poor	Yes
C	Commoner	Poor	No
D	Rare	Poor	Uncertain
E	Rare	Poor	No

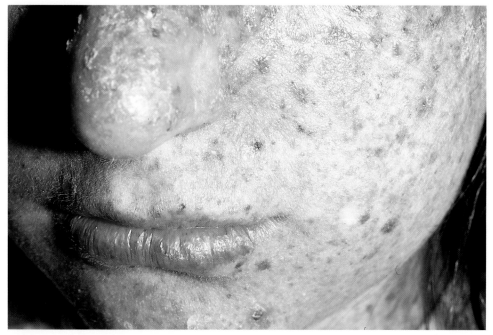

Figure 4.1 Facial appearance of an 8-year-old girl with xeroderma pigmentosum. Note atrophy and freckling.

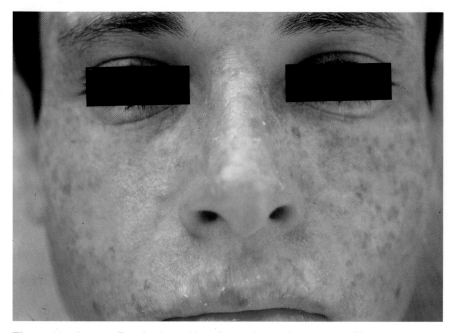

Figure 4.2 A young Egyptian boy with early xeroderma pigmentosum. (Photograph courtesy of Dr M El Sayed.)

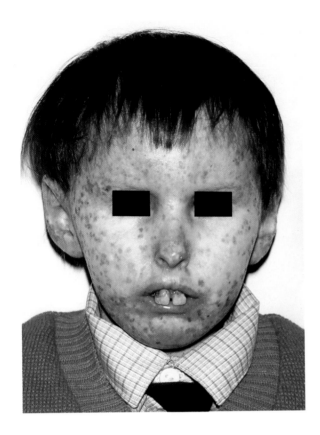

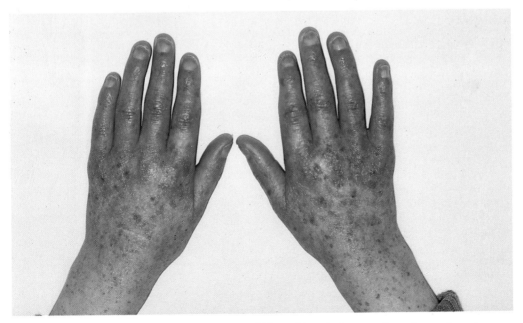

Figures 4.3 and 4.4 Face and hands of a 4-year-old boy with early features of xeroderma pigmentosum. (Photographs courtesy of Dr WN Morley.)

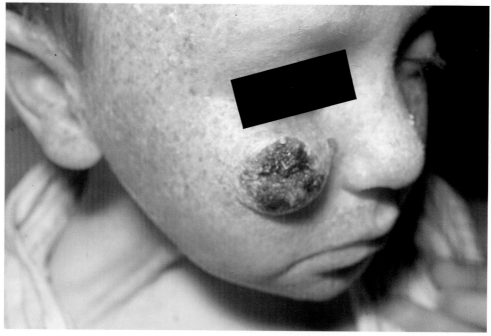

Figure 4.5   The 10-year-old brother of the girl illustrated in Figure 4.1, showing a large squamous cell carcinoma on the cheek.

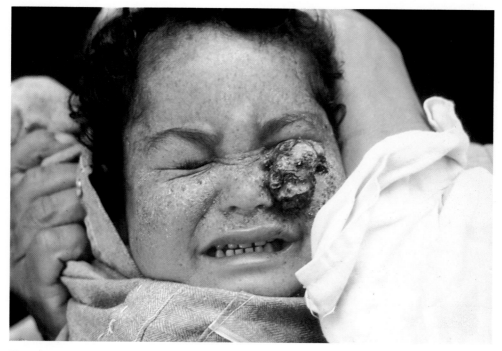

Figure 4.6   A tumour on the cheek of a young Egyptian child with xeroderma pigmentosum. (Photograph courtesy of Dr M El Sayed.)

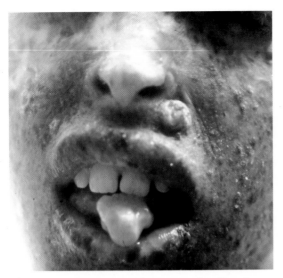

Figure 4.7 A tumour on the tongue of an Egyptian patient with xeroderma pigmentosum. (Photograph courtesy of Dr M El Sayed.)

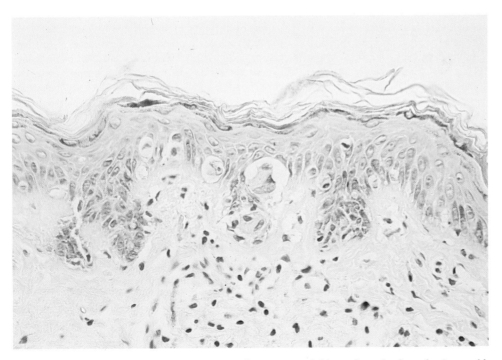

Figure 4.8 Pathological features of xeroderma pigmentosum. A biopsy from the face of a 4-year-old. There is epidermal thinning and loss of normal polarity.

causes and were due to severe neurological involvement and terminal infection. There have been reports in the past suggesting an increased incidence of non-cutaneous malignancy in these individuals and it is of interest to note that there is a high mutant frequency in circulating T-lymphocytes.[10]

Laboratory findings

The basic abnormality in fibroblasts in xeroderma pigmentosum was reported by Cleaver to be due to a low level of unscheduled DNA repair activity after UV exposure.[11,12] Repair of damage caused by DNA exposure after X-ray is normal, but certain drugs, including psoralens, chlorpromazine, and a number of cytotoxic drugs, are also associated with DNA damage and will accelerate cellular damage. In vitro studies of cultured fibroblasts from xeroderma pigmentosum patients have demonstrated varying degrees of unscheduled post-UV DNA repair defect in the groups.[13] The incidence of associated neurological problems also varies in the different complementation groups. Groups A–E are arranged in order of decreasing DNA repair defect. To date the largest numbers of patients studied are found in complementation groups A and C, and groups A and D are associated with the highest incidence of neurological problems. The human DNA repair gene *Xpac* corrects defective repair in cells from group A patients,[14] and the mouse *Xpac* gene has been cloned.[15] More recently the gene ERCC 2 has been shown to be the gene responsible for group D.[16] Thus the possibility now exists for gene therapy in this serious and disabling condition.

Diagnosis and management

Clinical diagnosis of sporadic cases should be made in the first year of life, although in practice about 5 per cent of cases are not diagnosed until puberty. In complementation groups A and D, clinical diagnosis can now be confirmed by detailed genetic studies, and prenatal diagnosis offered by studies of DNA repair in cultured fibroblasts obtained at amniocentesis or chorionic villus biopsy. In an affected infant in whom the diagnosis of xeroderma pigmentosum is considered possible on clinical grounds, a skin biopsy should be taken and sent to the appropriate laboratory for full DNA repair studies. The biopsy must be placed in tissue culture medium for transport, and prior contact with the laboratory is essential. The appearances on light microscopy are non-specific (Figure 4.8). The sophisticated DNA repair studies now required in a suspected case of xeroderma pigmentosum demand prior liaison with appropriate laboratories.*

Once the diagnosis is confirmed, sun avoidance and the use of total sunblocks at all times of the day throughout the year should be instituted. The infant or child should be dressed in clothing designed to minimize exposure of the skin to UV radiation and a shady hat and total sunblock preparation worn at all times. Liaison with the school authorities is essential to ensure that the child is allowed to sit well away from a sunny window, and that the child is excused participation in outdoor activities. Appropriate career advice must be offered with regard to avoidance of UV irradiation.

The use since the mid-1970s of extremely effective sunblocks on the skin of children with xeroderma pigmentosum has resulted in a substantial number now living through puberty into early adult life. This creates the new problem of genetic counselling and advice as to whether or not the affected individuals should produce their own children and thus increase the frequency of the gene that causes xeroderma pigmentosum in the community. Clearly, sophisticated professional genetic advice is needed in puberty and early adulthood.

All affected patients should be under regular dermatological supervision. The frequency of examination will vary with the environment. A patient living in Australia will obviously require more frequent total body examinations for developing cutaneous malignancy than one living in a less sunny environment. Once one cutaneous malignancy develops, the pattern is that multiple primary tumours, which may be basal cell carcinomas, squamous cell carcinomas, keratoacanthomas, or melanomas, tend to follow with increasing frequency. Thus, once one cutaneous malignancy is diagnosed, the intervals between follow-up visits should be shortened. Regular ophthalmological supervision and provision of appropriate spectacles or contact lenses are also essential to minimize UV-induced ocular damage.

Cutaneous actinic keratoses and malignancies should be treated as appropriate. In the case of multiple actinic keratoses, liquid nitrogen or topical 5-FU cream may be the most suitable approach if multiple lesions and

---

* In the UK this is the MRC Cell Mutation Unit at the University of Sussex, and in the USA the XP Registry can give helpful advice (address: Dr K. Kraemer, c/o Department of Pathology, Room C520, Medical Science Building, New Jersey Medical School, 100 Bergen Street, Newark, NJ 07103).

large areas of skin are involved. In the case of suspected invasive malignancies, excision for pathological confirmation should be carried out wherever possible. In general, radiotherapy is not recommended for these children, although their fibroblasts are not unduly sensitive to X-ray damage. At present there is considerable interest in the use of oral retinoid therapy to prevent or delay the development of cutaneous lesions. The value of this approach remains to be established.

Xeroderma pigmentosum variant or pigmented xerodermoid

This condition should be distinguished from true xeroderma pigmentosum. It was first recognized shortly after the excision repair defect in classical XP was described by Cleaver.[17–19] Patients with xeroderma pigmentosum variant have normal excision repair but have impaired postreplication or daughter strand repair.[20] Only 50 or so of these patients are described in the world literature. This disease is usually not recognized until early adult life. Affected individuals may have skin type 3 or 4 and give a history of easy tanning with no obvious evidence of dryness atrophy or freckling in childhood. They are frequently recognized by the development of multiple non-melanomatous and melanomatous malignancies on exposed skin in early adult life (Figure 4.9).

To make the diagnosis, if the condition is suspected on clinical grounds, a skin biopsy should be put in tissue culture medium, and the appropriate DNA repair studies carried out. As with xeroderma pigmentosum, the most effective treatment is complete and constant avoidance of all UV exposure.

Naevoid basal cell carcinoma syndrome

Introduction and genetics

Many names are eponymously used to describe this syndrome, most commonly that of Gorlin, who generously states

> I am personally opposed to eponyms since they say nothing about the disorder, frequently give rise to arguments regarding priority of discovery, and may be chauvinistic and unfair to those whose contributions to knowledge of the syndrome far exceed those of the individual for whom the disorder is named.[21]

This is a sentiment with which the author concurs.

However, to give some credit to the individuals who have brought this relatively common genodermatosis to our attention, it was first described as a genodermatosis by Gorlin and Goltz in 1960,[22] although Howell and Caro gave an excellent account of it in 1959,[23,24] and in 1951 Binkley and Johnson described the triad of basal cell naevi, dental cysts and agenesis of the corpus callosum.[25]

The naevoid basal cell carcinoma syndrome is a relatively common genodermatosis transmitted by autosomal dominant inheritance. A high proportion of cases have, however, no family history, suggesting a high rate of spontaneous mutation. Three recent studies published almost simultaneously have mapped the gene for Gorlin's syndrome to chromosome 9q31.

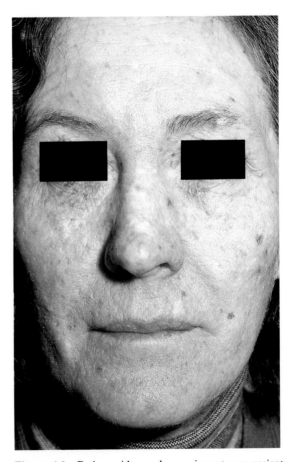

Figure 4.9 Patient with xeroderma pigmentosum variant or pigmented xerodermoid.

Farndon and colleagues[26] identified 10 informative families, and Reis[27] found that 9 of 14 European families who were suitable for analysis had the same defect. Gailani and colleagues[28] found allelic loss at chromosome 9q31 in five Gorlin's syndrome families, and also in some cases of sporadic basal cell carcinoma. Further work has confirmed the exact site of the gene on 9q.[29]

Clinical features (Figures 4.10–4.14)

This is a true syndrome in that abnormalities are found in the skin, in bone, in optic tissue, and in the central nervous system and other body sites. The cutaneous changes include the development of multiple basal cell carcinomas. These are not present at birth and the earliest reported basal cell carcinomas in affected children occur at the age of 2 years. The majority of lesions, however, make their appearance during the second decade. The basal cell carcinomas are clinically somewhat atypical in that the lesions are multiple but very small. On clinical inspection they frequently appear as small, pink, fleshy, pedunculated lesions, often rather like skin tags. The other cutaneous feature that tends not to appear until the second decade is the presence of small pits on palmar and plantar skin. Biopsy of these pits shows a relative reduction in the thickness of the stratum corneum.[30]

The bony changes associated with the syndrome are the presence of bony cysts, especially of the mandible, which may be associated with malaligned dentition. Abnormalities of the ribs are common and a short fourth metacarpal is frequently found on X-rays of the hands. Ophthalmological changes are relatively common and may present at birth with coloboma or later in life with cataract.

Neurological changes found in this syndrome include intracranial calcification and an increased risk of both medulloblastoma and meningioma. Mental deficiency is also recorded.

Diagnosis and treatment

This condition may be suspected in childhood if there is a positive family history. Some affected individuals have a typical facies with considerable frontal bossing. In suspected cases, early X-ray of the jaw, the hands, and the ribs may help confirm the diagnosis. A full dental assessment may also be of diagnostic value.

Once the diagnosis is made, careful surveillance for the development and early treatment of multiple basal cell carcinomas is essential. The lesions may be unremarkable basal cell carcinomas on histological examination, or may be of the morphoeic type (Figure 4.15). One published study suggests that UV-induced DNA repair synthesis decreases in affected individuals.[31] Because of this, and the recognized effect of UV on basal cell carcinomas in individuals without the full basal cell naevus syndrome, it is suggested that sun avoidance and the use of a total sunblock is a sensible approach. Recent studies of the distribution of lesions in affected patients give further suggestive information that UV exposure plays a part in the development of individual basal cell naevi.[32]

Once basal cell carcinomas appear, surgical excision is the treatment of choice. A proportion of the basal cell carcinomas in affected individuals are of

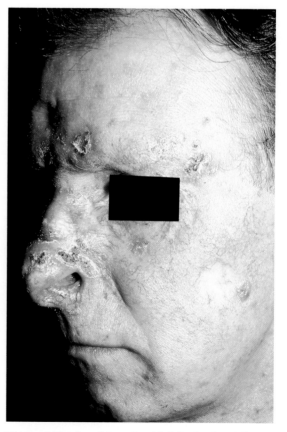

Figure 4.10 An adult male with fully developed features of naevoid basal cell carcinoma syndrome on the face.

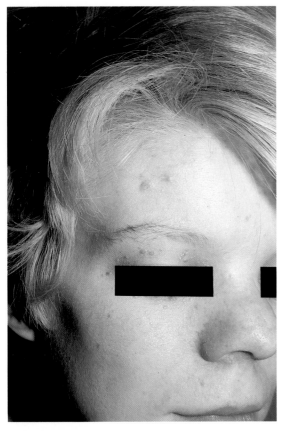

Figure 4.11 A young boy with naevoid basal cell carcinoma syndrome and two early basal cell carcinomas on the forehead.

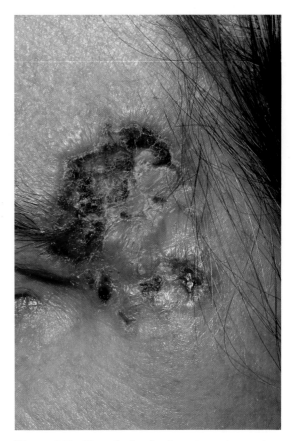

Figure 4.12 Extensive basal cell carcinoma in a patient with naevoid basal cell carcinoma syndrome.

the morphoeic variety, and for these micrographic control of completeness of excision by the Mohs or a similar technique may be helpful. It is important that X-ray therapy should not be used to treat these basal cell carcinomas. Although radiotherapy is an appropriate modality of treatment for basal cell carcinomas arising sporadically in individuals who do not have the basal cell naevus syndrome, there are a number of reports of the development of very large numbers of basal cell carcinomas in the area exposed to X-irradiation in patients with the syndrome.[33]

Familial atypical mole syndrome

This disorder was first recognized almost simultaneously by Clark and his associates, and the group of Lynch et al.[34,35] Clark suggested the name BK mole syndrome after the initials of two patients, while Lynch preferred the term familial atypical multiple mole malignant melanoma syndrome (FAMMM syndrome). The current preferred term is the atypical mole syndrome. Terminology has perhaps caused confusion and delayed comparison of findings between groups, but a recent NIH consensus conference has made sensible recommendations.[36] Sporadic melanoma with or without atypical moles is discussed in Chapter 9.

Genetics

Genetic studies of familial atypical mole patients who also have melanoma in several generations are a very active area of molecular genetic research at the present

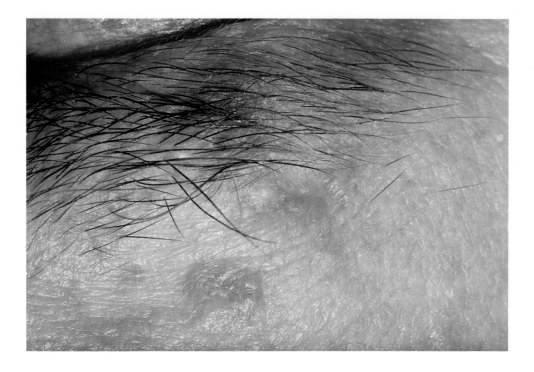

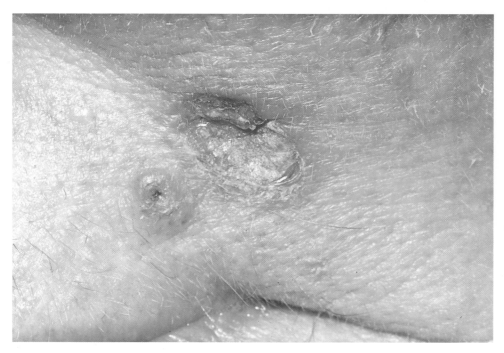

Figures 4.13 and 4.14   Early basal cell carcinomas in naevoid basal cell carcinoma syndrome.

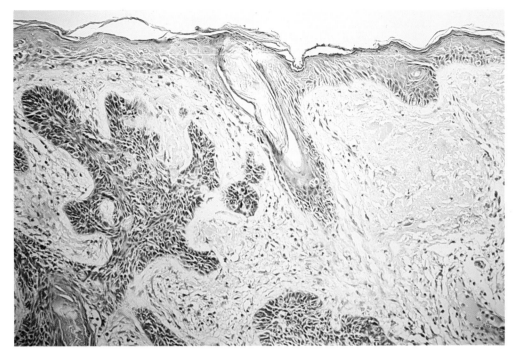

Figure 4.15 The pathological appearance of the lesion illustrated clinically in Figure 4.14. A typical basal cell carcinoma pattern is present.

time. Studies from both the USA and the Netherlands suggested that this syndrome is inherited by the autosomal dominant route, and American workers suggested that the gene was located on chromosome 1p.[37] No other group could confirm this finding, but both cytogenetic and family studies have now located an alternative genetic locus on chromosome 9p13–22.[37] Groups in Utah, Australia and the Netherlands have all confirmed this observation, and reanalysis of the patients originally suggesting a locus on chromosome 1 has shown that some of these families do also have chromosome 9 abnormalities.[38–40] It is currently hypothesized that there is on chromosome 9q a tumour suppressor gene involved in melanoma, and possibly also in other tumours,[41] and attention is currently focused on p16a tumour suppressor gene which inhibits cyclin-dependent kinase. This gene maps to 9p21, and is deleted in a high proportion of melanoma cell lines.[42]

Clinical features (Figures 4.16 and 4.17)

The original affected families were identified because of the presence of numerous large, irregular melanocytic naevi on the skin, a history of multiple primary malignant melanomas, and a family history of malignant melanoma. The atypical naevus pattern is visible by puberty, and primary melanomas develop one or two decades earlier than would be expected in patients with no such family history. The majority of melanomas that develop, but not all of them, do so in pre-existing naevi. While there are some reports of affected families also having an increased incidence of ocular melanoma, this has not been confirmed in all families studied. Similarly, although Lynch has suggested that there is a high incidence of non-melanoma malignancies in affected families,[43] it has not yet been established conclusively by appropriate case–control studies whether or not non-melanoma malignancy is higher in affected families than would be expected by chance.

Pathology

The precursor atypical mole, previously called a dysplastic naevus, will show architectural, cytological and host response features that allow the diagnosis of

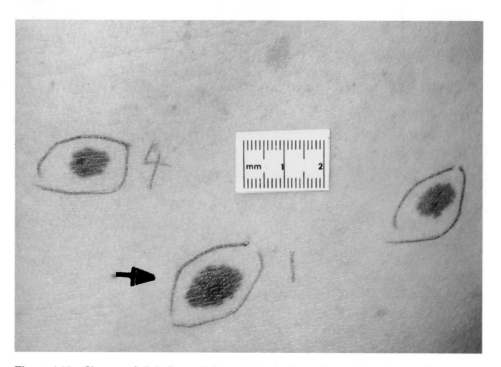

a dysplastic melanocytic naevus to be made.[44] The architectural features include lentiginous melanocytic hyperplasia, and bridging by melanocyte nests of rete pegs. The main cytological feature is nuclear hyperchromatism and occasional mitotic figures are seen in naevus cells. The host response features include elongation of epidermal rete pegs, the presence of a lymphocytic infiltrate, concentric or lamellar collagen fibroplasia, and angiogenesis at the base of the lesion. These features are not specific for the familial variant of the atypical mole syndrome and are seen also in lesions in sporadic cases.

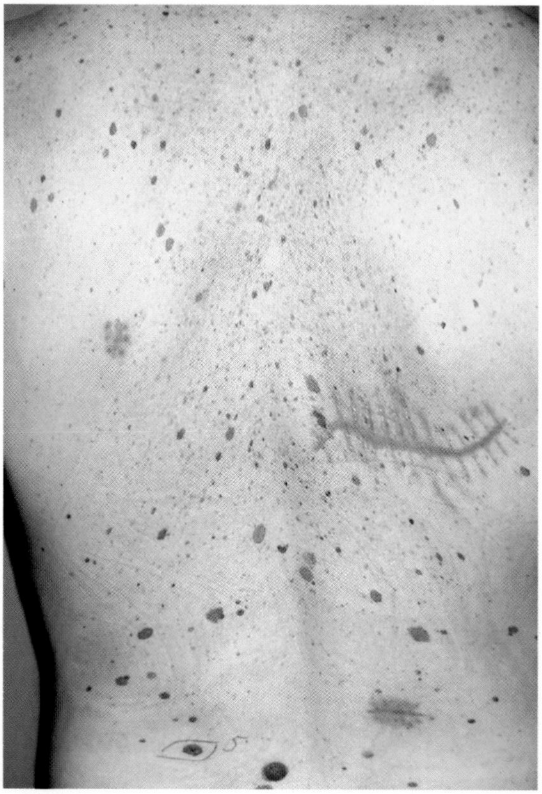

Management

The condition should be suspected in all cases of familial malignant melanoma, and considered in patients with multiple primary melanomas. When the

Figure 4.16   General view of a 40-year-old male with familial atypical mole syndrome. This patient had had four primary melanomas and his father died of melanoma.

Figure 4.17   Close-up of clinically atypical naevi, showing large size and irregular margin.

diagnosis is confirmed, all first-degree relatives should be examined if possible. Those with large numbers of melanocytic naevi 5 mm or greater in diameter, with an irregular outline and irregular pigmentation, should have at least two representative naevi biopsied for histological examination. The remaining lesions should be charted on body maps and photographed with an adjacent centimetre scale. The patient should be reviewed with this photograph and maps at appropriate intervals, possibly every 3–6 months. There is recent clear evidence from the Dutch studies that this type of screening and subsequent supervision results in identification and excision of early primary malignant melanomas while they are thinner and therefore of better prognosis.

It has been calculated that for the patient with multiple atypical moles and two or more relatives who have already had melanoma, the likelihood of developing melanoma during a lifetime is virtually 100 per cent.[45] Thus, although prevention of development of primary tumours may be impossible, early diagnosis and prompt surgery of thin curable lesions is feasible.

In view of the known effect of sun exposure on the development of sporadic melanoma and the history of more than average sun exposure in melanoma-bearing members of some of the affected families,[46,47] it is suggested that those with familial melanoma should be counselled against sunbathing and advised to use appropriately high SPF sunscreens.

As yet there are no reports of an increased incidence of primary tumours in women in the familial melanoma families who use oral contraceptives. However, in view of the known effects of oestrogens on the melanocyte system, other contraceptive techniques may be safer and more appropriate.

Multiple self-healing epithelioma of Ferguson-Smith[48]

Definition and genetics

An autosomal dominant condition in which affected individuals develop crops of raised nodules, the majority of which subside spontaneously to leave irregular, depressed scars. The gene has recently been mapped to chromosome 9q and appears to lie between 9q22 and 9q31,[49] the same locus as that associated with Gorlin's syndrome patients. Thus these two family cancer syndromes may be caused by different mutations of the same gene.

Clinical features (Figures 4.18–4.20)

This is a rare genodermatosis. Two large Scottish families have been carefully identified by the son of the individual who first recognized the entity.[50] Sporadic cases do occur, but some of these on more detailed history will be found to be related to the original families.

The great majority of lesions first develop in early adult life and will be found on the light-exposed skin of the face, around the ears, nose, and mouth. Lesions tend to develop in crops, and if untreated will usually resolve spontaneously over a period of 10–14 weeks, leaving a very unsightly scar with a crenellated edge.

On biopsy the lesion will be indistinguishable from invasive squamous carcinoma (Figures 4.21 and 4.22). Although the clinical history resembles that of keratoacanthoma, the histology is quite distinct. The characteristic raised shouldered lateral margin of the keratoacanthoma is absent, and the epithelial strands at the base have a more irregular and infiltrative pattern.

Management

The condition to date is usually diagnosed in family members who recognize the lesions themselves. Sporadic cases may be suspected on the basis of a young person developing rapidly growing lesions with the classic histology.

Although the great majority of lesions do 'self-heal', as the name of the condition suggests, a small number of case reports exist of patients in the affected families who did develop true invasive squamous carcinoma, which proved fatal.

For this reason, and because of the unsightly quality of the scars, excision of early lesions may be the preferred treatment. Cryotherapy may also abort lesions if administered at a very early stage in the growth pattern.

Group 2

Torre's syndrome

Both Muir and Torre deserve credit for recognizing the association between multiple sebaceous gland neoplasms and visceral malignancy.[51,52]

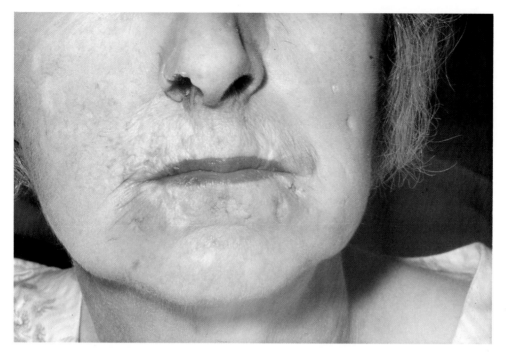

Figure 4.18   Facial appearance of a female patient with multiple self-healing epithelioma of Ferguson-Smith. Note multiple scars around mouth.

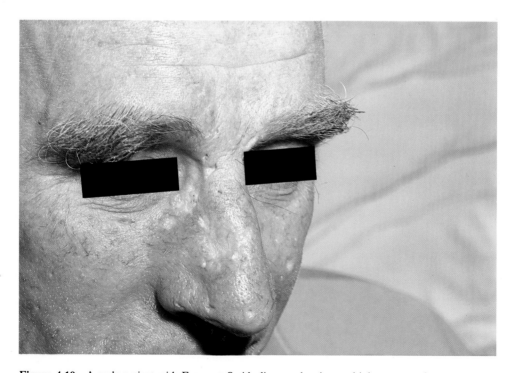

Figure 4.19   A male patient with Ferguson-Smith disease, showing multiple scars on the nose.

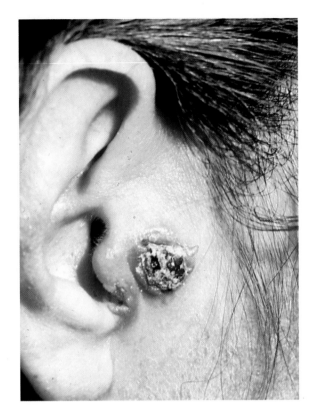

Figure 4.20   Typical keratoacanthoma-like clinical appearance of a Ferguson-Smith disease lesion. The pathology is not similar to that of keratoacanthoma.

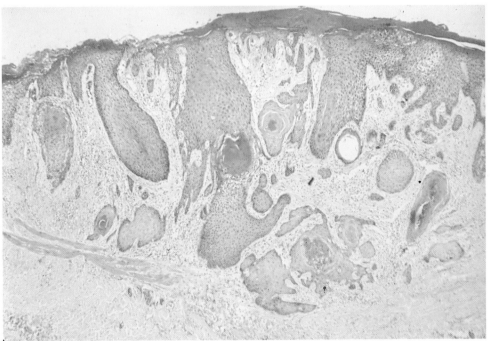

Figure 4.21   Low-power view of a Ferguson-Smith disease lesion. The appearance is very similar to that of invasive squamous cell carcinoma.

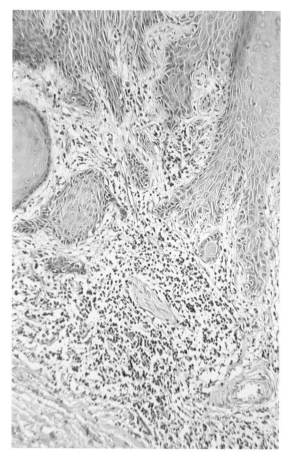

Figure 4.22 High-power view of a Ferguson-Smith disease lesion, showing an invasive tongue of epithelium and surrounding infiltrate.

Aetiology and genetics

The aetiology is unknown. The roles of growth factors and altered oncogene products are currently under active investigation. Inheritance is by the autosomal dominant route.

Clinical features

Patients may present first with either the cutaneous lesions or visceral malignancy.[53] The cutaneous lesions may be single or multiple sebaceous gland

tumours (Figure 4.23).[54] These may be adenomas, epitheliomas, or carcinomas. Keratoacanthomas are also reported with increased frequency.

A study of 59 patients with sebaceous gland proliferation revealed that 25 (42 per cent) had between them a total of 49 primary visceral malignancies.[55] The majority of these were in the colon (25), 9 were of the urogenital system, and 5 were haematological. Eighteen out of 25 patients (72 per cent) in a recent series had a family history of malignancy, predominantly of the colon. Patients may also have non-malignant thyroid disease and prostatic hyperplasia.

The hyperplastic lesions of the sebaceous gland elements may be single or multiple and range from adenoma to carcinoma. Sebaceous gland tumours of all types are relatively rare, and the Muir–Torre syndrome should be considered in any patient with such lesions.

Investigation and management

If the condition is suspected, full colonoscopy is required, as the majority of the colonic malignancies reported are proximal to the splenic flexure. It should be borne in mind that multiple primary colonic malignancies may develop, and that they may develop some years after the presentation of the facial lesions. Careful long-term follow-up is therefore required.

Cowden's syndrome (multiple hamartoma syndrome)

Definition and genetics[56]

A syndrome associated with multiple hair follicle tumours, mainly trichilemmomas (Figure 4.24), oral papillomas, and breast carcinoma. Studies of affected families to date suggest autosomal dominant transmission.

Clinical features

This condition bears the name of the patient first described by Lloyd and Dennis in 1963.[57] They identified a patient with facial nodules, thyroid adenoma, scrotal tongue, oral papillomas, and advanced fibrocystic disease of the breast. Early breast

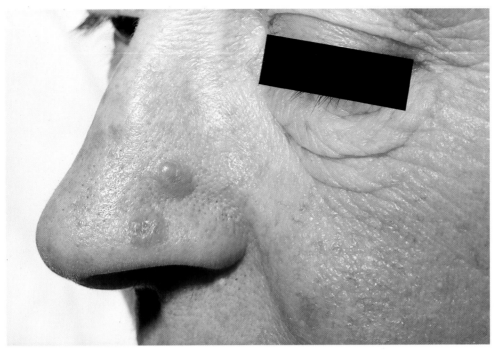

Figure 4.23   A sebaceous adenoma in a patient with carcinoma of the colon. Torre's syndrome.

cancer was also present in the propositus, and her mother and sister had similar problems. Two aunts had died of breast cancer.

In subsequent series, males and females appeared to be affected about equally, and half gave a positive family history. Cutaneous nodules frequently thought by affected individuals to be warts are seen on the face, palms of the hands and soles of the feet. Large numbers of these lesions may be present around the mouth and eyes (Figure 4.24). On biopsy they will be found to be tumours arising from the hair follicles (Figure 4.25).[58] Macular, brown-pigmented lesions may also be present on the skin, and 85 per cent of patients have striking involvement of the oral mucosa. Usually, this is first seen in the second decade and precedes the cutaneous lesions. The oral mucosa may show a cobblestoned appearance. Diagnosis of the condition is rarely feasible before the age of 20 years.

Non-cutaneous lesions associated with the syndrome include thyroid adenomas, found in 70 per cent, and breast lesions in 75 per cent of affected females. Gastrointestinal polyps and other gastrointestinal problems are reported in 40 per cent, and

skeletal abnormalities in a similar percentage. Ocular and neurological abnormalities are also seen.[59–61]

Carcinoma of the breast is to date reported only in females but is seen in 50 per cent of affected women. Thyroid carcinoma is reported in 10 per cent of both sexes affected.

Management

The diagnosis may be suspected in the late teens and early twenties because of the facial and oral lesions. Biopsies should be carried out to confirm the presence of hair follicle tumours. A full family history should be taken and first-degree relatives should be examined. The patient should be investigated for thyroid, breast, and gastrointestinal abnormalities. The frequency with which such investigations need to be repeated if no malignancy is found on first examination will vary according to local circumstances. The risk of breast carcinoma in affected females is obviously very high and in the past, because of this, prophylactic mastectomy has been suggested.

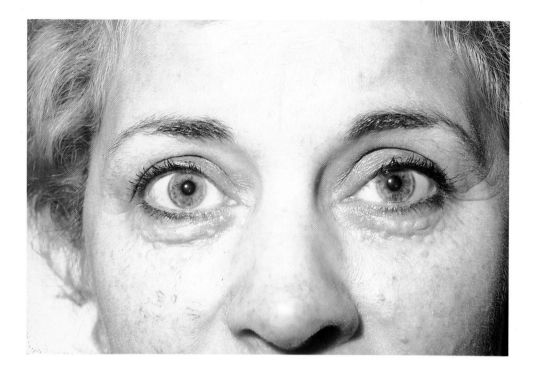

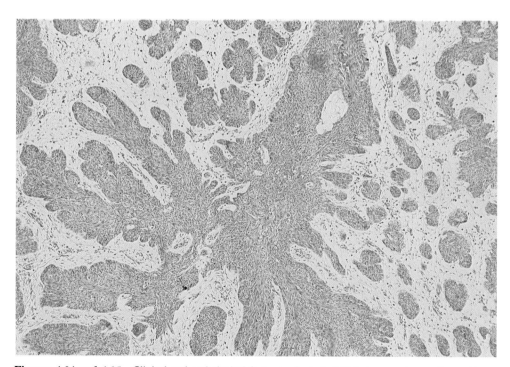

Figures 4.24 and 4.25   Clinical and pathological features of a hair follicle tumour in a patient with Cowden's syndrome.

Gardner's syndrome[62,63]

Definition and genetics

An autosomal dominant condition associated with cutaneous cysts, particularly on the scalp, bony abnormalities, and colonic polyps that progress to colonic carcinoma.

Clinical features[64]

These patients frequently present first with cutaneous or bony lesions. The cutaneous lesions may be epidermal cysts, or true sebaceous cysts, and may be found in very large numbers on the scalp. A pilomatricoma-like change is reported in some of these cysts.[65,66] Soft tissue tumours are also common, particularly desmoid tumours. Dental abnormalities may be noted in childhood, and also skeletal abnormalities of the skull and facial bones.

The more serious aspect of this syndrome is the presence of very large numbers of colonic polyps. These may cause problems with anaemia because of haemorrhage or intussusception, and up to 60 per cent of affected patients develop colonic malignancy, often at a relatively young age. Other malignancies are also reported in Gardner's syndrome, including adrenal, thyroid and ovarian carcinoma, and also carcinoid.

Management

Once the syndrome is diagnosed, all family members should be screened and regular barium enemas performed. The risk of malignancy of the colon is so high that some authorities would consider prophylactic colectomy justified.

The Peutz–Jeghers syndrome

Definition and genetics

A syndrome complex of perioral macular pigmentation and polyps of the small intestine associated with malignancy in other sites. Once again, inheritance is by autosomal dominant transmission.

Clinical features

Peutz first described this entity in 1921, and it was further described by Jeghers, McKusick and Katz in 1949.[67,68] Affected individuals are usually first recognized by the presence of large numbers of brown macules on and around the lips and also on the oral mucosa (Figure 4.26).[69] The gastrointestinal lesions are usually asymptomatic, although they may give rise to intussusception. Barium studies reveal large numbers of polyps in the small intestine.

Pathology

Pathology of the facial lesions is that of a benign lentigo. There is focal overproduction of melanin pigment by benign melanocytes. These lesions are not premalignant. The polyps are hamartomatous and adenomatous.

Associated malignancies

There has been some confusion in the literature over the relationship of the Peutz–Jeghers syndrome to non-cutaneous malignancy. Initial studies concentrated on investigation of the polyps of the gastrointestinal tract, and the overall results suggested that the polyps themselves were not premalignant.[70] More recently, however, attention has focused on non-cutaneous malignancies arising outside these polyps.[71] Linos et al reported a 29 per cent incidence of malignancy in 6 of 21 patients.[72] A recent review by Giardiello and colleagues concentrates on 31 patients from 13 families followed over 12 years.[73] Of these individuals, 15 have developed malignancies over the 12-year period, a relative risk compared with the general population of 18. Tumours developed include 4 pancreatic malignancies, 2 breast carcinomas, and 2 lung, 1 uterine and 1 ovarian cancer. All malignancies occurred when the patients were relatively young. The most outstanding increased rate of malignancy in this series is shown by pancreatic cancer, which is 100 times more common than would be expected in the population at large.

Management

The diagnosis may be suspected on the perioral pigmentation and should be confirmed by barium studies. Malignancies in non-intestinal sites should be excluded by CT scan of chest and abdomen and both abdominal and gynaecological ultrasound. As with other conditions in this group, the exact frequency of repeat investigations will vary according to clinical features and

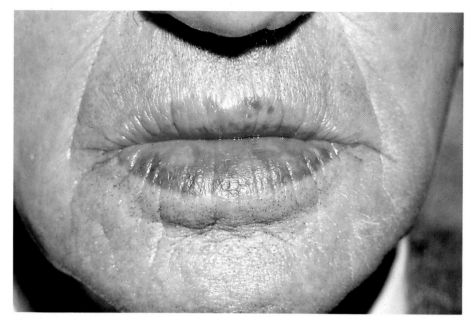

Figure 4.26   The Peutz–Jeghers syndrome – appearance of lip in an elderly male.

initial findings at first examination. It must be remembered with all these conditions that the cutaneous features may precede the malignancy by many years.

Dyskeratosis congenita (Zinsser–Engman–Cole syndrome)[74,75]

Definition and genetics[76]

Dyskeratosis congenita is a syndrome complex involving the skin, oral mucosa, and immune system. It is an X-linked disorder with, to date, only a small number of affected females reported.

Clinical features

The affected individual is likely to be male and will present in the first decade of life.[77] The children develop reticular pigmentation on sun-exposed sites and this becomes hyperpigmented. Blisters may also develop on these sites. There may thus be clinical confusion with Rothmund–Thomson syndrome or porphyria. In dyskeratosis congenita, however, the child will have nail abnormalities, which are not seen in the latter two conditions. Initially the fingernails and then the toenails develop ridging, become brittle, and eventually virtually disappear. Oral and genital leukoplakia are usually present and dentition is frequently incomplete and of poor quality.

Defects in both humoral and cell-mediated immunity have been reported in about 50 per cent of patients and this is likely to account for the multiple infections from which some children suffer.[78]

Marrow failure is also relatively common, beginning with a progressive and resistant anaemia. Malignancy may supervene on the oral mucosa abnormalities and gastrointestinal malignancies are also relatively common.

Recent studies on photosensitivity in these children have reported an increased incidence of sister chromatid exchange.[79]

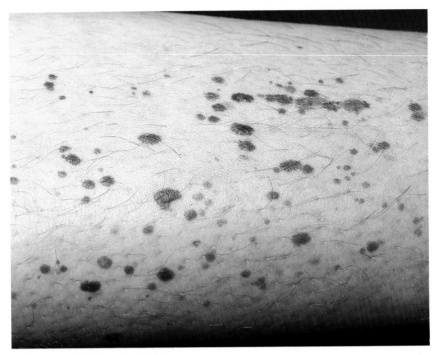

Figure 4.27 Multiple lentigines and blue naevi on arm of a young girl with multiple endocrine dysfunction and malignancy.

Carney's syndrome[80]

Definition and genetics

A syndrome complex of myxomas, endocrine dysfunction, and pigmentary abnormalities associated with breast and endocrine malignancies. At present only 40 cases of this syndrome are reported in the world literature. Of these 11 have a positive family history but the exact mode of inheritance is not yet firmly established.

Clinical features[81,82]

Affected individuals have striking facial lentigines similar to those seen in Peutz–Jeghers syndrome but more diffuse. Other sites are also involved (Figure 4.27). In addition to the lentigines, however, they also have more deeply set blue naevi. These are darker and palpable lesions. Myxomas of the cardiac muscle, the breast and the dermis are common, and adrenal cortical hyperfunction is also seen. Testicular tumours and pituitary adenomas are seen.

Management

The condition may present with cardiac myxomas, Cushing's syndrome, or sexual precocity. The characteristic pigmentary lesions may suggest the diagnosis. Echocardiography should be performed. The condition is probably the same entity as the NAME syndrome[83] (naevi, atrial myxomas, and ephelides) and also as the LAMB syndrome (lentigines, atrial myxomas and multiple blue naevi).[84]

5
Benign epidermal lesions and cysts

The lesions discussed in this chapter are relatively common. In contrast to those discussed in Chapter 6, they are a group of lesions in which malignant change is hardly ever recorded. However, because of their frequency it is important that family doctors, dermatologists and oncologists are able to recognize these lesions clinically, as they may give rise to considerable concern among patients and may be confused with aggressive and potentially fatal malignant lesions. This is particularly true in the case of the patient who has already had a cutaneous malignancy, such as a melanoma, and who is particularly conscious of new or changing lesions of any type on his or her skin.

The lesions discussed in this chapter are:

Verrucous epidermal naevi
 Linear lesions
 Inflammatory linear verrucous epidermal naevus (ILVEN)
 Naevi with Darier's like or epidermolytic hyperkeratosis-like histology
 The epidermal naevus syndrome
Becker's naevus
Seborrhoeic keratosis (basal cell papilloma)
 Acanthotic, hyperkeratotic and reticular types
 Irritated basal cell papilloma
 The sign of Leser–Trélat
Inverted follicular keratosis
Birt–Hogg–Dubé syndrome
Clear cell acanthoma of Degos
Kyrle's disease
Flegel's disease
Cysts (pilar and epidermal varieties)

Verrucous epidermal naevi[1]

The term naevus literally means 'maternal impression', but in the dermatological and pathological literature it is frequently used without definition to define a melanocytic naevus. This is, of course, an incorrect use of the word, which should always carry a qualifying term, such as epidermal or melanocytic.

An alternative name for these lesions is the term 'hamartoma', which means a non-neoplastic malformation.

Epidermal naevi are relatively common entities, being recorded in approximately 1 in 1000 of the population. They may be seen at birth or in early infancy, and, if visible at this stage in life, may be a pale, coffee-coloured, macular-pigmented area with little, if any, hyperkeratosis. As the child matures and reaches puberty these areas may become grossly hyperkeratotic with considerable disfigurement and continual shedding of greasy scales from the surface (Figures 5.1–5.5). Naevi may also become visible for the first time in childhood or in the second decade, and in this situation more rapid development of hyperkeratosis tends to be seen.

On pathological examination, it will be seen that while the lesions are generally hyperpigmented, this is not because of an excess of melanocytes, but because of a build-up of melanin pigment in the excessive numbers of keratinocytes (Figure 5.6).

The lesions of the simple verrucous type of epidermal naevus are usually asymptomatic, but may give rise to considerable cosmetic concern, particularly if on the face and neck. They may be painful if the lesions involve the nailbeds, and may give rise to

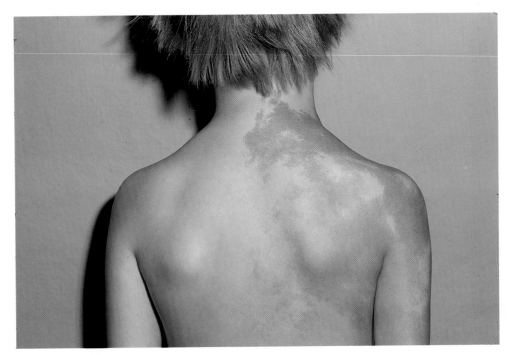

Figure 5.1   An epidermal naevus on the shoulder and right arm of a young boy.

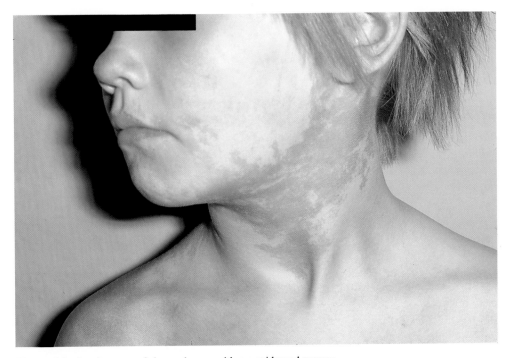

Figure 5.2   Involvement of the neck area with an epidermal naevus.

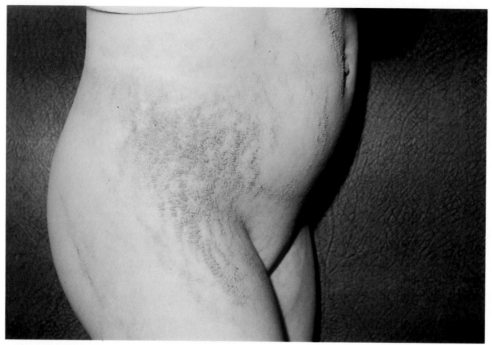

Figure 5.3 An epidermal naevus involving the right groin.

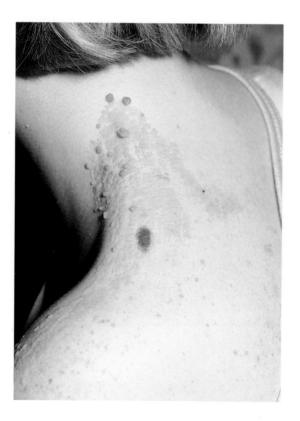

Figure 5.4 A patient in the second decade with an epidermal naevus becoming hyperkeratotic.

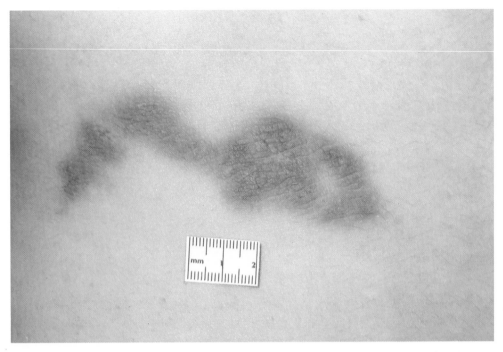

Figure 5.5 An epidermal naevus on the flank of a 17-year-old that had appeared for the first time 6 months before the photograph was taken.

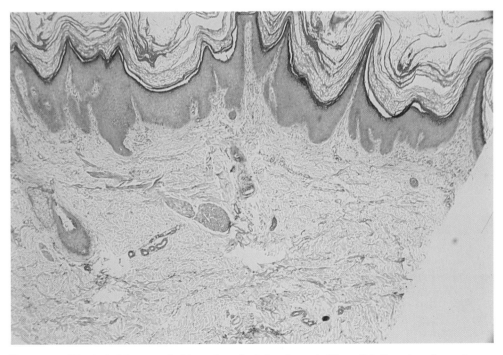

Figure 5.6 Histological features of a biopsy from the lesion shown in Figure 5.4. Gross hyperkeratosis is evident.

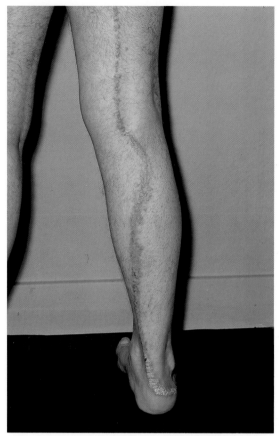

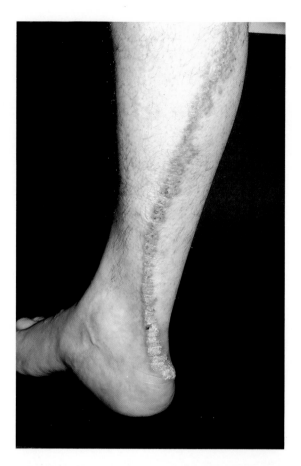

Figures 5.7 and 5.8   Linear epidermal naevus.

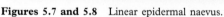

problems with appropriate footwear if they involve the foot. If the lesions are grossly hyperkeratotic and involve body flexures or the feet, secondary infection and bacterial colonization may cause problems with malodour from the lesions.

Diagnosis and management

The diagnosis is usually self-evident, with the presence of a frequently rather sworled area of hyperkeratotic, hyperpigmented skin more commonly on the upper than the lower part of the body. If the lesions are on the trunk and asymptomatic, the value of treatment is very doubtful.

Epidermal shaving may reduce the hyperkeratosis but this almost invariably recurs. Deep excision of the lesions will result in complete clearance, but will of course leave a scar. Some individuals find that freezing or electrodesiccation with cautery is of some value, but once again regrowth frequently occurs. Some patients find the use of an abrasive pad of the 'Buf Puf™ type or the use of emery paper on the lesions useful, but this is not generally medically recommended.

Linear epidermal naevus

This lesion is simply a verrucous epidermal naevus occurring in a clear linear pattern, usually involving one of the limbs (Figures 5.7–5.9). The linear pattern does not follow an obvious dermatome distribution, and if the lesion extends down the leg and over the

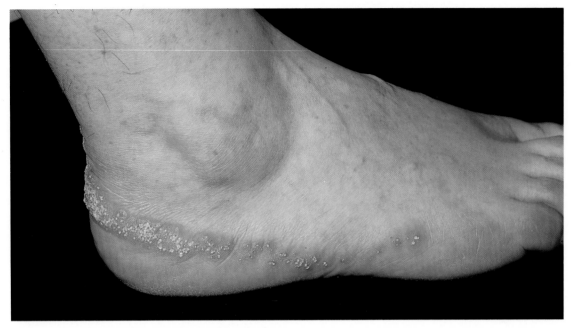

Figure 5.9 A linear epidermal naevus involving the foot.

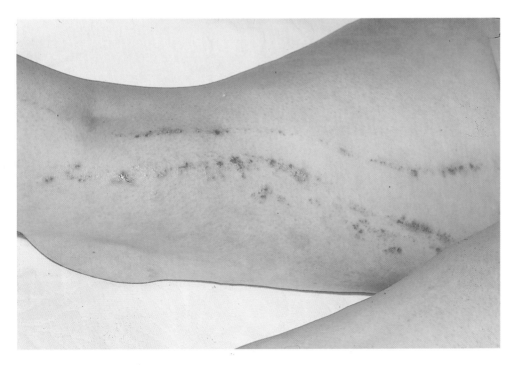

Figure 5.10 An inflammatory linear verrucous epidermal naevus (ILVEN) on the upper leg area of a young girl.

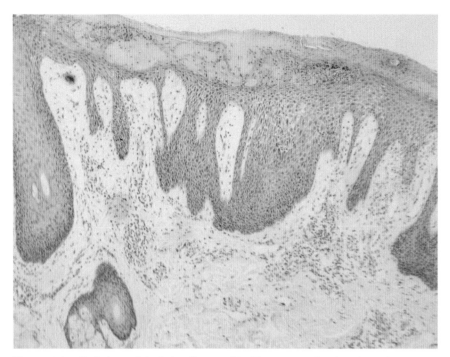

Figure 5.11   Pathology of the lesion illustrated in Figure 5.10, showing alternating orthokeratosis and parakeratosis.

heel may give rise to considerable problems with footwear (Figure 5.9). Malignant change is very rarely reported in these lesions, but usually in coexisting sebaceous naevi (Chapter 6).[2]

Inflammatory linear verrucous epidermal naevus (ILVEN)

This interesting lesion may be mistaken clinically for a chronic patch of dermatitis (Figure 5.10).[3,4] The condition should be suspected in any child who has a persistent hyperkeratotic dermatitic patch on the skin, but who is not obviously atopic. The lesions appear to be a simple verrucous naevus with the addition of an inflammatory response in the form of a brisk lymphocytic infiltrate. It is speculated that this is due to lymphokine secretion by the overabundant epidermal cells.

An intriguing pattern is seen on histological examination, with layers of parakeratotic stratum corneum alternating with layers of normal orthokeratotic stratum corneum (Figure 5.11).[5]

Management

These lesions are pruritic, and the patient tends to scratch the area, thus causing secondary infection. Control of symptoms is difficult and requires potent steroids, which are not generally recommended for young children. Excision of these lesions is therefore justified if they are of a size and on a site which makes this a practical approach.

Epidermal naevi with unusual histological features[1]

A small number of epidermal naevi have histological features similar to those seen in Darier's disease (keratosis follicularis) and other lesions have in patches histology indistinguishable from that seen in the non-bullous form of congenital ichthyosiform erythroderma (Figure 5.12) (epidermolytic hyperkeratosis). These differential diagnoses should cause no confusion if there is good collaboration and

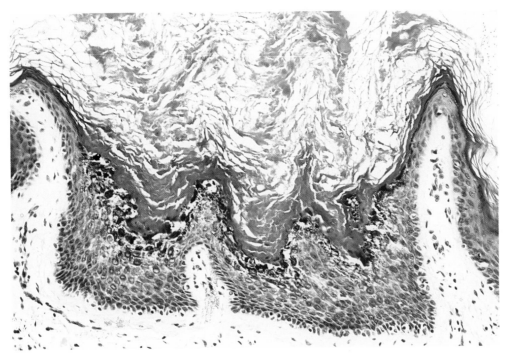

Figure 5.12 Pathological features from an epidermal naevus biopsy very similar to those seen in epidermolytic hyperkeratosis.

communication between clinician and pathologist. If, however, this is not the case the pathologist should delay reporting Darier's disease on an isolated hyperkeratotic lesion biopsied from a child and seek further clinical information.

The epidermal naevus syndrome[6]

This condition has given rise to some confusion. The terms systematized and segmental epidermal naevi have in the past both been used to describe this entity. There is involvement of large parts of the body surface with a gross verrucous epidermal naevus. A striking feature of many affected individuals is that their lesions are confined predominantly to one side of the body with a relatively sharp cut-off in the midline (Figure 5.13). Close inspection of the entire surface of the skin will, however, reveal that there are frequently areas of involvement on the minimally affected side. In addition to suffering the gross disfigurement caused by this large epidermal naevus, these unfortunate individuals frequently have significant skeletal abnormalities, with involvement of the spine, skull, mandible and clavicle, dental abnormalities, focal phocomelia, abnormalities of the central nervous system, including mental retardation, convulsions and tumours, and involvement of the eyes, ears and oral mucosa. In any young child with a large verrucous epidermal naevus, careful assessment of the skeleton, the dentition, the central nervous system, hearing and sight is advisable.

Becker's naevus (pigmented hairy epidermal naevus)[7]

This relatively common problem tends to present in young adults and involves mainly the shoulder girdle and upper limb area. It is seen in many different racial types, and there is frequently a history of preceding sunburn.[8] Following this trauma, the macular pigmentation becomes obvious on the affected limb, and is associated with, at times, significant overgrowth of

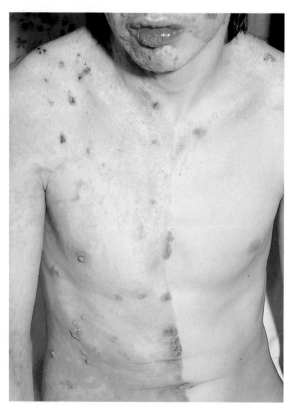

Figure 5.13 A 14-year-old male with epidermal naevus syndrome. This boy also had mental retardation.

hair on the affected site (Figure 5.14). In general, the pigmentation is relatively pale and uniform but there may be some darker areas within the lesion.

Biopsy will show surprisingly little abnormality. There is slight hyperkeratosis and no increase in melanocytes, but an increase in visible melanin pigment in the basal layer, and it is necessary to postulate that the increase in pigmentation is due to increased activity of a normal number of melanocytes (Figure 5.15). Hair follicles are present in increased numbers and the diameter of individual hairs is somewhat thicker than would be expected for the site in question.

Management

These lesions are usually easily recognized but difficult to manage. The area of skin involved is usually large, and complete excision is not practical. Some individuals are more concerned about the hair growth than the pigmentary change, and for these individuals regular epilation or even electrolysis may be worthwhile. Cosmetic cover of the pigmented area is usually unsatisfactory because of the associated hypertrichosis.

There have recently been a number of reports of benign smooth muscle hamartomas underlying these lesions of Becker's naevus.[9] These would appear to have no adverse prognostic significance.

The term 'naevus spilus tardus' has in the past been used as an alternative to Becker's naevus. This alternative terminology is not recommended. In the author's opinion, the true naevus spilus is an abnormality of the melanocyte system, and is better termed speckled lentiginous naevus. It is discussed in Chapter 9.

Seborrhoeic keratosis (basal cell papilloma)[10]

Acanthotic, hyperkeratotic and reticular types – definition, incidence and aetiology

This lesion is a benign overgrowth of epidermal keratinocytes. The term 'basal cell papilloma' is used by some individuals because a large proportion of the cells are small cells with dark nuclei and relatively small quantities of cytoplasm, thus resembling basal cells of the epidermis. They are seen mainly on the skin of the trunk in individuals in the fourth decade and older. They may become extremely numerous. Their aetiology is unknown, although on occasion large crops have been seen to develop after skin damage such as sunburn. Very similar lesions develop on the skin of experimental animals after the application of croton oil.[11]

Clinical features

Basal cell papillomas may have a large range of clinical presentations. One of the most common types is a solid, warty, acanthotic pigmented lesion, which grows on the surface of the skin.[12] The term seborrhoeic wart is often used to describe this lesion, which is confused by non-medical individuals with a melanocytic naevus, or even malignant melanoma. The lesions tend to grow to 1–3 cm in diameter,

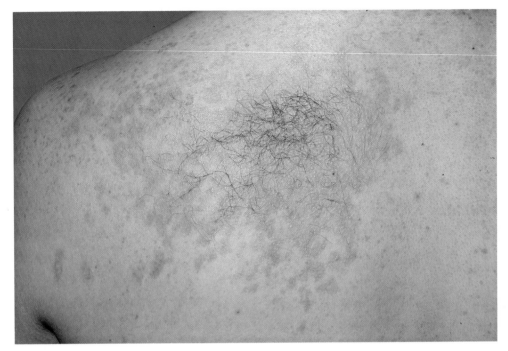

Figure 5.14 Clinical appearance of Becker's naevus, showing pale pigmentation and hypertrichosis.

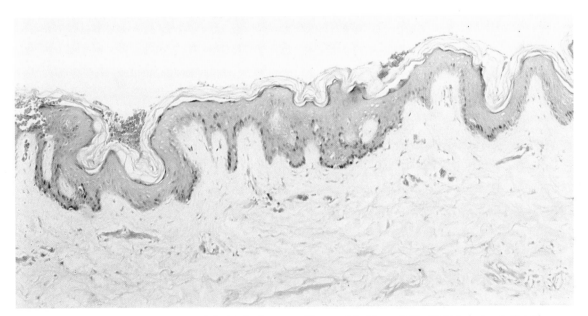

Figure 5.15 Pathological appearance of the Becker's naevus illustrated in Figure 5.14. Slight hyperkeratosis and increased melanin pigment are visible.

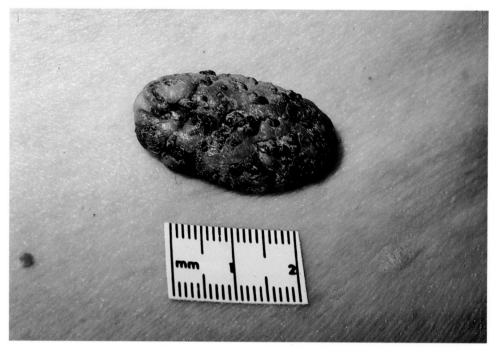

Figure 5.16   A solid basal cell papilloma with dense pigmentation and cerebriform appearance.

although a few may become much larger. The lesions are asymptomatic in general, although some patients complain of minor pruritus and irritation, particularly when they are on sites which are traumatized by clothing.

The solid pigmented basal cell papillomas are usually relatively easily distinguished on clinical grounds from benign melanocytic naevi and also from malignant melanoma, but occasionally there may be clinical doubt because of the intensity of pigmentation (Figures 5.16–5.19). The most helpful features are the profile of the lesion, virtually all of which is above the normal skin surface, and the irregular verrucous superficial surface of the lesion, on which a number of horn cysts can be seen clearly.

The flat type of basal cell papilloma is usually paler in colour than the solid type (Figures 5.20–5.22). Pigmentation in these lesions is not due to any specific involvement of the melanocyte system. The pigment is present merely because the melanocytes associated with the keratinocytes involved in the process have donated pigment to the cytoplasm of the keratinocytes and thus there is a greater volume of pigment, but not

of melanocytes, present (Figures 5.23–5.25). The flat type of seborrhoeic keratosis is seen most often on the cheek and may be a sandy brown irregular plaque. The most common cause of clinical confusion in these lesions is an early lentigo maligna, and in many cases a small biopsy may be necessary to confirm the histological nature of the lesion.

A number of seborrhoeic keratoses show gross scaling and hyperkeratosis, and these lesions may cause clinical confusion with actinic keratoses. A smaller number may, on pathological study, have a reticulate or adenoid appearance. These usually appear clinically as raised, pale brown plaques on the skin surface.

Irritated or inverted basal cell papilloma[13]

On occasions the seborrhoeic keratosis will become irritated. These lesions may be clinically similar to an early squamous cell carcinoma and may be both large

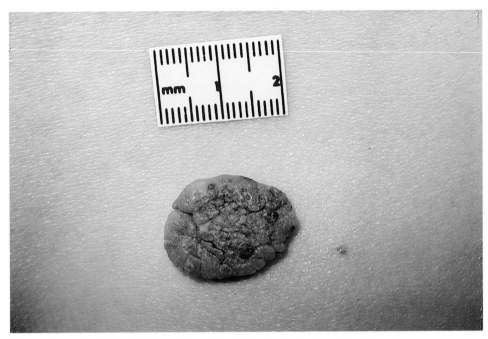

Figure 5.17 A solid basal cell papilloma. The lesion is clearly above the skin surface.

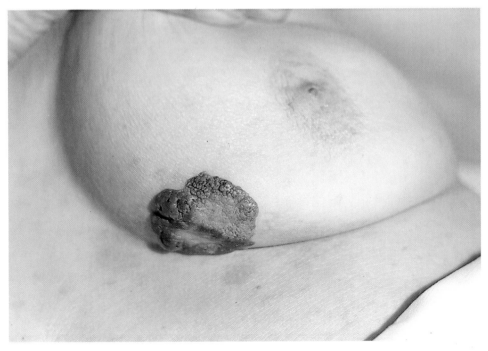

Figure 5.18 An extensive basal cell papilloma under the breast. The hyperkeratotic nature of the pigment is clearly seen.

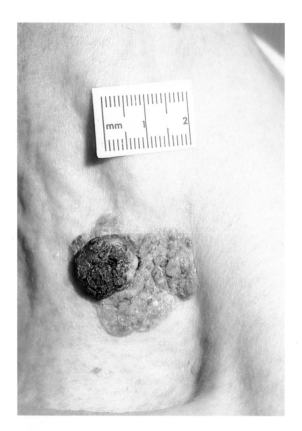

Figure 5.19 Nodular basal cell papilloma on top of a flat basal cell papilloma base.

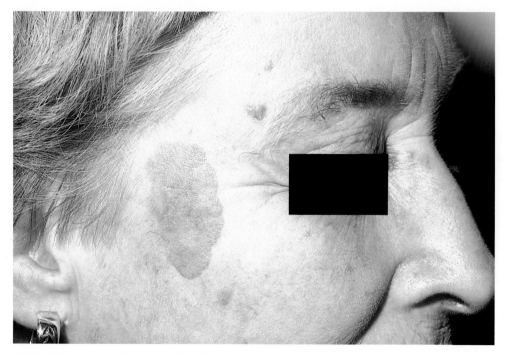

Figure 5.20 A large, flat, basal cell papilloma on the right cheek.

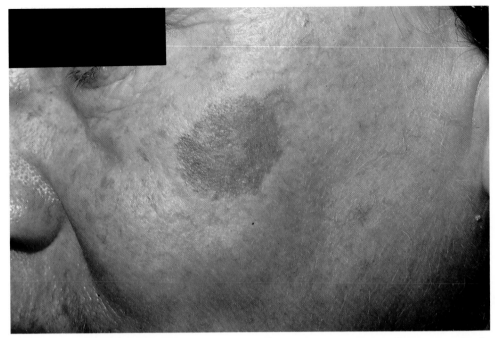

Figure 5.21 A flat basal cell papilloma on the left cheek. Clinically, a lentigo maligna was suspected.

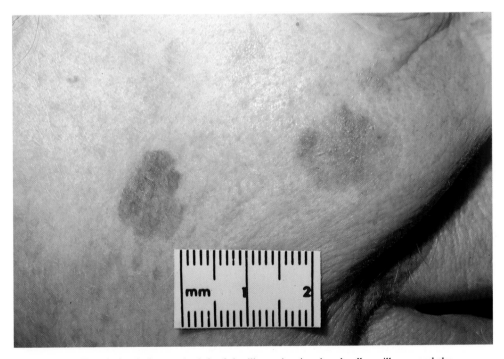

Figure 5.22 The darker lesion to the left of the illustration is a basal cell papilloma, and the inflamed lesion on the right is an early lentigo maligna.

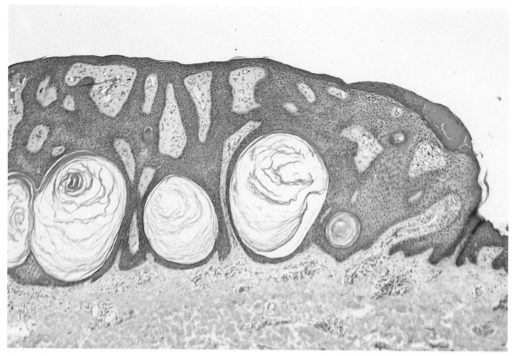

Figure 5.23   Pathological features of a basal cell papilloma, showing hyperkeratosis and horn cysts.

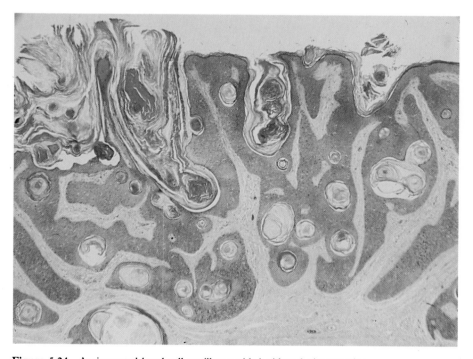

Figure 5.24   A pigmented basal cell papilloma with incidental pigmentation.

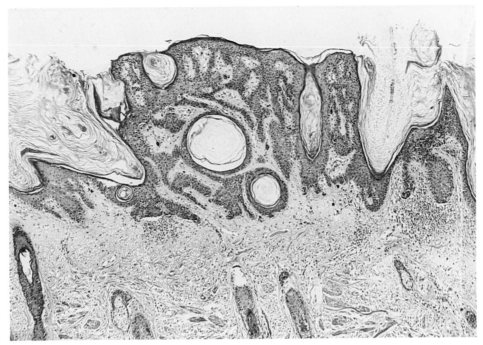

Figure 5.25   Pathology of a basal cell papilloma, showing hyperkeratosis and a reticular pattern.

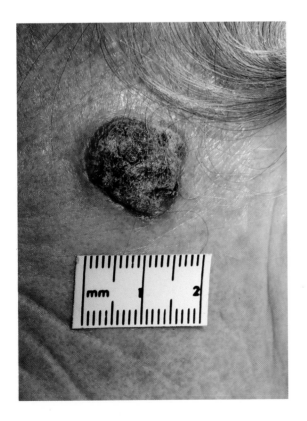

and inflamed (Figure 5.26). On biopsy it will be seen that there is a considerable inflammatory infiltrate around the body of cells involved in the process. These irritated basal cell papillomas frequently appear to have a larger proportion of their cell mass below the normal skin surface rather than above it, and this may account for the different clinical appearance and the inflammatory reaction that they provoke.

For the pathologist there may be difficulty in distinguishing between an extremely irritated seborrhoeic keratosis and an early squamous cell carcinoma. The cytology of the seborrhoeic keratosis should be reassuring, and mitotic figures are rare. The squamous eddies that are the hallmark of the seborrhoeic keratosis should be identified in these lesions (Figures 5.27 and 5.28).

Figure 5.26   An irritated basal cell papilloma.

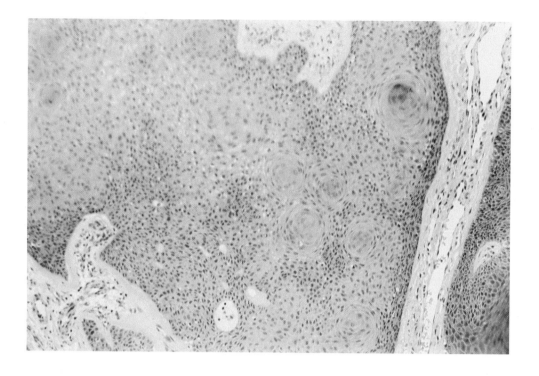

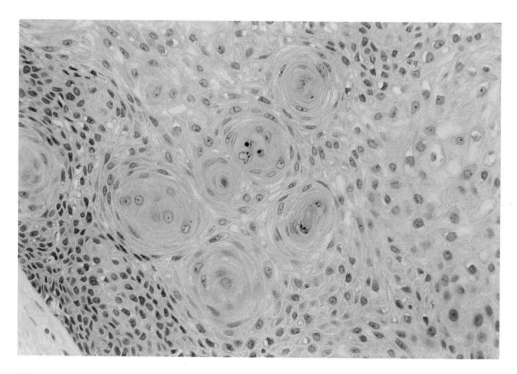

Figures 5.27 and 5.28 Pathology of irritated basal cell papillomas. Note the squamous eddies but lack of cytological signs of malignancy.

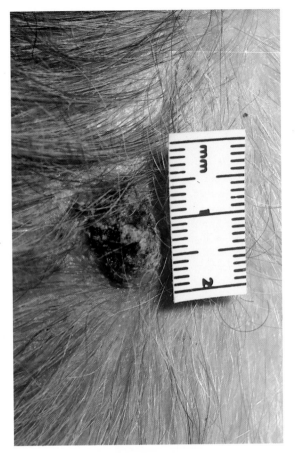

Figure 5.29 Inverted follicular keratosis. Note the clinical similarity to Figure 5.26.

on a number of occasions and the association should therefore be considered in a patient who reports the very sudden appearance of large numbers of seborrhoeic keratosis lesions. The most common site of any malignancy found appears to be the gastrointestinal tract.[16]

The mechanism for this association is not known. It would seem reasonable to postulate that growth factors are playing a role both in the malignancy and in its cutaneous marker.

Management of seborrhoeic keratoses

Benign seborrhoeic keratoses do not require specific management. If the lesions are asymptomatic, removal is not essential. If they are giving rise to symptoms or are cosmetically unacceptable they may be destroyed by coagulation diathermy or by cryotherapy. If there is clinical diagnostic doubt about any lesion, and in particular if there is any possibility that the lesion could be of melanocytic origin and possibly melanoma, a diagnostic biopsy and histological examination rather than destruction is the appropriate method of treatment.

Inverted follicular keratosis

Definition

This lesion was first described by Helwig in 1955, as an epidermal, usually facial, lesion.[17] Many individuals find it impossible to distinguish it, on either clinical or pathological grounds, from the irritated basal cell papilloma, which is the reason for its inclusion at this point in the text.

The sign of Leser–Trélat

In a small number of case reports there has been an association between the sudden appearance of very large numbers of seborrhoeic keratoses and internal malignancy. This observation was first made by Edmund Leser and Ulysse Trélat and is thus sometimes referred to as the sign of Leser–Trélat.[14,15] As with many cutaneous markers of internal malignancy, there is not convincing statistical proof of an association, but the phenomenon has been reported

Clinical features

The great majority of all reported lesions to date are on the face, and present clinically as firm, grey, non-inflamed lesions (Figure 5.29).[18] The most common clinical differential diagnosis is a verruca vulgaris, but the majority of patients are middle-aged or older. This clinical appearance may, however, explain the belief of Spielvogel et al that the lesion is of viral origin.[19] As yet no type of human papilloma virus has been identified in these lesions.

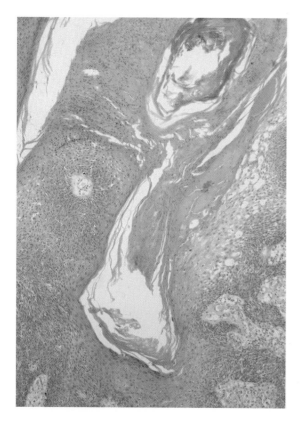

Pathology

This lesion, if it is indeed an entity, may be a proliferation of the keratinocytes of the follicular infundibulum or intraepidermal part of the hair follicle, and thus is the equivalent in the pilosebaceous follicle of the eccrine poroma in the eccrine sweat duct.

A papillomatous mass of keratinocytes is seen, which may on low-power examination resemble a keratoacanthoma. The typical shouldered edge of the keratoacanthoma is, however, lacking. The deepest margin of the lesion is composed of a mass of keratinocytes with a broad, blunted profile, unlike the tongues of invading keratinocytes which are seen in invasive squamous carcinoma.[18,20] The cellular detail is also reassuring, and mitotic figures are rare. The squamous eddies seen in the irritated basal cell papilloma are present, and at times, in the author's view, the two conditions are quite indistinguishable. If an obvious hair follicle is seen in the centre of the lesion, this clearly suggests inverted follicular keratosis rather than irritated basal cell papilloma (Figure 5.30).

Figure 5.30   Pathology of inverted follicular keratosis.

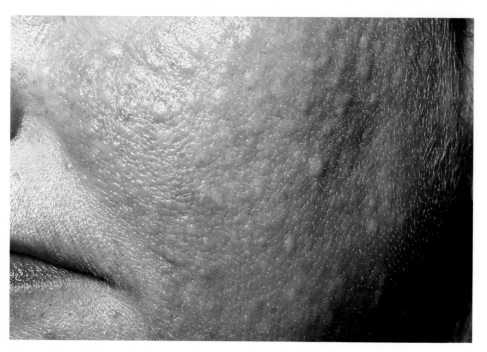

Figure 5.31   Multiple trichodiscomas.

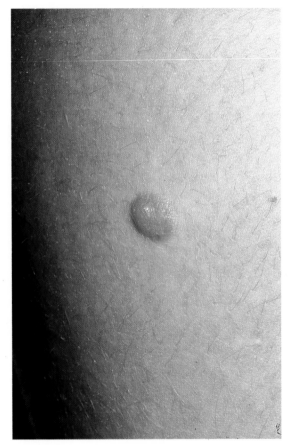

Figure 5.32 Clear cell acanthoma of Degos.

Management

The lesion is usually removed surgically to obtain a histological diagnosis, and because of concern that it may be a basal or squamous cell carcinoma.

Trichodiscoma, fibrofolliculoma and acrochordon – the Birt–Hogg–Dubé syndrome[21]

This triad was first reported in 1977 from a family with 15 affected members.[21] Subsequent reports have confirmed that the lesions appear to be transmitted by the autosomal dominant route.[22,23]

Clinical features

Family members have large numbers of asymptomatic flesh-coloured papules, almost exclusively on the face, and mainly around the nose. The majority of reported cases to date have been in young adults (Figure 5.31).

The pathological features will depend on the type of lesion biopsied. The trichodiscoma is a benign epidermal lesion related to the superficial parts of the hair follicle, and has been described by Pinkus.[24] The acrochordons are simple fibrous skin tags, and the fibrofolliculomas are benign proliferations of the dermal component of the hair follicle.

Although one of the first reported family members had a medullary carcinoma of the thyroid, this association has not been reported in any other family.

Management

A diagnostic biopsy and examination of first-degree relatives is appropriate. Thereafter the lesions require removal only on cosmetic grounds.

Clear cell acanthoma of Degos[25]

Definition and incidence

A raised, scaly nodule, usually on the lower leg, composed of large keratinocytes with an unusually clear cytoplasm. The aetiology of this entity is unknown.

Clinical presentation[26]

The lesions usually present as isolated, raised, pink nodules on the lower leg (Figure 5.32). Multiple lesions are occasionally reported.[27] Some oozing from the surface of the lesion is not uncommon. The lesions are otherwise asymptomatic.

If the lesions are excised it will be seen that the pathology is that of a proliferation of a population of keratinocytes with large quantities of clear cytoplasm.[28] The margination between normal keratinocytes and those composing the lesion is striking and abrupt. Staining with periodic acid–Schiff stain will reveal that these cells are rich in glycogen (Figures 5.33–5.35).

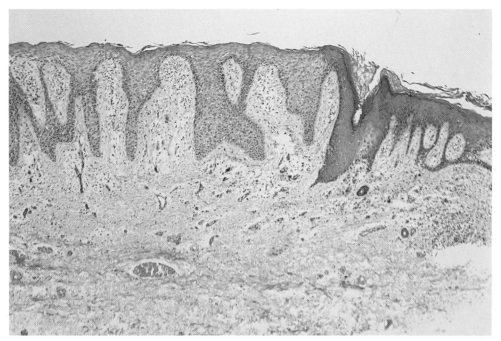

Figure 5.33   Low-power view of the histological features of a clear cell acanthoma of Degos. Note the sharp division at the left side of the slide between normal epidermis to the left and lesion to the right.

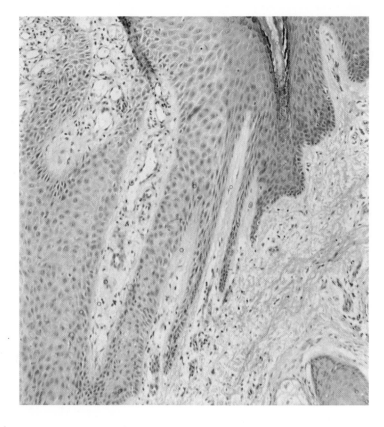

Figure 5.34   High-power view of a clear cell acanthoma. On this slide the lesion is to the left and normal epidermis to the right.

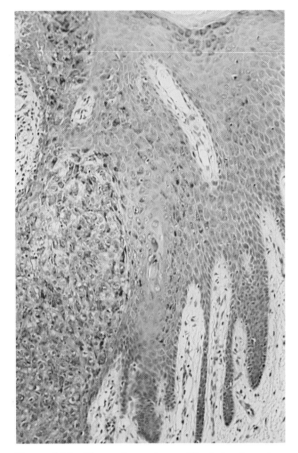

Figure 5.35 Clear cell acanthoma. The lesion is to the left, and cells positive on periodic acid–Schiff staining are clearly seen.

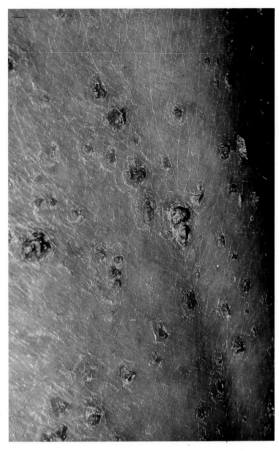

Figure 5.36 Clinical features of Kyrle's disease, showing discrete hyperkeratotic lesions.

Management

These lesions are usually surgically excised to obtain a diagnosis.

Kyrle's disease (hyperkeratosis follicularis et parafollicularis in cutem penetrans)[29]

Definition

The lesions are multiple hyperkeratotic plugs occurring mainly on the lower limbs. The aetiology is unknown. In some patients a family history of similar lesions is obtained. The lesions are reported more often in those with diabetes and with renal failure than in the normal population.[30]

Clinical features[31]

Patients with this condition tend to present with multiple hyperkeratotic lesions on the lower limbs (Figure 5.36). Occasionally the upper limbs, trunk and soles of the feet are involved but the face is very rarely, if ever, affected. The lesions can reach a considerable size, and removal of them can leave a crater.

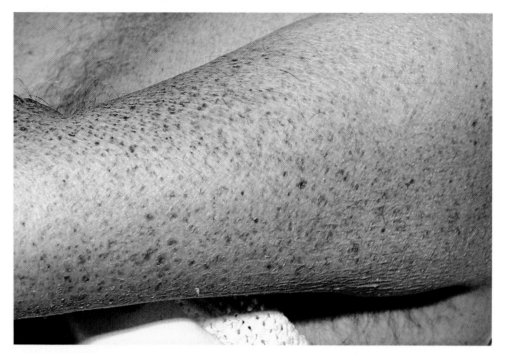

Figure 5.37 Clinical features of Flegel's disease.

The pathology of the lesion shows an area of gross hyperkeratosis mainly based around hair follicles.[32] A lichenoid tissue reaction is seen around the area, together with a considerable lymphocytic infiltrate. The base of the parakeratotic plug may stimulate a foreign body giant cell reaction in the underlying dermis.

There is some dispute in the literature as to exactly how many true cases of Kyrle's disease have been reported, and this may relate to the absolute histological criteria required. In particular, the need for epidermal intrusion into the dermis is a subject of controversy.

Management

The lesion needs to be differentiated on clinical grounds from actinic keratosis and squamous cell carcinoma. Frequently this will require a biopsy and histological examination. If the patient has multiple similar lesions, a positive family history, and the diagnosis is not in doubt, cryotherapy may be of value. The use of both topical and systemic retinoids is currently under investigation.

Flegel's disease (hyperkeratosis lenticularis perstans)[33]

Definition

A scaling plaque of unknown aetiology, commonly occurring on the lower legs.

Clinical features

There is some doubt as to whether Kyrle's disease and Flegel's disease are separate entities or the one hyperkeratotic disorder at different stages in evolution. Its importance in the context of cutaneous tumours lies in the fact that clinically they may be confused with both premalignant and malignant disorders. These lesions have been reported in families.[34,35] Both sexes are affected, and vertical transmission is seen, indicating autosomal dominant inheritance.

Rough scaly plaques occur, mainly on the legs and feet of middle-aged adults (Figure 5.37).[36] Biopsy is frequently necessary to confirm the clinical diagnosis.

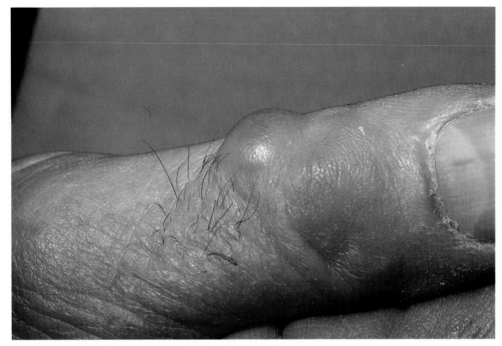

Figure 5.38 An epidermal inclusion cyst on a topical site on the finger.

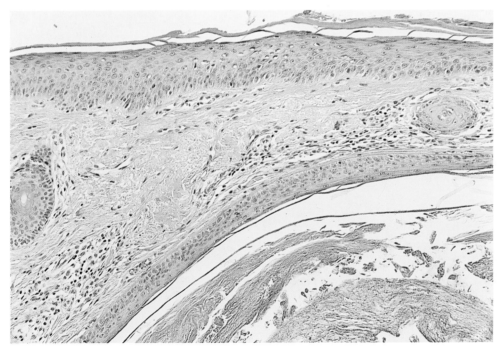

Figure 5.39 Pathology of the epidermal inclusion cyst shown in Figure 5.38. The lining of the cyst has a granular layer.

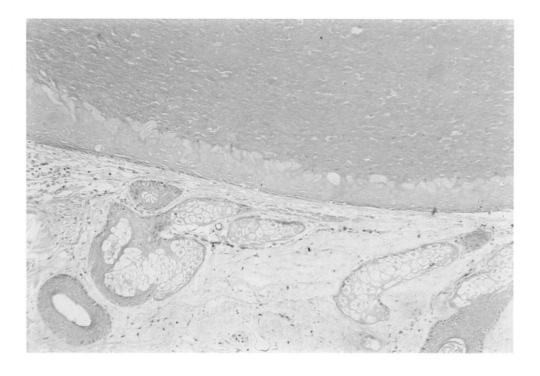

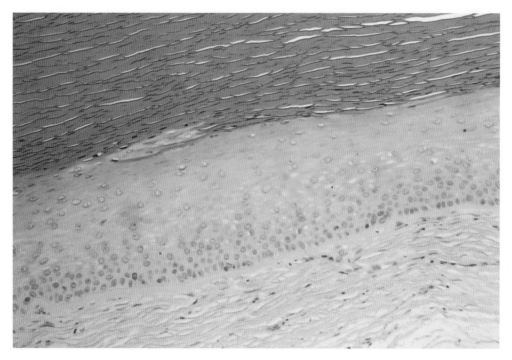

Figures 5.40 and 5.41   Low- and high-power views of a pilar trichilemmal cyst, showing the absence of a granular layer.

A parakeratotic epidermis is present and the underlying layers of the epidermis appear atrophic. Beneath this, a fairly dense and well-circumscribed lymphocytic infiltrate is seen.[37]

Management

These lesions require histological differentiation from actinic keratoses. The absence of any inflammation is a particularly useful clinical feature, but a biopsy and histological examination will usually be required for confirmation. Liberal use of emollients and selective cryotherapy will minimize the discomfort caused. Retinoids are also being used in an experimental approach to this situation.[38]

Cysts

Cysts within or just beneath the epidermal surface are not uncommon. They may expand relatively rapidly, and therefore patients may be inappropriately concerned.

The two main groups of cysts are epidermoid and trichilemmal cysts. The term sebaceous cyst is inappropriate on pathological grounds for either lesion.

Epidermal cysts[39]

These are seen commonly on the fingers, and are usually translucent lesions. There may be a history of a penetrating injury, and the pathology suggests that a small portion of epidermis has been implanted in the dermis (Figure 5.38). Biopsy will reveal a lesion which does not usually have a connection with the epidermis (Figure 5.39). The wall of the cyst is composed of epidermal tissue, with reproduction of the layers seen in the true epidermis. The presence of a granular layer is important in differentiating this lesion from a trichilemmal cyst. If the lesion is composed of proliferating cells, there may be some difficulty in differentiation from an early squamous cell carcinoma. These lesions are best excised.

Trichilemmal cysts[40]

These are relatively common, particularly on the scalp. There may be a positive family history.[41] They are lesions that are lined by epithelium resembling the hair root sheath, and can be pathologically distinguished from the epidermal cyst by the absence of a granular layer (Figures 5.40 and 5.41).[42] As with the epidermal cysts, a population of benign proliferating cells in these cysts should not be confused with a squamous cell carcinoma. Clinically, these lesions present as large – sometimes very large – pedunculated lesions, mainly on the scalp. Secondary infection is relatively common, and removal is therefore recommended. Although it is possible to curette out the contents of these lesions, recurrence is relatively common if this approach is used, and formal excision is therefore a more satisfactory definitive procedure.

6

Premalignant or in situ malignant conditions and lesions of the epidermis

The decision as to whether to include certain lesions under the headings of Chapter 5 or in this chapter has not been a straightforward one. Some readers will inevitably question the inclusion of the epidermal naevus, in which malignancy has occasionally been reported to develop, in Chapter 5, and the inclusion of keratoacanthoma, which is usually a benign self-resolving lesion, in this chapter. The criterion for inclusion in this chapter is that there are a number of papers in the literature reporting malignant changes in up to 5 per cent of the particular condition.

Good-quality epidemiological studies on relatively large series are needed to clarify the currently confused borderline between conditions in which malignant change is a coincidental finding and those in which there is evidence of a causal association between the pre-existing condition and the malignancy. An excellent example of a field in which this approach is being applied is the work of Dr Robin Marks and colleagues in Australia on the incidence of solar keratosis and non-melanoma skin cancer.[1] Similar work on a large series of keratoacanthomata and porokeratoses would clarify the situation greatly in what are at present confused and confusing areas. There is a natural tendency to report in the literature positive events, such as malignant change occurring in lesions, and to regard situations in which malignant change does not occur as 'non-events'. This fact may well relate to the reported incidence versus true incidence of malignant change in, for example, the porokeratosis group of lesions.

The following conditions are discussed in this chapter:

Actinic or solar keratosis
Large-cell acanthoma
Chondrodermatitis nodularis helicis
Cutaneous horn
Radiodermatitis
Bowen's disease
Erythroplasia of Queyrat
Bowenoid papulosis
Paget's disease
Organoid or sebaceous epidermal naevi and syringocystadenoma papilliferum
Keratoacanthoma
The porokeratoses
Fibroepithelioma of Pinkus

Actinic keratosis

Definition

An area of epidermal dysplasia giving rise to cutaneous scaling usually seen on light-exposed Caucasian skin.

Clinical features[2]

Actinic or solar keratoses are seen predominantly on the face, hands and forearms of white-skinned individuals. Recent work from Australia has shown that in that particular climate, 40 per cent of individuals over the age of 40 will have one or more actinic or solar keratoses, and 2–3 per cent will have

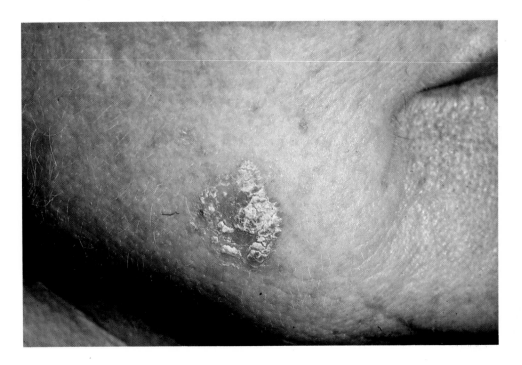

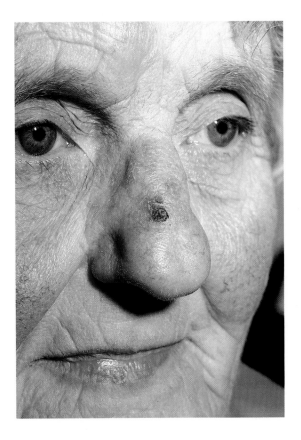

a non-melanoma skin cancer.[3] Recent epidemiological work carried out by Marks and Selwood has indicated that only a small change in solar exposure in two towns 110 km apart is associated with a 14 per cent higher rate of solar keratoses in the town nearer the Equator.[4]

Actinic keratoses are recognized as scaling erythematous lesions on light-exposed skin (Figures 6.1–6.3). To the patient they may appear as non-healing wounds. Inflammation is usually present and is important in the clinical differential diagnosis from seborrhoeic keratosis and other benign lesions discussed in Chapter 5. Actinic keratoses are rarely solitary lesions, and frequently the patient will present with an area of field change covering the whole of the forehead or back of the hand (Figures 6.4 and 6.5). The lower lip is also a common site (Figure 6.6).

In the Australian setting, men are affected more frequently than women, and this may reflect an outdoor occupation, although in the UK there are an increasing number of individuals with large numbers of actinic keratoses, and a history of recreational rather than occupational sun exposure.

Figure 6.2 Actinic keratosis on the nose. Crusting and pigment are present.

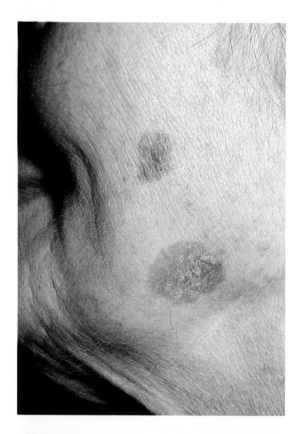

Figure 6.3 Two pigmented actinic keratoses on cheeks. On occasion, clinical differentiation from lentigo maligna can be difficult.

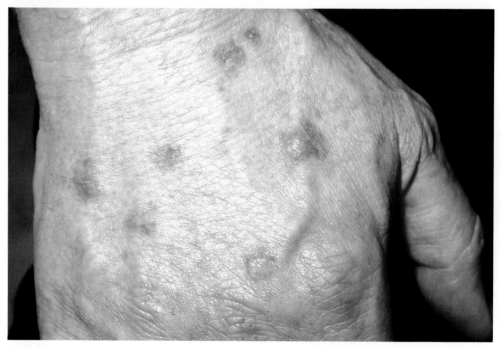

Figure 6.4 Actinic keratoses on the back of the hand.

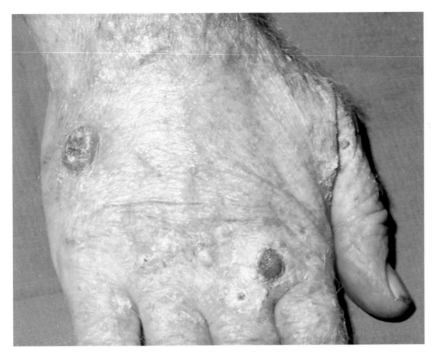

Figure 6.5 Extensive actinic keratoses on the back of the hand.

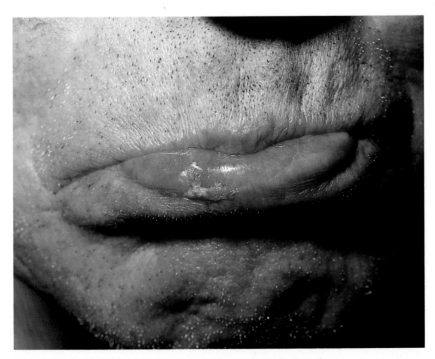

Figure 6.6 Actinic keratosis on the lower lip of an outdoor worker.

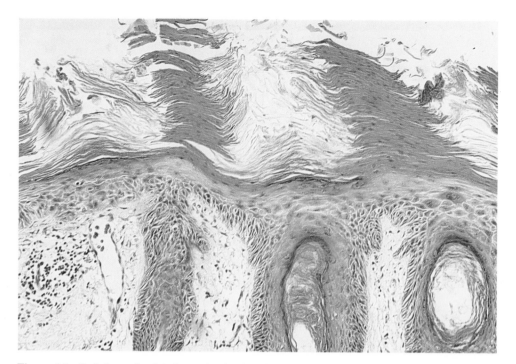

Figure 6.7   Pathology of actinic keratosis, showing alternating parakeratosis and orthokeratosis.

In Australia, those of Anglo-Saxon descent born in Australia have a higher incidence of solar keratosis at an earlier age than those who migrated there in early adult life, emphasizing the importance of total lifetime sun exposure, and the importance of events in childhood and early adult life.[2]

Pathology

The pathology of actinic keratosis is that of epidermal dysplasia. Patches of regular orthokeratotic epidermis will alternate with patches of epidermis in which there is striking parakeratosis. It has been pointed out by Pinkus that the areas of epidermis overlying skin appendages are the orthokeratotic areas and therefore tend to show less evidence of actinic damage than adjacent areas (Figure 6.7). He has suggested that this is due to the fact that the putative stem cells in the epidermis adjacent to skin appendages may be situated more deeply and therefore may be more protected against the sun.

Within the epidermis the normal maturation pattern and polarity of the epidermal cells is lost and the individual keratinocytes will show keratinization. In more advanced lesions, a lymphocytic infiltrate will be present in the dermis, which presumably correlates with the inflammation seen on clinical examination. Frequently, the surrounding dermis shows signs of actinic damage in the collagen with a rather grey and fragmented appearance. This material stains strongly using conventional elastic tissue stains.

A number of additional pathological features may be seen in actinic keratosis. Some lesions show focal acantholysis (Figure 6.8). This is a loss of the normal desmosomal cohesion of one keratinocyte to another, and is seen also in the autoimmune blistering disorder pemphigus. It may be seen also in squamous cell carcinoma. A second feature is a rather lichenoid tissue reaction pattern similar to that seen in lichen planus. The pathologist should beware of diagnosing true lichen planus on a biopsy from a patch of light-exposed skin with surrounding evidence of UV damage.

A number of lesions may also show pathological features similar to those seen in Bowen's disease (see below, Figure 6.9). These include gross epidermal dysplasia and individual cell keratinization with giant

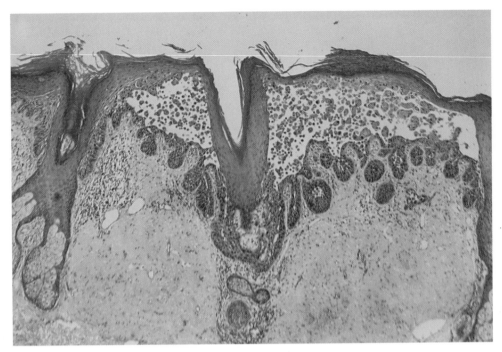

Figure 6.8   Epidermal acantholysis in an area of actinic keratosis.

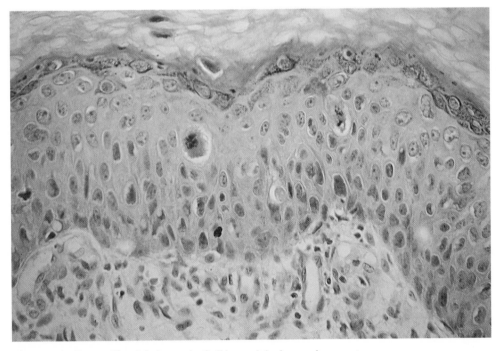

Figure 6.9   Bowenoid actinic keratosis. Striking actinic damage is present.

atypical keratinocytes. There is no convincing evidence that this Bowenoid pattern seen in actinic keratosis has any particular prognostic significance.

Management

In the normal healthy individual, the identification of multiple actinic keratoses is a sign that that individual has had UV exposure in excess of that which his or her epidermis can tolerate. Advice about protection from further exposure to noonday sun and from Mediterranean or hotter sun and the use of a hat and an appropriate sunscreen with an SPF of 15 or greater are well worthwhile.

Marks has shown that, in Australia, 36 per cent of 1040 individuals had remission of at least one actinic keratosis over a year of follow-up.[5] Resolution of lesions after protection from further actinic damage can therefore occur, and it should never be assumed in the case of the patient with actinic keratosis that the damage is done and that there is no point in offering advice about further exposure to sun. Mathematical modelling of the true risk of malignant transformation over a 10-year period appears to suggest a range of 6–10 per cent.[6]

The management of the existing keratoses can be by cryotherapy, topical 5-FU, or surgery. Cryotherapy is effective in this situation but may result in some unsightly pigmentary changes. Topical 5-FU (Efudix) can be used with great benefit. The best results are seen on the face, with the backs of the hands and the lower legs showing less satisfactory results. Topical 5-FU is applied to the affected area daily (using gloves to protect the hands) for a period of 2–3 weeks. The duration of therapy will depend on the response observed in the treated skin, and the patient must be warned that it is necessary to produce a fairly striking inflammatory reaction in both the actinic keratosis and the surrounding skin if any lasting benefit is to be achieved. Recent studies have suggested that the addition of a topical retinoid such as 0.05 per cent tretinoin will enhance the activity of the 5-FU on extrafacial sites.[7] Once the inflammatory reaction is fully developed, therapy should be discontinued and the area observed over a further 2–3 week period. Any lesion that does not show complete response to cryotherapy or 5-FU should be observed closely and the possibility of invasive squamous cell carcinoma considered. A biopsy may be necessary to establish the pathological nature of such a residual lesion.

Complete surgical removal of actinic keratoses is not always practical because of the widespread nature of the actinic damage in the skin of individuals with these lesions. It may, however, be the best method of dealing with multiple lesions on some sites; for example, complete resurfacing with excision and grafting of the skin of the back of the hand may produce an excellent result.

Two situations in which actinic keratosis must be regarded with greater concern are in the rare patients with xeroderma pigmentosum (Chapter 4) and in-patients who are on long-term immunosuppressive therapy. These are usually patients who have received a transplanted kidney, and current studies from many centres show clearly that these patients are at greater risk of developing both actinic keratosis and squamous cell carcinoma (see Chapter 8). These patients should be advised against exposure to strong sunlight and have a topical sunscreen prescribed from the time of transplantation. All lesions with a clinical resemblance to actinic keratosis should be examined carefully and preferably biopsied, as squamous cell carcinoma can develop rapidly in these immunosuppressed individuals and can look deceptively benign on clinical examination.

The exact incidence of development of squamous cell carcinoma in actinic keratosis is at present a matter of debate. In the past it has been suggested that as many as 20 per cent of patients with actinic keratosis went on to develop invasive squamous cell carcinoma on the affected sites. Work from Australia has suggested, however, that less than 1 per cent of actinic keratoses are genuinely premalignant lesions.[5] Further epidemiological work in varying climates and among varying racial types is needed. At the present time it is suggested that the patient with actinic keratoses should be regarded as an individual who has had more UV exposure than his epidermis can tolerate and is therefore at risk of future squamous cell carcinoma and basal cell carcinoma, which may not necessarily develop on the actinic keratosis already present, but may be seen on sun-damaged surrounding skin.

Large-cell acanthoma

This interesting entity was first described in 1978.[8] Clinically it is indistinguishable from an actinic keratosis and is seen on the epidermis as a scaling lesion with associated erythema.

On biopsy a striking pattern will be seen, with a sharp demarcation between surrounding normal epidermis and an apparent clone of epidermal cells that are

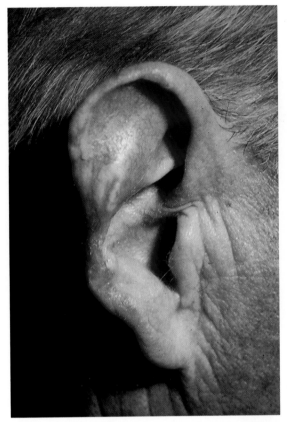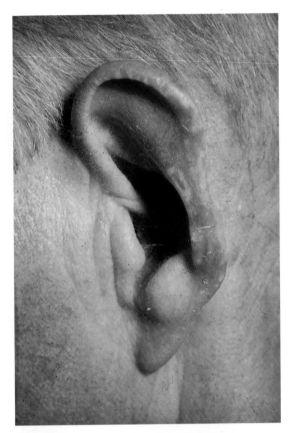

Figures 6.10 and 6.11   Extensive chondrodermatitis nodularis helicis, showing destruction of ear tissue.

approximately twice the size of their adjacent normal neighbours. These lesions show rather less loss of polarity and general dysplasia than the actinic keratoses described above. It would appear to be a relatively rare condition, with 38 cases identified among 34 000 specimens in a large, specialized dermatopathology laboratory. The management is as for actinic keratosis.

Chondrodermatitis nodularis helicis

This condition is by definition seen on the ears, and is most common in males who have worked in an outdoor environment. It was first described by Winkler in 1915.[9] However, as with actinic keratoses, these lesions are now being seen more frequently on those who have an outdoor recreation rather than occupation.

The typical patient is an elderly Caucasian male who has a short hairstyle and complains of painful ears (Figures 6.10 and 6.11). This frequently results in discomfort when sleeping at night, and scaling lesions with inflammation, ulceration and tethering of the epidermis to the underlying cartilage are seen on examination. In advanced cases there is clearly significant cartilage destruction, resulting in an abnormal distorted appearance of the external ear.

Pathology

Biopsy of these lesions will show striking actinic damage in the epidermis, with ulceration and surrounding pseudoepitheliomatous hyperplasia. The essential feature for diagnosing this condition is, however, the inflammatory damage to the underlying collagen. Destruction of large areas of collagen with a lymphocytic infiltrate may be seen, and there may be actual extrusion of cartilage through the ulcerated epidermis.[10,11]

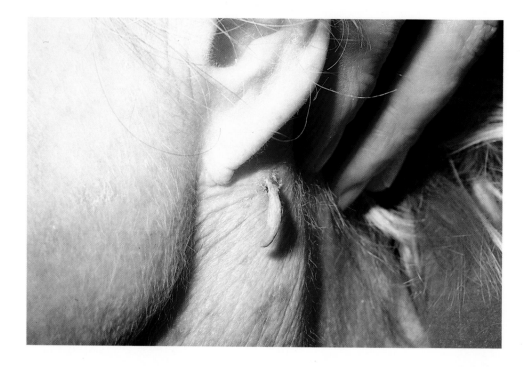

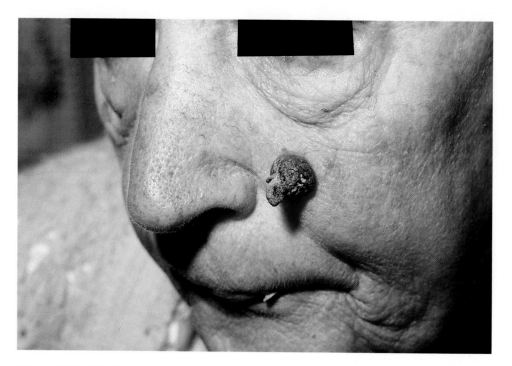

Figures 6.12–6.15 Four types of cutaneous horn. All need pathological examination of the base to establish the underlying cause.

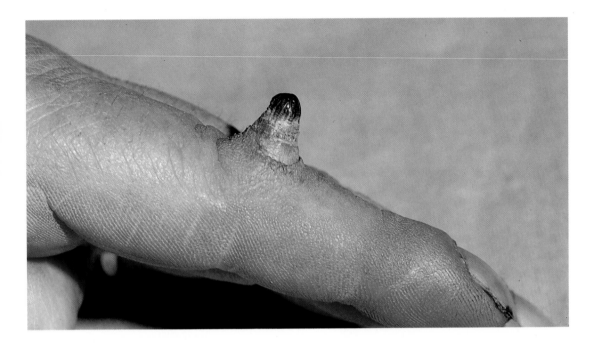

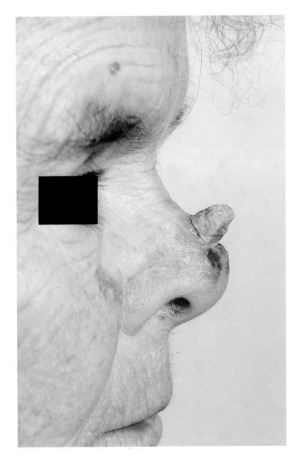

Management

Once the diagnosis is made, the patient may be managed by topical treatment or surgical excision. In the past, extensive surgery has been the treatment most commonly used for this condition, but there are recent reports of good results using potent steroids either applied topically or by intralesional injection. It may therefore be appropriate to give patients a trial of topical steroid prior to considering extensive surgical excision. Surgical excision may involve removing a wedge of cartilage from the ear, with cosmetic repair, or in extensive cases removal of the outer ear and replacement with an artificial ear.

A proportion of patients with chondrodermatitis nodularis helicis will, if untreated, progress to develop invasive squamous cell carcinoma (see Figure 8.7).

Cutaneous horn

Cutaneous horns may overlie an area of epidermis that is dysplastic or is frankly neoplastic. It is, therefore, a clinical marker that the underlying epidermis is abnormal rather than a diagnosis in itself.

Cutaneous horns are usually seen on light-exposed skin such as the face or the hands (Figures 6.12–6.15). The lesions should be biopsied and a

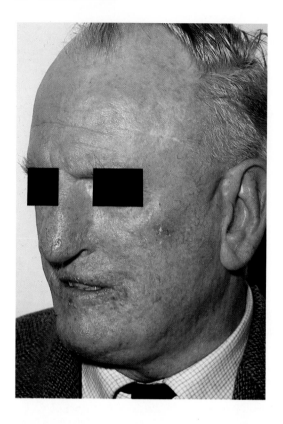

portion of the base excised to determine the nature of the underlying epidermal damage. If this has a similar pathology to that of actinic keratosis, the treatment is the same (see page 84). However, if frank invasive squamous cell carcinoma has developed, the lesion will require appropriate wide excision (Chapter 8).

Radiodermatitis[12]

Definition

An area of skin damaged by excessive exposure to X-irradiation.

Figure 6.16 Clinical appearance of chronic radiodermatitis.

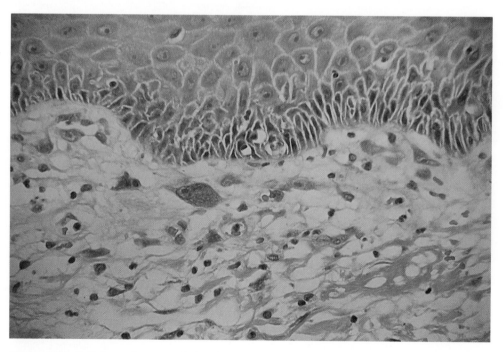

Figure 6.17 Pathology of recent radiation damage, showing plump fibroblasts.

Clinical features

Affected individuals will usually give a history of exposure to X-rays, either in their occupation or therapeutically. In the past, X-ray therapy has been used for a number of benign skin conditions, such as sycosis barbae, acne vulgaris, atopic dermatitis, and even plantar warts. Radiodermatitis may also develop on skin overlying a malignancy that has received therapeutic radiation, such as breast carcinoma.

The affected skin is thin, dry due to the destruction of the sebaceous glands, and discoloured. There is a loss of elasticity and the epidermis frequently looks as if it is tethered to the underlying dermis. This skin is particularly uncomfortable in extremes of ambient temperature (Figure 6.16).

Pathology

The epidermis is atrophic and there is a loss of polarity of the epidermal keratinocytes. The underlying dermis shows thickened collagen, and if the radiation exposure is relatively recent, abnormal plump fibroblasts will be seen (Figure 6.17).

Management

Obviously, the best approach is prevention. Once radiodermatitis has developed, regular use of emollients will minimize discomfort. Topical steroids are not recommended, as they will increase the atrophic change. Basal cell carcinoma, squamous cell carcinoma and malignant melanoma have all been reported in areas of radiodermatitis, and careful follow-up is therefore essential. In animal models, soft tissue tumours develop in irradiated sites. This is not commonly recorded in humans.

Bowen's disease (intraepidermal carcinoma in situ)

Definition

Bowen's disease is an in situ carcinoma derived from the epidermal keratinocytes, and was first described by Bowen in 1912 as a precancerous dermatosis.[13] It is considered that two of the causes are exposure to UV light and a history of previous ingestion of arsenic, either from well-water or from medicinally administered tonics.[14] This, however, does not entirely explain the Bowen's lesions that occur on covered sites in younger people with no history of arsenic ingestion. A small proportion of patients having Bowen's disease go on to develop frank invasive squamous cell carcinoma on the lesion, and there is debate as to whether or not Bowen's disease should be regarded as a possible marker of internal malignancy (see below).

Clinical features

Bowen's disease presents as an isolated red, scaling lesion, most often on the trunk (Figures 6.18–6.21). These lesions may be 2–5 cm in diameter by the time they are recognized, and a common error amongst those who see relatively little skin cancer is to mistake them initially for an isolated patch of psoriasis. Psoriasis is rare as an isolated plaque, and the absence of any psoriatic lesions on the knees, elbows or scalp should arouse suspicion. A second differential diagnosis that needs to be made is that of the multifocal or extrafacial basal cell carcinoma. The Bowen's lesion does not have the raised, rolled edge characteristic of basal cell carcinoma (Chapter 7). The fact that the lesion is on a habitually covered site should help to differentiate it from a solar keratosis, although clinically the lesions may be rather similar, and frequently a biopsy is needed to establish that squamous cell carcinoma has not developed in a pre-existing patch of Bowen's disease.

Very large lesions may be seen on occasion (Figures 6.22 and 6.23) and there is a higher than expected incidence of Bowen's disease and multiple lesions in patients with a history of arsenic ingestion (Figure 6.24).

Pathology

This lesion shows very gross dysplasia of the upper layers of the epidermis. The basal layer appears relatively normal but there is complete loss of polarity in the overlying keratinocytes, and the lesions show striking individual cell keratinization and the presence of giant keratinocytes with grossly atypical mitoses (Figures 6.25–6.27). The overlying stratum corneum frequently shows parakeratosis. This is a situation

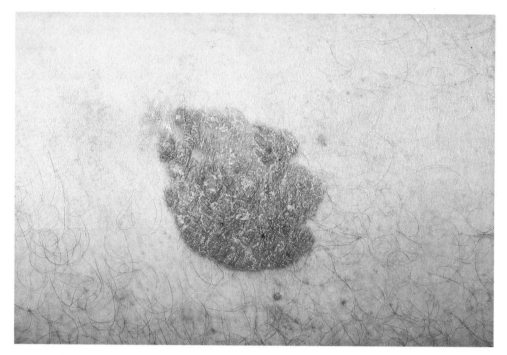

Figure 6.18

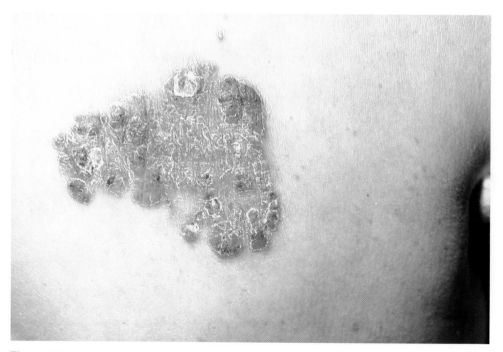

Figure 6.19

Figures 6.18–6.21   Classic lesions of Bowen's disease. Figure 6.21 shows considerable pigmentation and may cause confusion with a superficial spreading melanoma.

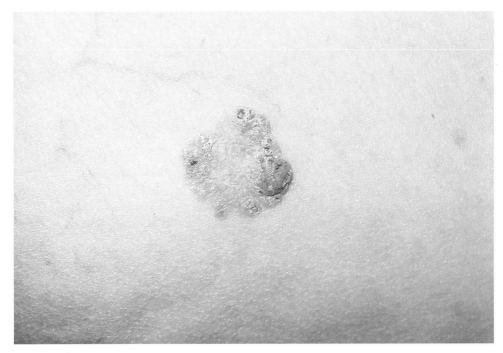

Figure 6.20

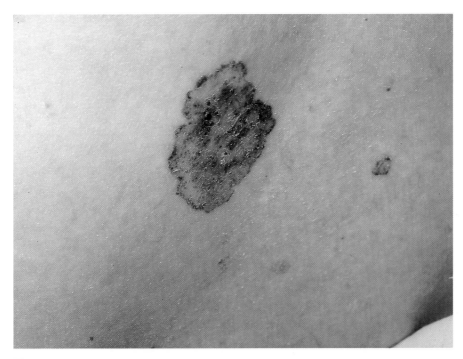

Figure 6.21

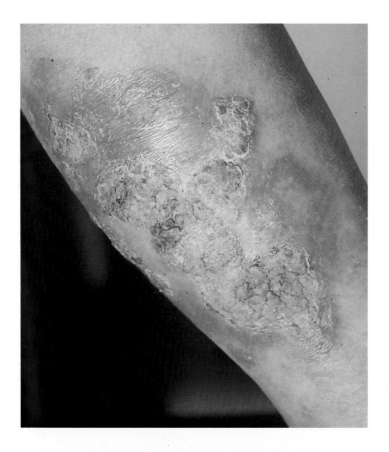

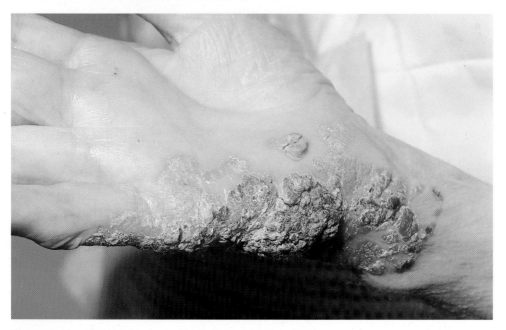

Figures 6.22 and 6.23   More extensive lesions of Bowen's disease.

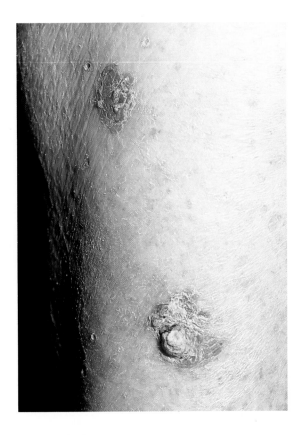

Figure 6.24   Multiple Bowen's disease lesions in a patient with a history of arsenic ingestion.

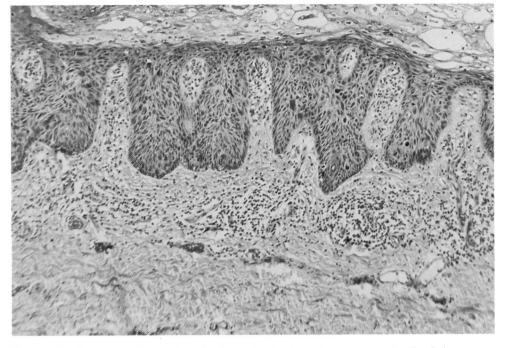

Figure 6.25   Low-power view of Bowen's disease showing loss of usual epidermal cell polarity.

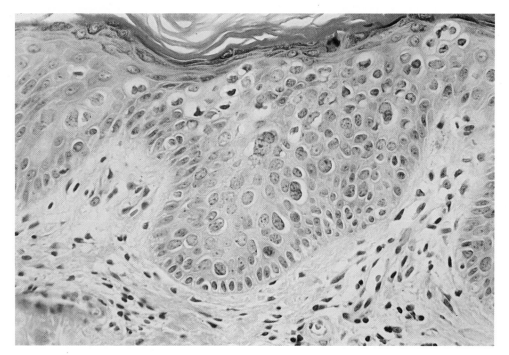

Figure 6.26   Medium-power view of Bowen's disease showing striking cellular atypia.

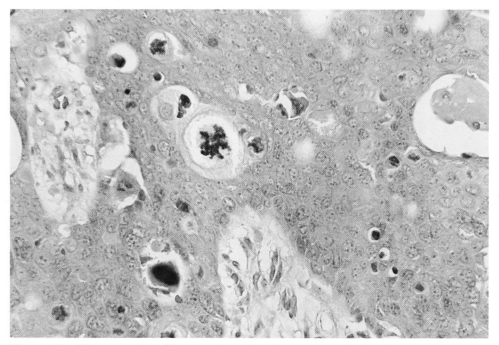

Figure 6.27   High-power view of Bowen's disease showing gross cytological atypia.

where the cellular cytology is more alarming than the biological behaviour of the lesion. The possibility of a viral cause of Bowen's disease has been postulated, and recently HPV 16 has been reported in a lesion from a renal transplant recipient.

Management

This is divided into three parts. These are the histological confirmation that the lesion is indeed Bowen's disease and that invasive squamous cell carcinoma has not developed, the treatment, and the consideration that Bowen's disease may be a marker of malignancy elsewhere.

A biopsy from the most indurated part of the lesion is essential to confirm the clinical suspicion that the lesion is Bowen's disease. This is a situation where an incisional biopsy, possibly a punch biopsy, is acceptable. Once the pathological nature of the lesion is confirmed, the lesion can be dealt with by cryotherapy, by topical 5-FU, by radiotherapy, or by complete excision. Complete excision is the treatment of choice if the biopsy, which should be taken from the apparently thickest part of the lesion, gives any suggestion that invasive squamous cell carcinoma has developed in a pre-existing Bowen's lesion.

The percentage of cases of Bowen's disease in which invasive squamous cell carcinoma develops is a subject of dispute.[15–17] It has been stated that, if untreated, 3–5 per cent of patients will develop an invasive, squamous cell carcinoma, but few individuals, having pathologically confirmed a diagnosis of Bowen's disease, would leave a lesion untreated. It is, therefore, anticipated that the incidence of squamous cell carcinoma developing on Bowen's disease will now be very much lower. It is stated in the literature that in patients with Bowen's disease in whom invasive cell carcinoma develops, 13 per cent of lesions metastasize, and death occurs in 10 per cent of these cases. These figures should be interpreted in the light of modern management.

A further problem, once the diagnosis of Bowen's disease is made, is whether or not Bowen's disease is an established cutaneous marker of malignancy in other body sites. An early report from the Armed Forces Institute of Pathology, Washington, suggested that as many as 80 per cent of the patients with Bowen's disease might have a non-cutaneous malignancy.[18] A study in 1980 suggested that up to 25 per cent of patients with Bowen's disease might develop an internal malignancy.[19] In this report, however, malignancies varied in site and type, and rarely developed simultaneously with the lesions of Bowen's disease. A recent review of seven published cohort studies suggests that in six of them there are major deficiencies, including the lack of an adequate control group.[20] It would therefore appear that at present the role of Bowen's disease as a marker of internal malignancy is disputed,[21–23] and a recent population-based study refutes any association.[24] In view of this uncertainty, it is suggested that a good clinical history be taken from every patient with Bowen's disease, a thorough clinical examination performed, and further examinations, including chest X-ray, barium studies, and so on, carried out as considered appropriate. It may be that the early high figures related to a population that had previously ingested arsenic, predisposing both to Bowen's disease and to the other malignancy.

Erythroplasia of Queyrat[25]

This name is used to describe Bowen's disease occurring on the glans penis (Figure 6.28). It is seen almost

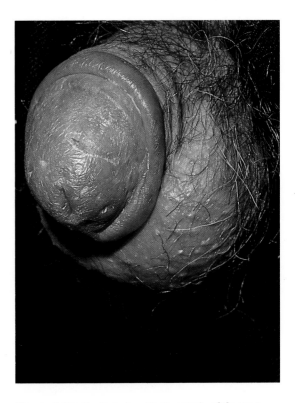

Figure 6.28   Penile lesion. Erythroplasia of Queyrat.

exclusively on uncircumcised males and presents as a smooth red velvety plaque on the glans penis.[26] The histology is identical to that seen in Bowen's disease.

Management

Circumcision and cryotherapy to the remaining lesions is a reasonable approach to treatment. Obviously, careful follow-up is needed.

Bowenoid papulosis

This condition has been described by Wade et al.[27] These lesions present on the genital, cutaneous, and mucosal surfaces of young adults as reddish-brown papules, almost always multiple. They are frequently clinically confused with genital warts.[28]

On biopsy the histology will be seen to be very similar to, if not indistinguishable from, that of classic Bowen's disease. The possibility that this condition is of viral origin has been suggested, and virus-like particles have been identified using electron microscopy.[29] Recently, human papilloma virus has been specifically identified in these lesions.

Management

A biopsy of a representative lesion is required to establish the diagnosis. A number of patients with Bowenoid papulosis have been followed and it has been observed that a high proportion of lesions regress spontaneously.[30] Provided that regular supervision is feasible, it is therefore suggested that, initially, careful regular clinical observation is an acceptable method of managing such patients. In the early days of Bowenoid papulosis, before it was recognized as a self-limiting disease distinct from Bowen's disease, a number of young females had radical vulvar surgery. Observation of these lesions suggests that this is inappropriate and that an expectant approach to treatment or local destruction is more appropriate.

Paget's disease[31]

Paget's disease is included at this point in the text as, clinically and pathologically, it may cause some

confusion with Bowen's disease. The cells involved are thought to be derived from the apocrine gland (Chapter 12).

Clinical features

Paget's disease of the breast is a predominantly female problem and is associated with an underlying intraduct carcinoma of the breast in the great majority of cases.[32,33] It presents as an oozing, eczematized erythematous area on the breast skin (Figures 6.29 and 6.30). The lesion is usually moister than that of classic Bowen's disease, but there is frequently a clinical similarity.

Extramammary Paget's disease is also most commonly seen in women and affects the vulvar area (Figure 6.31).[34] The male genital area is affected less often, and in both sexes the perianal area may be involved (Figure 6.32).[35] As with Paget's disease involving the female breast, Paget's disease in the genital and perianal region is commonly a marker of an adenocarcinoma of underlying structure. The lesion will be seen in the genital area as a red, moist, oozing plaque.

Pathology

The pathology of extramammary or mammary Paget's disease shows a striking colonization of the epidermis by large epithelioid cells showing cytological atypia with dark hyperchromatic nuclei and frequent mitotic figures.[36] There is controversy as to the origin of these cells, and there is an absence of desmosomes between them and the surrounding keratinocytes. The cells may lie singly or in nests, and the overall epidermal picture on staining with haematoxylin and eosin may be very similar to that seen in superficial spreading malignant melanoma. However, in Paget's disease there is usually a very brisk lymphocytic infiltrate in the underlying dermis which is proportionally greater than in melanoma (Chapter 10). There are continuing and unresolved arguments as to whether or not the cells in Paget's disease are an upward extension of in situ adenocarcinoma in the sweat glands, or whether Paget's disease represents a multifocal primary tumour and the malignant cells in the epidermis have developed de novo.

The large epidermal cells in Paget's disease are periodic acid–Schiff-positive and mucin-positive

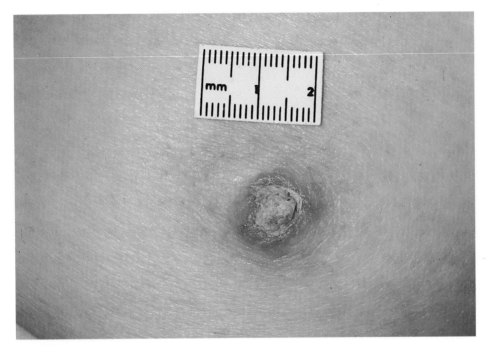

Figure 6.29 Close-up view of Paget's disease of the nipple.

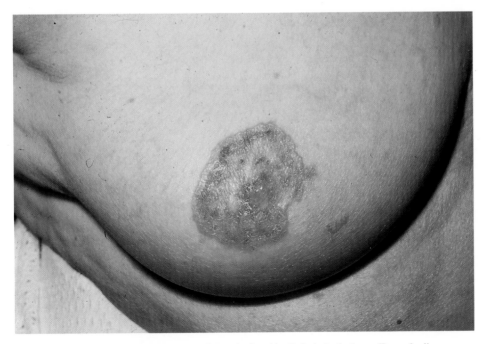

Figure 6.30 Extensive Paget's disease of the nipple with clinical similarity to Bowen's disease.

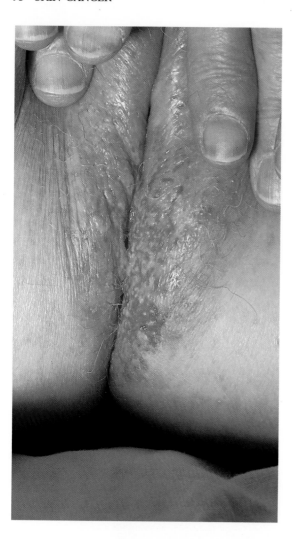

Figure 6.31   Paget's disease of the vulva.

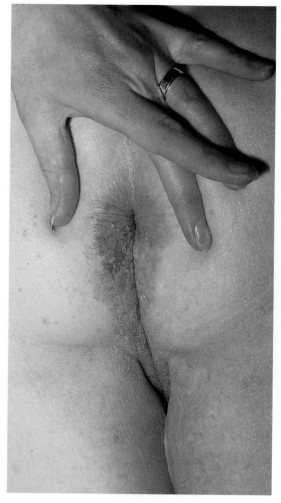

Figure 6.32   Perianal Paget's disease.

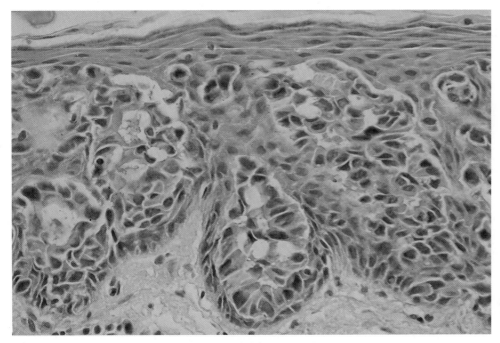

Figure 6.33 Pathology of Paget's disease, showing mucin positivity.

(Figure 6.33) and stain strongly with carcinoembryonic antigen.[37] This is a useful differentiation marker between Paget's disease, usually of extramammary type, and superficial spreading malignant melanoma.

Management

If the clinical diagnosis of Paget's disease of the mammary or extramammary type is suspected, a diagnostic biopsy should be performed. When the condition is confirmed a thorough search should be carried out for an underlying malignancy of the breast or appropriate tissue if on an extramammary site. If this is identified, the cutaneous lesion may well be removed as part of the definitive treatment of the underlying malignancy. If no such underlying malignancy is identified, the lesion should be locally excised, and the patient followed up carefully.

Organoid or sebaceous epidermal naevi

Definition

Naevi composed of an abnormal number of skin appendages that have a propensity to develop basal cell carcinoma.

Clinical features

The naevus sebaceous of Jadassohn is a relatively common condition.[38] It is usually present at birth and most frequently involves the scalp.[39] Initially it may be

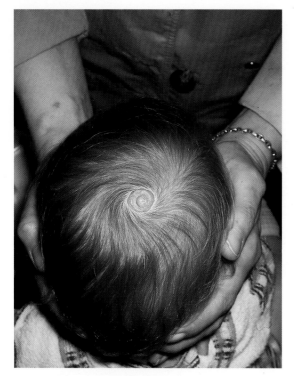

Figure 6.34 An organoid naevus on the scalp of a 2-year-old.

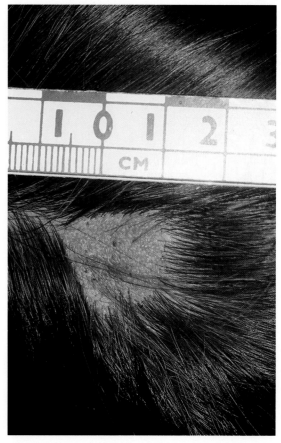

Figure 6.35 An organoid naevus on the scalp of a 13-year-old.

seen as an area of relatively light hair growth with a raised papular yellow area (Figure 6.34). As the child matures and reaches puberty, the lesion becomes much more papillomatous (Figure 6.35), and at this time the patient may present because of repeated trauma to the lesion as a result of brushing or combing of the hair. This may give rise to continuous trauma and secondary infection. In a proportion (up to 10 per cent) of cases, basal cell carcinoma has been reported to develop (Figure 6.36). As stated at the beginning of this chapter, it is likely that this is a higher percentage than the true incidence because of the tendency to report positive events.

The lesion of syringocystadenoma papilliferum, which is derived from the apocrine gland, is sometimes also associated with the organoid naevus (Figure 6.37), and once again basal cell carcinoma may develop in association with this lesion.

Pathology

The term organoid naevus is more appropriate than sebaceous to describe the lesion. The skin appendages are present in increased numbers. Sebaceous glands may well be present in large numbers, but so also may eccrine sweat glands, and straps of smooth muscle. The hair follicle element of the pilosebaceous apparatus is generally under-represented in these lesions.

Syringocystadenoma papilliferum develops in a proportion of these lesions and is recognized by the

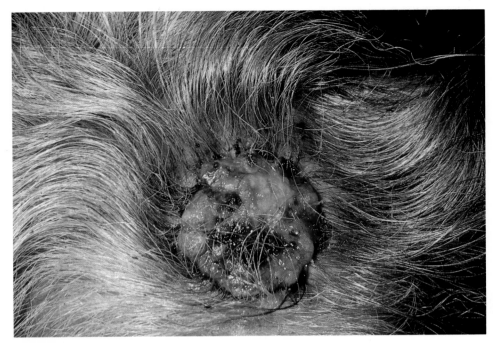

Figure 6.36   Basal cell carcinoma on a pre-existing organoid naevus.

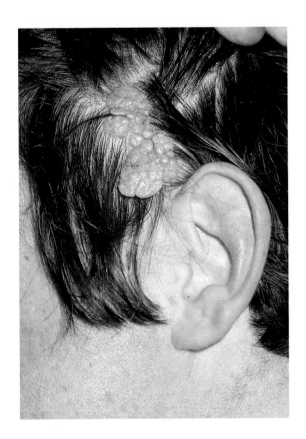

presence of large numbers of plasma cells underlying a cystic invasion of the epidermis, which is lined by a double layer of columnar epithelium showing decapitation secretion.[40] This pattern is, of course, highly suggestive of an origin from the apocrine gland (see Chapters 1 and 12).

Management

These lesions are frequently identified around puberty. A biopsy is often necessary to establish the diagnosis and it is suggested, in view of the relatively common development of basal cell carcinoma (Figure 6.36)[41] and the very rarely reported development of squamous cell carcinoma, that complete local excision of these lesions is the most appropriate method of management.

Figure 6.37   Syringocystadenoma papilliferum associated with organoid naevus.

Keratoacanthoma (previously called molluscum sebaceum)

Definition

A normally self-limiting, rapidly growing, hyperkeratotic papule.

The 'typical' or classical keratoacanthoma will regress spontaneously but as the diagnosis cannot always be made with confidence until this phenomenon is observed, and as both clinical and at times very considerable pathological doubt is present about the differentiation between an 'atypical keratoacanthoma' and an early invasive squamous cell carcinoma, this lesion is felt to merit inclusion as a possibly premalignant lesion rather than being confidently regarded as always benign. This premalignant potential is realized in patients who are immunosuppressed (see below).

Clinical features

Keratoacanthoma is a most interesting and relatively understudied problem. In terms of the current interest in regulation of growth control and the interaction between oncogenes and growth factors, it is clearly a most important natural model. It may well be that on other body sites, such as the gastrointestinal tract, there are similar self-limiting lesions, but obviously these are not visible for regular observation.

Keratoacanthoma is usually an isolated lesion, although there are examples of multiple lesions. It was first described in 1936 by MacCormack and Scarff as 'molluscum sebaceum',[42] and in 1950 the feature of spontaneous regression was described by Musso.[43] Lesions are seen more frequently than can be attributed to chance on the exposed skin of those who handle tar or pitch.[44]

The most common sites involved in the case of solitary lesions are sun-exposed skin of the face, head and neck areas and the backs of the hands of individuals aged 40 or older (Figures 6.38–6.41).[45,46] There appears to be a clear association with UV exposure in that the numbers of keratoacanthomas excised annually are highest in Australia, and the numbers excised within Australia vary according to the hours of UV exposure recorded in the geographic area in question. The lip may be involved.[47]

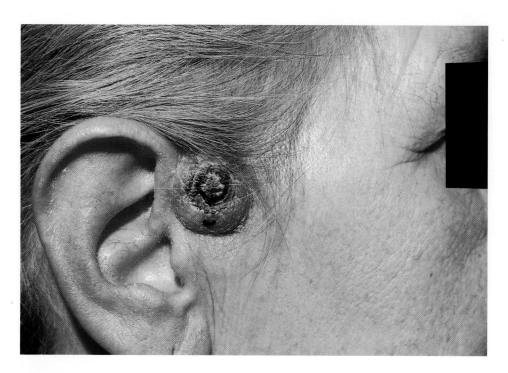

Figure 6.38   Keratoacanthoma in front of the ear.

Figure 6.39   Keratoacanthoma on the cheek.

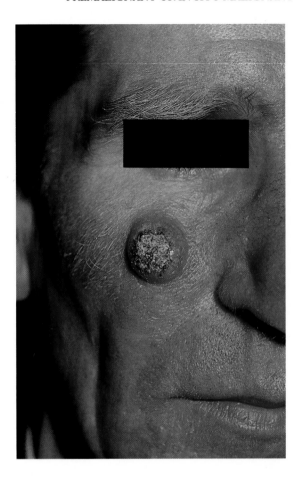

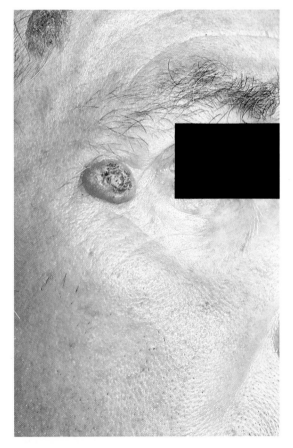

Figure 6.40   Keratoacanthoma at the outer canthus.

Figure 6.41 Close-up view of a typical keratoacanthoma.

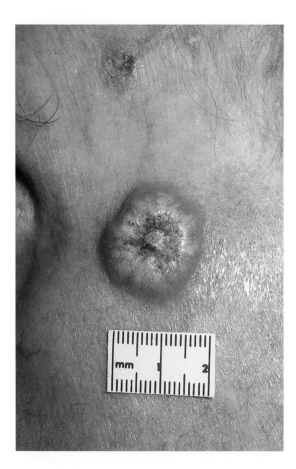

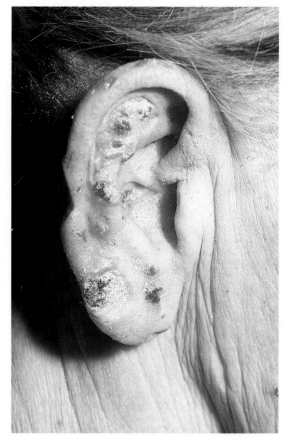

Figure 6.42 Multiple keratoacanthomas on the ear.

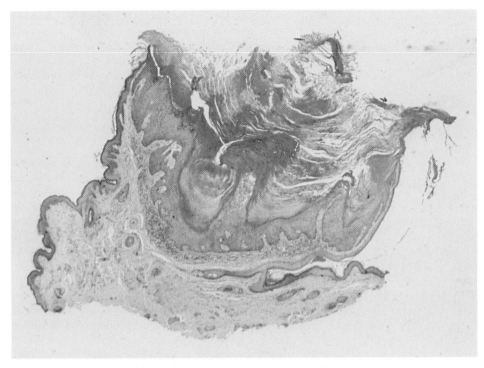

Figure 6.43   Low-power view of the architecture of a keratoacanthoma.

The lesions present as rapidly growing pink papules. Over a period of days the lesions may double or treble in size. After reaching approximately 2–4 cm in diameter, the lesions generally stop growing and remain static for 2–3 months, after which time they regress spontaneously. At the end of the growth phase the lesion is a firm, domed, pinkish papule on the skin and over the period of regression the central part of the lesion becomes hyperkeratotic and a core of keratinous debris can be shelled out. If the lesion resolves spontaneously, the end result is a rather ugly scar. In a small proportion of normal non-immuno-suppressed individuals, lesions that begin with this growth pattern go on to become invasive squamous carcinoma.

Multiple keratoacanthomas are relatively rare but may occur on any body site. They may, if not excised, reach a considerable size, and leave very disfiguring scars (Figure 6.42). In some textbooks they are confused with the multiple self-healing epitheliomas of Ferguson-Smith (Chapter 4, page 43). They are quite distinct lesions on both clinical and pathological appearance, and the Ferguson-Smith patient will usually give a positive family history. Patients with xeroderma pigmentosum may develop keratoacanthomas in the first and second decade, but this is most unusual and the average age of presentation is 40 or older. Keratoacanthomas occur more frequently than would be expected by chance in those on immuno-suppressive therapy following renal transplantation, and in this group in particular clinical care must be exercised, as lesions with the clinical appearance of keratoacanthoma may be found on biopsy to be invasive squamous cell carcinomas. This observation may well give an important clue to the importance of the host response in the spontaneous involution of the keratoacanthoma.

Pathology[48]

If a biopsy of a keratoacanthoma is planned, a punch biopsy is not the optimal method of obtaining the

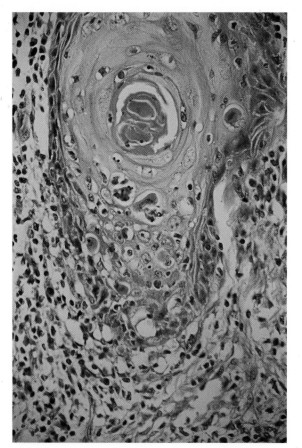

Figure 6.44 High-power view of leucocyte infiltration at the base of a keratoacanthoma.

most useful specimen for critical examination. The lesion should either be excised in toto, or a large scalpel biopsy taken through the widest diameter of the lesion, including both lateral margins, the central area, and the deepest part of the lesion. Low-power microscopic examination of the specimen will reveal a lesion, the bulk of which is above the normal epidermal surface. A distinct shoulder of epidermal keratinocytes with a central crater of keratin and debris can be seen (Figure 6.43). The cells in the depths of the lesion are not as deep as the underlying eccrine sweat glands, and there is no subtle infiltration of the dermis as would be seen in an invasive squamous cell carcinoma. Nevertheless, mitotic figures and a lymphocytic infiltrate may be seen, and if a punch biopsy is taken and the high-power objective of the microscope used, the appearance of a

keratoacanthoma would be very difficult to distinguish from that of an invasive squamous cell carcinoma. Polymorphonuclear leucocytes are seen in the stroma of a keratoacanthoma, a feature which would be unusual in a squamous cell carcinoma (Figure 6.44).

Management

Histological confirmation that the lesion is indeed a keratoacanthoma is essential. As has been emphasized above, such a large portion of a lesion needs to be removed to provide an adequate specimen for the pathologist that a complete excision biopsy is often most sensible, both as a diagnostic and a therapeutic procedure. If this is not done, and an incisional biopsy carried out, the lesion may be either observed for spontaneous remission or excised. If the expected spontaneous remission does not take place within a 3–4 month period, complete excision of the remainder of the lesion is recommended, because of the possibility of squamous carcinoma developing in the lesion, and many patients are in fact happier with a shave excision of the lesion at an earlier stage. Such a procedure will frequently give a more satisfactory cosmetic result than the scar obtained from spontaneous resolution.

The porokeratoses

Definition

A group of epidermal disorders that share a common dyskeratotic pattern. The name was originally used because the early workers believed that there was an involvement of the sweat glands. This is now known to be incorrect but the name persists.

Clinical features

The earliest description of a type of porokeratosis was that given by Mibelli in 1893–95.[49] This variety usually begins in childhood as a keratotic papule, commonly on the extremities, and may be clinically mistaken for a viral wart. This papule slowly expands and develops a characteristic, and almost diagnostic, thread-like raised rim around a central area of slightly atrophic epidermis, which does not sweat on exposure to high temperatures (Figure 6.45).[50] The lesions are

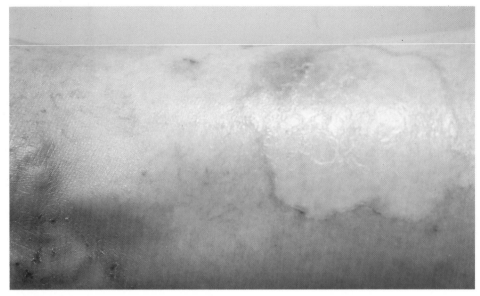

Figure 6.45   Classic porokeratosis of Mibelli.

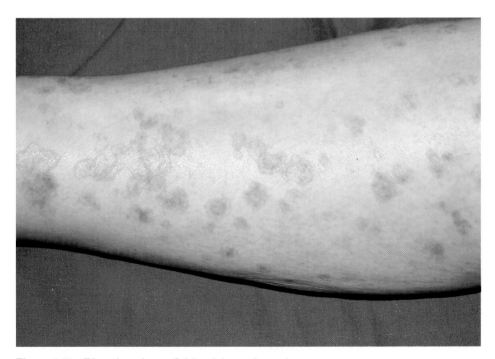

Figure 6.46   Disseminated superficial actinic porokeratosis.

seen on all body sites. A linear variant of porokeratosis was described intermittently in the literature throughout the early part of this century and definitively in 1972 when Eyre and Carson published their paper.[51] The linear lesions may cause clinical confusion with linear epidermal naevus, as they involve the limbs and are frequently grossly hyperkeratotic.

In 1967 Chernosky and Freeman described disseminated superficial actinic porokeratosis, and in 1969 Chernosky and Anderson demonstrated autosomal dominant inheritance in nine affected families in Texas.[52–54]

Although it is stated in the majority of textbooks that all the porokeratoses are genodermatoses, a negative family history is, in the author's experience, more common than a positive one, and this certainly applies to reported cases in the literature in which malignant change has developed, thus explaining the inclusion of this group of disorders in this section rather than in Chapter 4.

The lesions of disseminated superficial actinic porokeratosis are seen on habitually exposed sites in older individuals (Figure 6.46). A large proportion are on the lower legs of females and are scaly circular patches about a centimetre in diameter with the same

typical raised, thread-like edge seen in the other variants of porokeratosis. Despite the name of the lesion, not all patients give a positive history of excessive sun exposure.

A further variant of porokeratosis is the disseminated palmo-plantar variety.[55] This is very similar in clinical appearance to the disseminated actinic variety, but the positive history of sun exposure is lacking and there is involvement of the palms of the hands and soles of the feet.

Recently, a number of case reports have indicated that porokeratosis is more common than would be expected in renal transplant patients, suggesting that immunosuppression may be a positive feature in the development of these interesting lesions.[56,57] A report of porokeratosis developing after chemotherapy for malignancy may lend this theory further support.[58]

Pathology

The diagnostic feature of all types of porokeratosis is the presence of the cornoid lamella. This is a striking plume of parakeratosis which appears to arise from

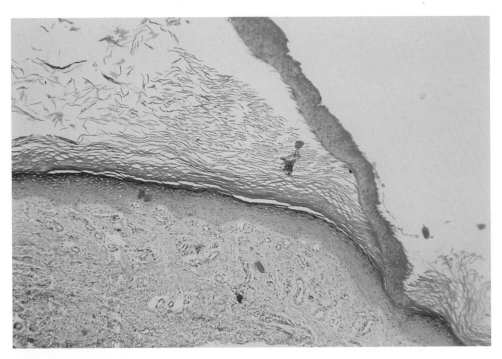

Figure 6.47   Cornoid lamella of porokeratosis.

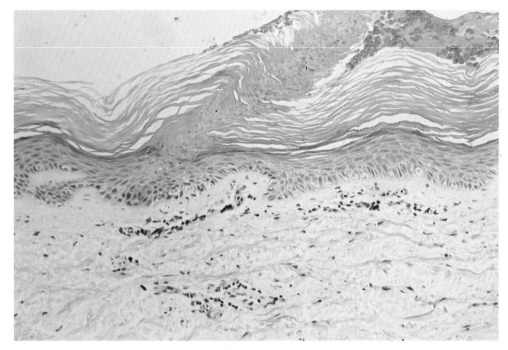

Figure 6.48   High-power view of the base of the cornoid lamella, showing loss of granular layer.

one or two underlying epidermal cells (Figures 6.47 and 6.48). If the plume of parakeratotic stratum corneum is followed down into the epidermis, it will be seen that there is an absence of granular layer at the point of origin of the parakeratotic plume. There is frequently a lymphocytic inflammatory infiltrate underlying this area, and the central areas of the lesions, which are clinically atrophic, also show pathological signs of atrophy.

This striking pathological picture is difficult to explain. Reed and Leone have suggested that this arises from a mutant clone of epidermal cells that expand peripherally.[59] Cultured fibroblasts have shown chromosomal instability, which may explain the underlying tendency to develop malignancy in lesions of porokeratosis.[60]

Management

Once the lesion has been confirmed pathologically, the individual lesions of disseminated superficial porokeratosis may be partially controlled by cryotherapy. The larger lesions of porokeratosis of Mibelli do not respond well to cryotherapy and require either observation or excision.

Various types of malignancy have been reported to develop in all types of porokeratosis. Squamous cell carcinoma, basal cell carcinoma and Bowen's disease have all been reported as developing in pre-existing lesions of porokeratosis.[61] A recent study reports that in 200 cases of porokeratosis malignant change developed in 7 per cent. Figures of this magnitude clearly suggest that careful follow-up of all patients in whom porokeratosis is diagnosed is essential.

Fibroepithelioma of Pinkus[62]

Definition

A tumour composed of strands of epithelial cells that are in contact with the overlying epidermis, admixed with a fibrous stroma.

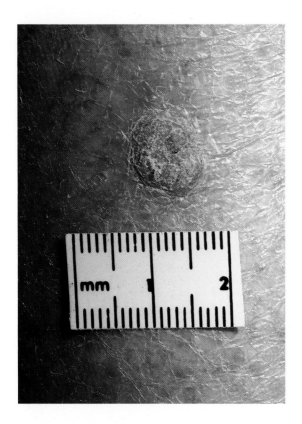

Figure 6.49   Appearance of fibroepithelioma of Pinkus.

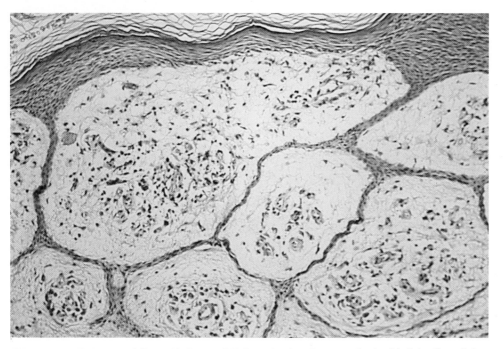

Figure 6.50   Pathology of fibroepithelioma of Pinkus, showing the network of epithelial cells and the associated stroma.

This lesion is frequently found adjacent to a basal cell carcinoma, and this contiguity, together with the dual component of epithelial cells and stroma, which is shared by the basal cell carcinoma (Chapter 7), is a reason for its inclusion, in some textbooks, in sections devoted to basal cell carcinoma. The fact that discrete individual lesions are seen is the justification for its inclusion in this chapter.

Clinical features

Fibroepitheliomas of Pinkus are often seen on the lower back, and clinically may appear similar to flesh-coloured skin tags (Figure 6.49).

Pathology

A network of anastomosing epithelial strands will be seen, with contact maintained between these and the overlying epidermis. This network may only be two cells thick in places, so that any suggestion of the palisading seen in basal cell carcinoma may be difficult to substantiate (Figure 6.50). There may be some acanthosis of the overlying epidermis, and horn cysts may be present, giving a superficial resemblance to a basal cell papilloma. This epidermal proliferation intermingles with the fibrous stroma in the dermis.

Basal cell carcinomas are reported to develop in a variable proportion of these fibroepithelial tumours. Management is usually local excision to obtain a histological diagnosis.

7

Basal cell carcinoma

This is the commonest skin tumour, and individuals working in a wide range of specialties will come across these in the course of their contact with patients. The term basal cell epithelioma is used by some as an alternative because of the relatively localized nature of spread characteristic of the majority of these lesions. However, the term carcinoma is preferable in view of the very striking local destruction which may develop if these lesions are neglected or regarded as benign and therefore as not requiring effective therapy. Even in the 1990s in a country such as the UK, where health care is free at the point of delivery, it is surprising to observe the quantity of destruction these lesions can cause, and the extent to which some elderly, often rather solitary individuals delay before seeking medical assistance.

Incidence and aetiology

As with most types of skin tumour, basal cell carcinoma is most common in Caucasian individuals, particularly those of Scottish and Irish descent. The earliest reports of the tumour are in fact from Ireland.[1] The work of Gellin and colleagues[2] emphasized the importance of a fair complexion, blue eyes, and fair hair, and a recent study from Australia[3] comparing the incidence of basal cell carcinoma, squamous cell carcinoma and melanoma in a study of 31 000 people indicated that the incidence of basal cell carcinoma was 652 new cases per year per 100 000 of the population. This compared with 160 cases of squamous cell carcinoma per 100 000 population and

19 cases of malignant melanoma. Thus, the ratio of basal cell carcinoma to squamous cell carcinoma in this series is just over 4 : 1 and the ratio of basal cell carcinoma to melanoma is 34 : 1. A recent study from the USA suggests that the annual incidence is currently 480 per 100 000 population per year for males and 250 per 100 000 per year for females,[4] with a study confined to Hawaii giving higher figures of 576 per 100 000 for males and 298 per 100 000 for females.[5] Current trends in Australia indicate a 5 per cent rate of increase per annum.[6] A study from Switzerland covering the period 1976–92 shows a steady increase in the incidence of basal cell carcinomas in the over-65 age group, even in a temperate climate.[7] A case–control study from Australia emphasizes that important and independent risk factors include inability to tan and large numbers of naevi on the back as features relatively specific for basal cell carcinoma as distinct from other cutaneous malignancies.[8,9]

Basal cell carcinomas are found virtually exclusively on hair-bearing skin, the only exceptions to this rule being tumours associated with the basal cell naevus syndrome and linear basal cell naevus.[10] In these situations, basal cell carcinomas are occasionally seen on the non-hair-bearing skin of the soles of the feet. It is doubtful whether basal cell carcinoma is ever seen on mucous membranes. This observation has given rise to the theory that basal cell carcinomas are derived from part of the hair follicle apparatus.

Although basal cell carcinomas are seen more frequently on those who have had significant sun exposure, the body sites on which basal cell carcinoma develops most commonly are not always the sites of maximum solar exposure.[11] Lesions are commonly seen adjacent to the inner canthus and in the nasolabial fold. Because of these observations, it has been suggested that, in addition to the undoubted effects of UV exposure, a relationship to embryological closure lines may exist.[12] When basal cell carcinoma spreads, it does so by direct extension, and tends to invade along embryological fusion planes, perhaps giving some support to this theory.

Trauma appears to play a part in the development of basal cell carcinoma and there are reports of basal cell carcinoma developing in sites of traumatic injury, on sites of smallpox vaccination, and on burn scars.[13–15] These observations have given rise to hypotheses concerning the permissive role of scar tissue in the development of basal cell carcinoma. An alternative theory would be to suggest that the temporary adjustment in growth control factors required for wound repair in the situations mentioned above is not under complete control, and the down-regulation required when a scar is completely healed is faulty on occasion, allowing development of either basal or squamous cell carcinoma.

Clinical features

In temperate climates, the majority of patients who have basal cell carcinoma are elderly individuals, with the exception of patients who have xeroderma pigmentosum, the basal cell naevus syndrome and linear basal cell naevi, who may develop basal cell carcinomas in the first and second decades. In countries such as Australia, white-skinned individuals otherwise in good health may develop their first basal cell carcinoma in the second or third decade of life. About half of all basal cell carcinomas are found on the face, and extrafacial lesions are more common in sunnier regions. In patients living in a temperate climate the lesions are usually solitary but 25 per cent of Australian patients will have multiple lesions.[16]

A large number of clinicopathological variants of basal cell carcinoma have been described. The broad divisions are into the solid, cystic, adenoid, pigmented, multiple superficial and morphoeic lesions. The basal cell carcinomas associated with the basal cell naevus syndrome and linear basal cell naevus have been described in Chapter 4, and the association between the fibroepithelioma of Pinkus and basal cell carcinoma has been discussed in Chapter 6.

An interesting and difficult tumour, which links basal cell carcinoma with squamous cell carcinoma, is the basisquamous or metatypical type of tumour.[17,18] These lesions have pathological features intermediate between the basal and squamous cell tumours and their biological behaviour appears to mirror this pathological ambiguity.

In view of the prevalence of basal cell carcinoma it is important to be able to recognize these lesions clinically. A recent survey of American residents, faculty and clinicians revealed that the accuracy rate of identification of basal cell carcinoma was 64 per cent for residents, 70 per cent for faculty, and 65 per cent for clinicians.[19] The lesions with which basal cell carcinoma was most often clinically confused were actinic keratosis, squamous cell carcinoma, and intradermal naevus. The fact that only two-thirds of basal cell carcinomas were accurately diagnosed on clinical grounds is a matter for some concern in view of the fact that they are regarded by many dermatologists as one of the easiest types of skin tumour to recognize.

The solid or nodular basal cell carcinoma occurs most frequently on the face, and is most likely to be seen around the inner canthus of the eye, on the nose, and on the forehead (Figures 7.1–7.4). Lesions on the chin (Figure 7.5) and on the outer surface of the cheek are less common. Basal cell carcinomas are initially seen as slowly growing, shiny, or translucent raised nodules (Figures 7.6 and 7.7). The lesion may reach a diameter of half a centimetre over a period of 1–2 years, and small dilated blood vessels may be on the surface of the lesion. If the lesion is not recognized and treated at this stage, the tempo of local growth may increase, and central ulceration will develop, giving rise to the nodulo-ulcerative type of tumour (Figure 7.8). This lesion has a raised, rolled border with the translucent appearance seen in the early nodular lesions, but has an ulcerated centre. Once again, the dilated capillaries may be seen coursing over the lateral margin of this lesion. A number of nodular basal cell carcinomas may contain some pigment, and these lesions may appear as variably pigmented lesions (Figure 7.7). They may be confused with malignant melanoma, but are usually fairly easily distinguished on clinical grounds. The pigment may in some cases be melanin trapped in the lesion, or may be altered blood due to haemorrhage into the lesion. A small proportion of basal cell carcinomas have a rather hyperkeratotic surface and these lesions may have a superficial scaly appearance, giving rise to clinical confusion with actinic keratosis or basal cell papilloma. A small number of basal cell carcinomas are found in the relatively sun-protected area behind the ear (Figures 7.9 and 7.10) and may occasionally be clinically confused with a granuloma,

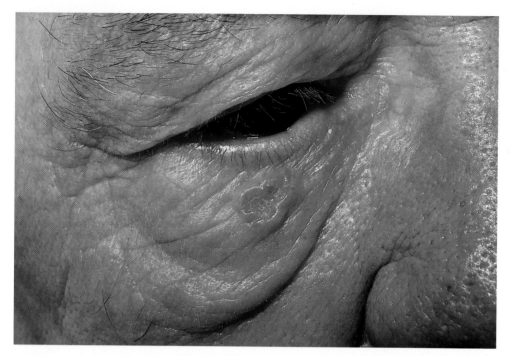

Figure 7.1 A basal cell carcinoma in the common site below the right eye, showing a typical raised, rolled edge.

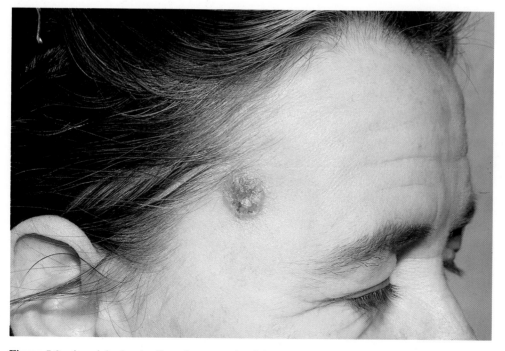

Figure 7.2 A nodular basal cell carcinoma on the right temple.

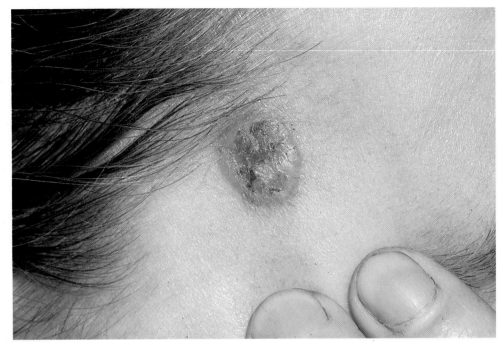

Figure 7.3   Close-up view of the lesion shown in Figure 7.2, to illustrate the raised border and dilated vessels.

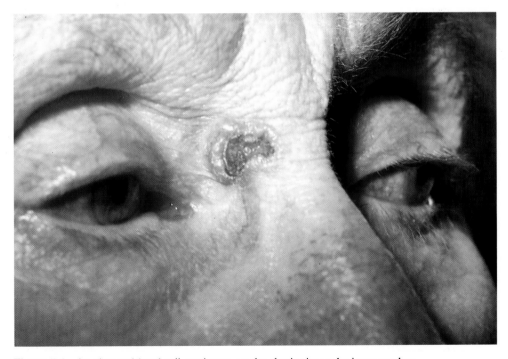

Figure 7.4   An ulcerated basal cell carcinoma on the classic site at the inner canthus.

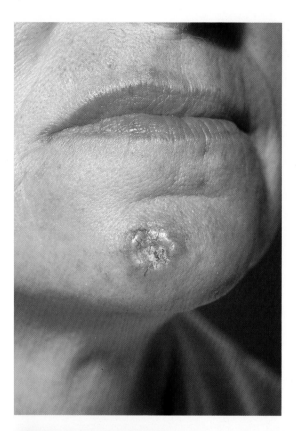

Figure 7.5 A large, ulcerated basal cell carcinoma on the chin. The site is a little unusual, but the clinical appearance is typical.

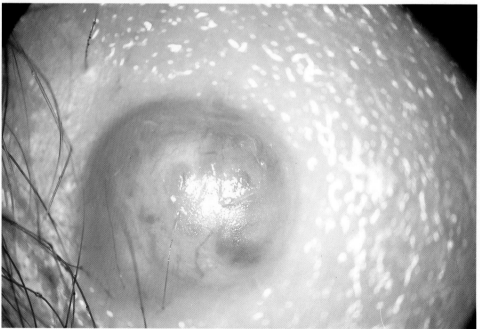

Figure 7.6 Close-up view of a nodular basal cell carcinoma, showing a cystic appearance with blue pigmentation due to deeply situated incidental melanin pigmentation.

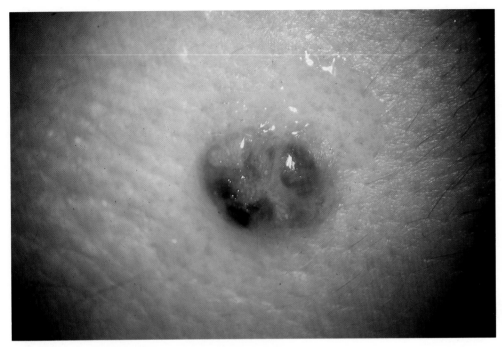

Figure 7.7   A heavily pigmented basal cell carcinoma. Clinically malignant melanoma was suspected, but the lesion is a cystic basal cell carcinoma containing altered blood.

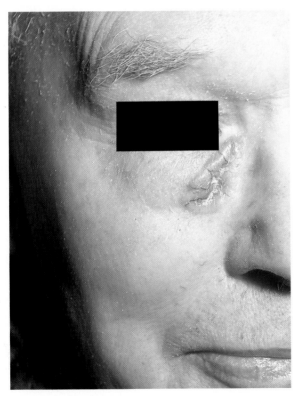

Figure 7.8   A larger basal cell carcinoma extending in a linear fashion below the eye.

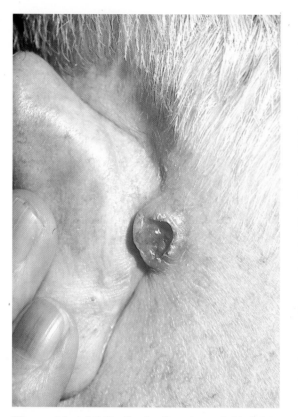
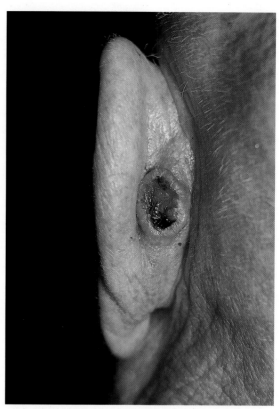

Figures 7.9 and 7.10   Basal cell carcinoma behind the ear. Occasionally, irritation caused by spectacle frames may cause a granuloma at this site. These granulomas usually occur in the crease between ear and scalp.

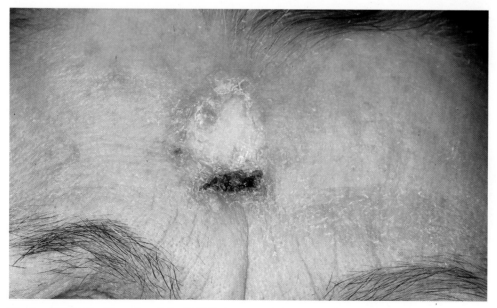

Figures 7.11–7.13   Examples of the 'field fire' or central healing basal cell carcinoma.

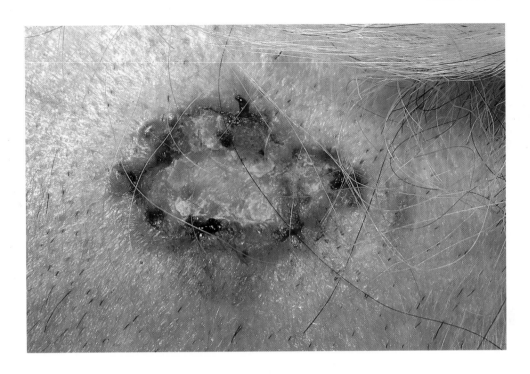

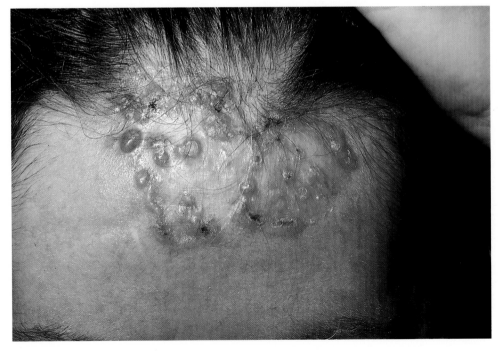

Figure 7.13

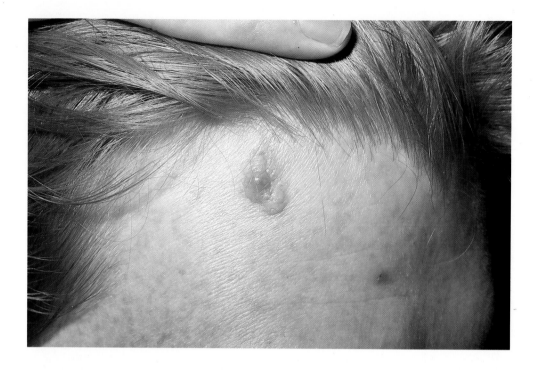

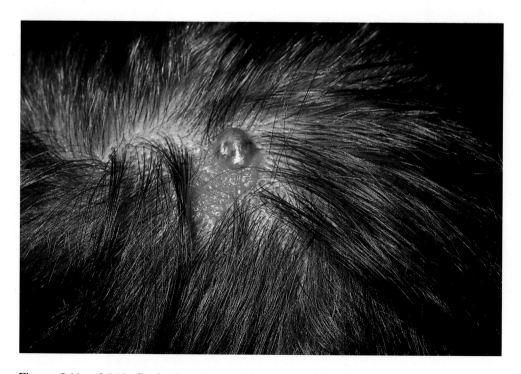

Figures 7.14 and 7.15   Basal cell carcinoma arising on organoid naevi.

which is sometimes seen in this site in spectacle wearers and is thought to be caused by friction from the leg of the spectacles.

Some basal cell carcinomas are seen on pathological examination to have a rather adenocystic appearance. These lesions usually appear as rather more diffuse plaques on clinical examination but the same translucent quality of the slightly rolled edge of the lesion is seen. A less common appearance is of a more rapidly expanding plaque, often with several raised nodular foci at the edges, but central healing. These lesions have in the past been referred to on occasion as the 'field fire' type of lesion (Figures 7.11–7.13).

Figures 7.14 and 7.15 illustrate basal cell carcinoma developing in an organoid or sebaceous naevus. This is usually seen as a nodular elevation on the already papillomatous lesion, and may occur as early as the second decade.

Basal cell carcinomas found on extrafacial sites tend to be large, plaque-like lesions. They are most likely to be mistaken for Bowen's disease, but on careful examination it will be seen that the erythematous scaling plaque of an extrafacial basal cell carcinoma retains the raised, rolled edge that is seen on the more classic facial lesions (Figures 7.16–7.20). In contrast, the plaque of Bowen's disease does not have this clearly marginated lateral border (see Figures 6.18–6.21 for comparison). In the past, these extrafacial lesions have on occasion been described as multifocal lesions, but complex and detailed three-dimensional reconstruction of the lesions following serial section has shown that the lesions are in fact unifocal despite their clinical appearance.[20]

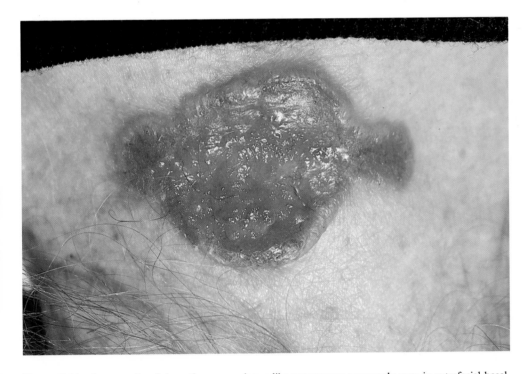

Figure 7.16 An example of the rather more plaque-like appearance commonly seen in extrafacial basal cell carcinomas. The raised, rolled edge is helpful in differentiation from Bowen's disease or an isolated patch of psoriasis.

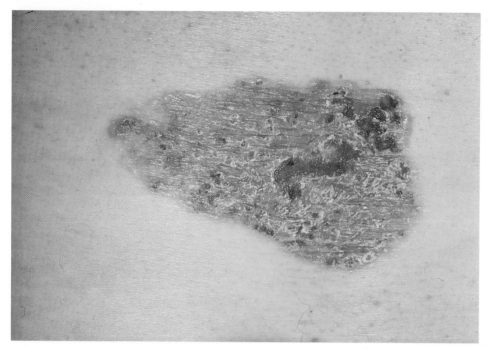

Figure 7.17

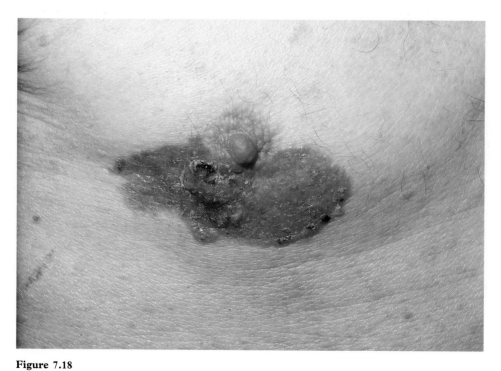

Figure 7.18

Figures 7.17–7.19   Plaque-like extrafacial basal cell carcinomas.

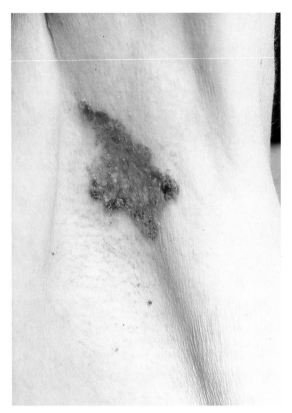

Figure 7.19

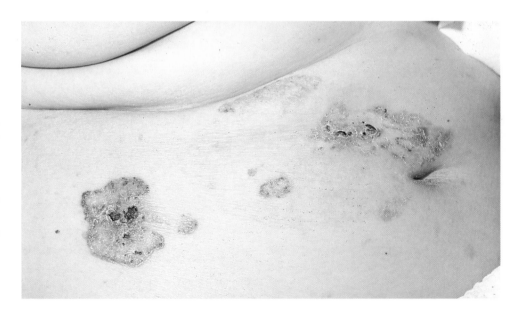

Figure 7.20   Multiple histologically confirmed basal cell carcinomas. The patient had a history of medicinal arsenic ingestion.

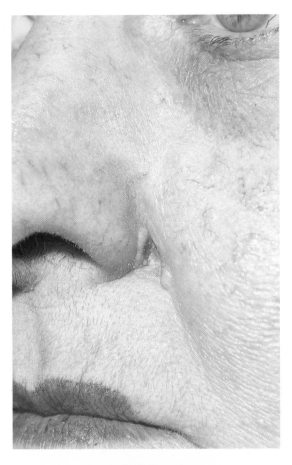

The morphoeic type of basal cell carcinoma is seldom diagnosed correctly. This lesion tends to develop in the nasolabial fold and may present as a firm, scar-like area (Figures 7.21 and 7.22). The translucent raised edge and central ulceration are rarely present. This lesion tends to be much more extensive on palpation than on inspection because of the large quantity of associated stroma found in the morphoeic lesions.

It is important to recognize this lesion clinically before surgery is undertaken; incomplete excision of morphoeic basal cell carcinoma is extremely common as a result of failure to recognize the extensive nature of the lesion.

The basisquamous or metatypical type of basal cell carcinoma frequently has some pathological features similar to the morphoeic lesion, and is clinically more like a squamous cell carcinoma than a basal cell lesion (Figure 7.23).[21]

The majority of patients present with relatively small lesions, 2–4 cm or less in diameter, but on occasion elderly individuals, particularly those who lead a solitary life, will delay for many years before seeking medical advice about their lesions. This may result in striking destruction of skin, soft tissue, cartilage and even bone.

Figure 7.21 and 7.22   Morphoeic basal cell carcinomas on the typical site in the nasolabial fold.

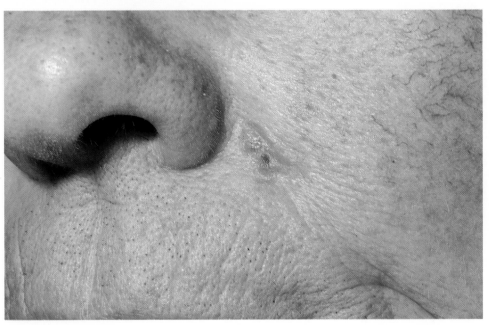

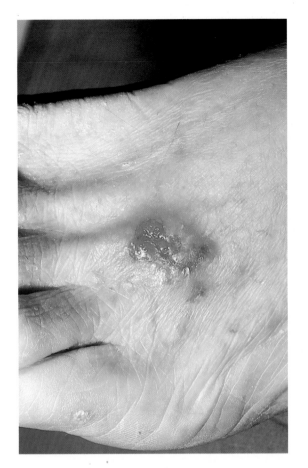

The erosive and destructive quality of untreated basal cell carcinoma should not be underestimated (Figure 7.24).[22]

Pathology and biology[23]

The essential feature in all types of basal cell carcinoma is a downgrowth from the epidermis of small, dark, epithelioid cells with the cytological characteristics of cells of the basal layer (Figures 7.25 and 7.26). Krompecher has suggested that these are indeed outgrowths of the basal cells of the epidermis and skin appendages.[24] He and others have suggested that basal cell carcinomas can be divided broadly on pathological grounds into differentiated and undifferentiated lesions. The former lesions show differentiation similar to that seen in skin appendages, while the undifferentiated tumours show no such differentiation.

The second essential component of the basal cell carcinoma is the stroma surrounding these downgrowths of dark epithelial cells (Figures 7.27 and 7.28). These two components of basal cell

Figure 7.23   Basisquamous carcinoma on the dorsum of the foot. The raised, rolled edge of the classic lesion is not seen in this lesion.

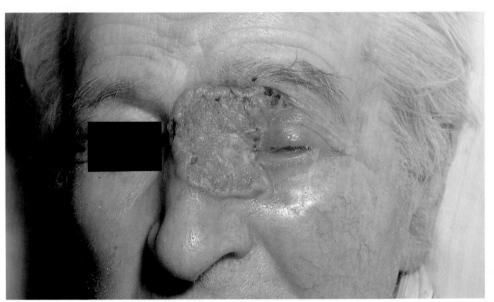

Figure 7.24   Neglected, and therefore extensive and destructive, basal cell carcinoma.

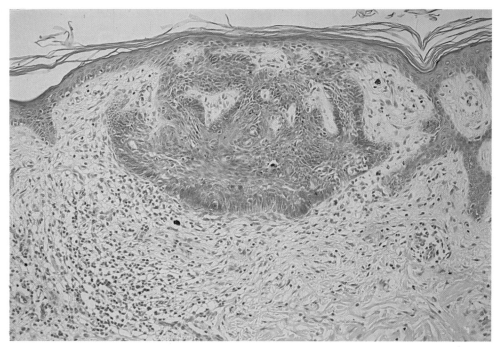

Figure 7.25 Low-power view of a basal cell carcinoma stained with haematoxylin and eosin, showing downgrowth of dark basaloid cells from the dermoepidermal junction.

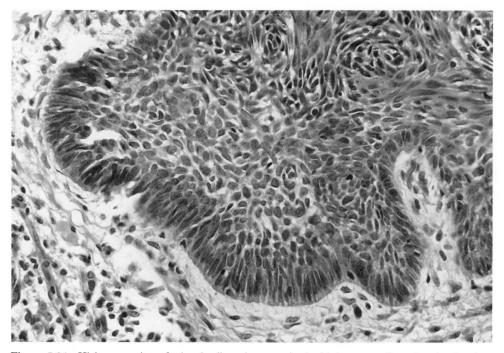

Figure 7.26 High-power view of a basal cell carcinoma stained with haematoxylin and eosin, showing the classic palisading pattern of cells at the periphery of the tumour nodules.

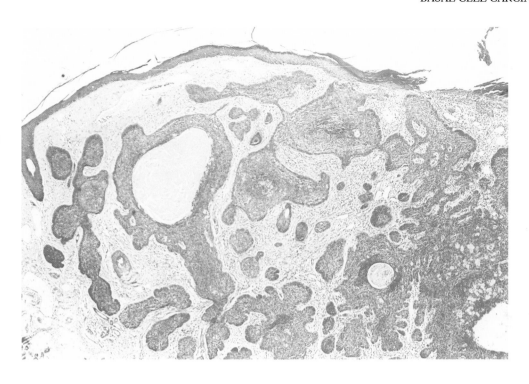

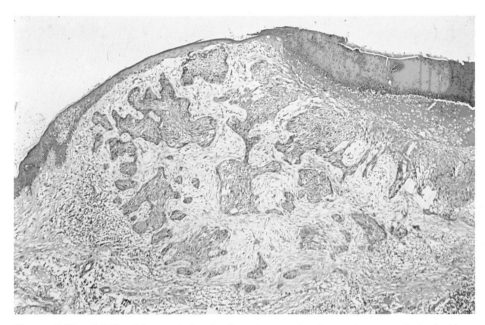

Figures 7.27 and 7.28 Adenocystic basal cell carcinomas, showing cystic spaces admixed with tumour nodules and dense fibrous stroma.

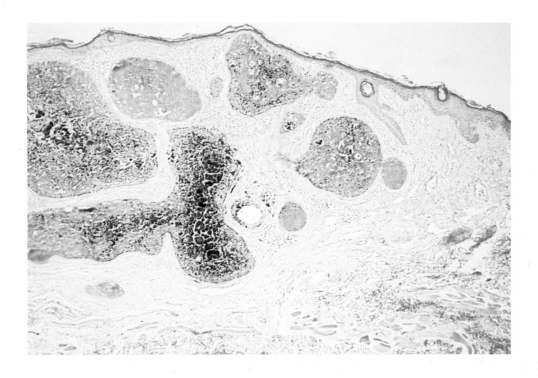

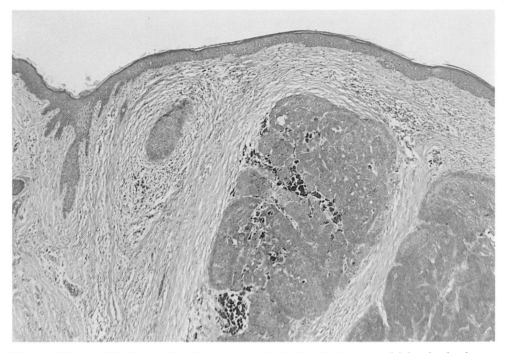

Figures 7.29 and 7.30   Basal cell carcinomas containing incidental pigment, explaining the deeply pigmented clinical appearance seen in some lesions.

carcinoma appear to interact, and attempts to grow basal cell carcinoma cells in culture in the absence of stroma have not been found to be successful.[25,26] There appears to be, therefore, a symbiotic relationship between these two components, and the pathologist examining sections from basal cell carcinoma for completeness of excision must examine not only the cells but also the surrounding stroma. Pigment may be seen, but is usually either incidental melanin or altered blood (Figures 7.29 and 7.30).

The nodular, cystic and adenoid types of basal cell carcinoma show very clear peripheral palisading of dark epithelial cells around the downgrowths of epithelial tissue. The nuclei of the palisaded cells are at right angles to the edge of the lesion and this appearance is almost diagnostic on low-power microscopic examination of the section. This palisading is not always seen uniformly throughout all parts of the tumour and is rarely present in such a marked way in the extrafacial, morphoeic and basisquamous lesions (Figure 7.31).

The most common differential diagnosis to be made is from the trichoepithelioma. This lesion frequently has a palisaded edge to nodules of tumour cells, but in addition numerous keratin cysts will be seen. These are not a feature of the basal cell carcinoma.

A second, less common, differential diagnosis is from the recently described desmoplastic trichoepithelioma, or sclerosing epithelial hamartoma.[27,28] These lesions affect individuals over a wide age range, are mainly on the face, and are composed of cysts and epidermoid cells infiltrating a very sclerotic stroma (Figures 7.32 and 7.33). The palisading of the true basal cell carcinoma is absent. A number of lesions found in children in the past and diagnosed as basal cell carcinoma may have belonged more correctly to this category.

Large numbers of mitotic figures will be seen within the cellular component of the basal cell carcinoma. This observation, of course, is at variance with the slow growth tempo of most basal cell carcinomas. Weinstein and Frost have calculated that the cell cycle

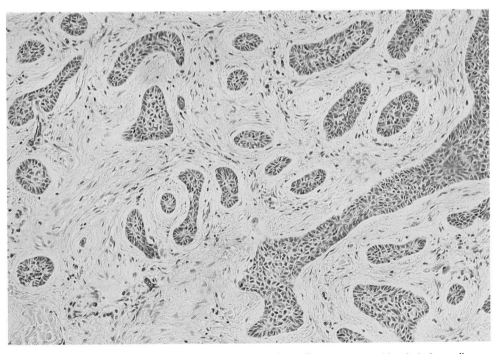

Figure 7.31 Morphoeic basal cell carcinoma. Note the dense fibrous stroma with relatively small numbers of cells embedded in it.

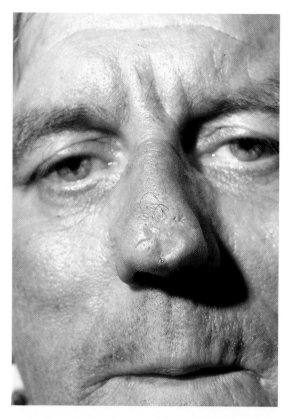

time in basal cell carcinoma is 217 hours.[29] With a cell cycle time in this range, basal cell carcinomas should theoretically double in size every 10 days. As, clearly, this does not occur, other methods of cell destruction or elimination must take place within these lesions. The phenomenon of apoptosis, or individual cell death and destruction within the epidermis, is thought to play a large part in the control of tumour expansion in basal cell carcinoma.[30,31] Basal cell carcinomas of all types may show small areas of amyloid deposition within the body of the lesion.[32] These have no diagnostic or prognostic significance. The clinically pigmented basal cell carcinoma may show large aggregates of melanin pigment within the body of the lesion. There is no associated proliferation of melanocytes and this melanin pigmentation appears to result purely from an aggregation of melanin in the epithelial cells. On occasion, clinical pigmentation

Figure 7.32 Desmoplastic trichoepithelioma, or sclerosing epithelial hamartoma – clinical presentation.

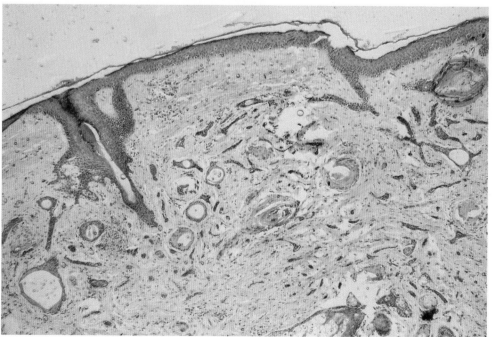

Figure 7.33 Histology of the desmoplastic trichoepithelioma shown in Figure 7.32. Note the presence of cysts, and ribbons of cells embedded in a dense stroma.

may be due to the presence of haemorrhage into the lesion, giving rise to a dense reddish or black coloration on clinical inspection.

The morphoeic basal cell carcinoma does not show the characteristic and diagnostically helpful palisading pattern. The striking component of the morphoeic lesion is the stromal change, and very large areas of dense fibrous stroma may be seen with relatively small numbers of epidermal cells apparently trapped within this stroma. The use of crossed prisms and polarized light may delineate more clearly the lateral margin of this stromal change from surrounding normal dermis (Figure 7.31).

The basisquamous type of tumour is recognized by the combination of a fibrous stroma, typical of that seen in basal cell carcinoma, with a downward proliferation of epithelial cells that lack peripheral palisading in some areas of the lesion and have many features more suggestive of squamous cell carcinoma, with frequent mitoses, individual cell keratinization and horn cysts present. Metatypical lesions are reported to be much more frequent among those lesions that metastasize than would be expected relative to their incidence, further emphasizing the importance of definitive and complete excision when the lesion is first diagnosed (Figure 7.34).

McNutt[33] has reported a relative lack of hemidesmosomes in basal cell carcinomas. This observation may explain in part the striking retraction pattern that is occasionally seen around the palisaded areas and that is a useful diagnostic aid on low-power microscopic examination. It has been suggested, but not confirmed, that morphoeic basal cell carcinomas have a higher number of microfilaments in their cytoplasm than non-morphoeic basal cell carcinomas.[34] This observation could correlate with clinical behaviour in that greater cell motility is associated with such a filament pattern and thus a greater capacity for local spread. A further observation has been the report of higher levels of collagenase activity in the morphoeic type of basal cell carcinoma, possibly indicating a more destructive type of lesion.[35]

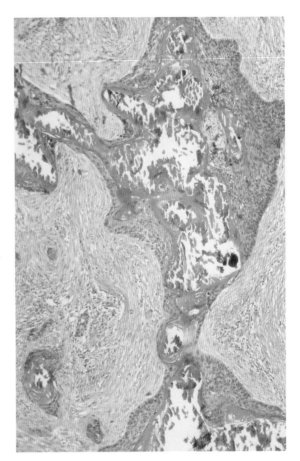

Figure 7.34 Histology of a basisquamous tumour. A little palisading is seen, and a fibrous stroma is present.

do those on other sites, and a high proportion of lesions on this site are of the infiltrative or morphoeic type.

Local recurrence

Sloane has suggested that lesions with a multifocal and infiltrative pattern are more likely to recur.[36] This, of course, may relate to the difficulty in ascertaining that excision is complete. Basal cell carcinomas in the central panel of the face recur more frequently than

Metastasis and basal cell carcinomas

The vast majority of basal cell carcinomas spread by direct extension from the primary tumour site, and although this direct extension may be extremely widespread, metastatic spread is extremely rare. To date, approximately 100 cases of metastatic basal cell carcinoma have been reported in the world literature.[37]

The incidence of metastasis among basal cell carcinomas in Brisbane has been estimated at 0.002 per cent.[38] The majority of lesions that do metastasize do so only as far as lymph nodes, but about one-third metastasize to the lungs and other organs.[39] The lesions that appear to show the greatest propensity for metastasis tend to be deeply invasive lesions occurring on the face or scalp. Morphoeic basal cell carcinomas appear to have a higher incidence of both relentless local spread and metastasis than other types,[17] and this is why it is so important completely to excise morphoeic basal cell carcinomas when they first present.

Management

Clinical suspicion of basal cell carcinoma should be confirmed pathologically. In the case of small tumours, an excision biopsy is an appropriate method of management. The width of excision should take into account the stromal element of the tumour, and in the case of lesions in the central panel of the face, adequate depth of excision is particularly important to avoid local recurrence.

In the case of large tumours, once pathological confirmation is obtained on an incisional biopsy, radiotherapy or further surgery can be selected for further treatment. The exception to this is the patient with the basal cell naevus syndrome, as discussed in Chapter 4. These patients tend to develop multiple new tumours in X-irradiated sites, and surgery is therefore the treatment of choice. The choice of treatment for other patients will depend on local availability, the patient's age, and the site of the lesions. There is currently some support for less aggressive treatment of basal cell carcinomas using topical 5-FU, and in some cases for cryotherapy. The author's personal view is that, if the patient is in otherwise reasonable health, definitive treatment with surgery or radiotherapy is more appropriate, as there is a risk that cryotherapy or localized chemotherapy will not completely eradicate the lesion, and there may be a local recurrence.

In patients with multiple basal cell carcinomas and the basal cell naevus syndrome, there have been recent studies on the use of oral retinoids. Continuous treatment and high-dose therapy appear necessary to prevent completely further development of new basal cell carcinomas.

The morphoeic basal cell carcinoma, and particularly the recurrent morphoeic basal cell carcinoma, is a tumour for which the use of micrographically controlled surgery using Mohs' fresh tissue technique is the treatment of choice. This is a totally appropriate situation for surgery using Mohs' technique in that the tumour spreads by direct extension, and therefore it should be possible to remove all tumour cells and all associated tumour stroma with minimal destruction to surrounding normal tissue. If a patient has a recurrent basal cell carcinoma of the morphoeic type, referral to a centre where this technique is available should be considered.

Follow-up

All patients who have had a basal cell carcinoma excised should be followed up for a minimum of 3–6 months to check that there is no local recurrence. If there is no sign of recurrence after this period, follow-up regimes may then vary according to the health care system and the patient's age and distance from a centre with an interest in these tumours. In the UK, patients who have had one classic basal cell carcinoma should be seen by their family doctor at least yearly for a general skin examination to check for local recurrence and further basal cell carcinomas as well as for actinic keratoses, squamous cell carcinomas and malignant melanoma, as an individual who has had one basal cell carcinoma is at increased risk of developing all types of skin cancer. Patients should also be shown illustrations of early skin cancer of all types and encouraged to seek medical advice between follow-up visits if they have any concern about an individual skin lesion.[40,41]

If an individual has had a morphoeic basal cell carcinoma or a recurrent basal cell carcinoma, follow-up at a specialist centre is recommended, as dealing with these recurrences can be technically difficult.

At these follow-up visits patients should be continually advised to restrict sun exposure, to avoid noonday sun, to wear a broad-brimmed hat and to use a broad-spectrum sunscreen with an SPF of 15 or over.

8

Squamous cell carcinoma

A squamous cell carcinoma is a malignant lesion derived from the epidermal keratinocytes, and is composed of cytologically malignant keratinocytes with the capacity for metastatic spread.

Incidence and mortality

As with basal cell carcinoma, squamous cell carcinoma is most frequently seen in white-skinned individuals who have migrated to tropical climates. The true incidence of basal and squamous cell tumours is difficult to determine with accuracy, in comparison to the figures available for malignant melanoma. This is partly because many cancer registries include basal and squamous cell carcinoma under one heading, and the exact contribution of each to the total is not known. A second problem is that in some health care systems a large proportion of non-melanoma skin cancers are removed in private offices and surgeries. Some of these may not be sent for histological examination, and thus no tissue diagnosis will be available for reporting to a local cancer registry. A further complication is that in some cases, particularly in the very elderly section of the population, destructive treatments such as cryotherapy or laser therapy may be considered the best treatment approach, and no tissue will be available for pathological examination.

For these reasons, it is widely accepted that published figures for non-melanoma skin cancer are likely to be significant under-representations of the true situation. This problem was emphasized by a group from Bristol in 1982, who estimated that for the year 1974 there was an under-recording of non-melanoma skin cancer of between 14 and 28 per cent.[1] This figure, obtained in a nationalized health care system with relatively small numbers of individuals engaged in private office practice, is disturbing and suggests that in other health care systems the figure could be very much higher.

In the Australian setting, Giles and colleagues, in their study of 31 000 individuals (see page 112), report an incidence of 160 squamous cell carcinomas per 100 000 population per year.[2] This compares with 19 melanomas for the same population over the same period of time, and is approximately one-quarter of the number of basal cell carcinomas recorded. This ratio of 3–4 basal cell carcinomas per squamous cell carcinoma is common on white or Caucasian skin, with the exception of certain unusual situations, such as patients receiving PUVA therapy. On coloured skin, however, the incidence is approximately equal. A more recent Australian survey reports a 51 per cent increase in the incidence of squamous cell carcinoma between 1985 and 1990,[3] and an American study calculates the current incidence of squamous cell carcinoma in males and females to be 136 and 59 per 100 000 population, respectively.[4] A European study documenting the changes in skin cancer incidence in Switzerland between 1976 and 1992 records a trebling in incidence of squamous cell carcinoma in females over this period.[5] Mortality from non-melanoma skin cancer is low by comparison with melanoma, and most of the non-melanoma skin cancer deaths are attributed to squamous cell carcinoma rather than to basal cell carcinoma, but in studying such figures it is important to exclude patients with Kaposi's sarcoma who may be classified in this group. In the USA in 1991, the age-adjusted mortality rate for non-melanoma skin cancer was 0.44 per 100 000 population.[6]

Aetiology

Epidemiological, experimental and clinical evidence suggests that excessive exposure to UV light is the main aetiological factor in the development of squamous cell carcinoma.[7,8] A study of World War II veterans showed a higher incidence of skin cancer among those who had served in the Pacific than in those who served in Europe,[9] and a study of the effect of cumulative sun exposure in Maryland watermen also showed that chronic lifetime sun exposure is a risk factor,[10] and that blue eyes and childhood freckling are additional risk factors. Squamous cell carcinoma can also arise from industrial or occupational exposure, and the classic historical example of this is the recording by Percival Potts of scrotal malignancy in chimney sweeps due to contact with carcinogens in soot.[11] This was followed by the observation of Paris that arsenic was a carcinogen, both for the skin and other organs.[12] In an excellent review of arsenic and carcinogenesis in 1947, Neubauer[13] listed pemphigus, pemphigoid, eczema, dermatitis herpetiformis, lichen 'ruber' and acne as indications for arsenic therapy in the pre-steroid era. Thus a high proportion of arsenic-induced malignancy was iatrogenic, although in certain areas well-water is heavily contaminated with arsenic.

Tar was identified as a proven carcinogen in 1925 and, following this, petroleum, shale oils and creosote oils were also recognized as causes of skin cancer.[14] Squamous cell carcinoma was recognized in the past as an occupational hazard among cotton spinners due to oil contact, and the modern problem is the exposure of individuals to cutting oils in an occupational setting.[15,16] The development of squamous cell carcinoma as a result of industrial exposure to such cutting oils is a proscribed industrial disease in the UK.

The first realization that exposure to sunlight might also be a cause of skin cancer was made by Unna in 1896, when he described 'seaman's skin', which showed actinic keratosis and squamous cell carcinoma.[17] Following this, Dubreuilh and Hyde both reported clinical associations between sun exposure and cutaneous malignancy.[18,19] In 1928 Findlay[20]

produced skin tumours on laboratory animals using UV radiation. In 1940 Blum[21] produced early epidemiological evidence of a higher incidence of skin cancer in the more southerly states of the USA, and in 1941 Rusch and colleagues[22] identified the UVB part of the spectrum as being responsible for skin cancer in laboratory animals. The work of Macdonald in 1950–59 showed that squamous cell carcinoma was eight times more common in Texas than in Connecticut.[23] This difference was ascribed to the different latitudes, and the resulting differences in exposure to sunlight.

As already discussed in Chapter 2, current work on the role of mutations in the $p53$ gene in initiating and promoting squamous cell malignancy strongly suggests that UV acts as both an initiator and a promoter,[24,25] and that early $p53$ mutations prevent the initiation of the process of apoptosis which appears to remove UV-damaged cells and thus prevent expansion of clones of UV-damaged cells which may then undergo a second mutation in the process of UV-induced tumour promotion.

Squamous cell carcinoma is more common in males than in females, and the postulated reason for this has been that in the past more males were employed in outdoor occupations than females. With the growing importance of outdoor leisure time, this ratio may well change in the future.

The classic patient with squamous cell carcinoma is an individual who is fair-haired and fair-skinned, who tans with difficulty, and whose skin already bears the signs of excessive sun exposure in the form of dryness, wrinkling, and actinic keratosis. Albinos are at greatly increased risk of squamous cell carcinoma, particularly in a tropical climate where fatal metastasizing tumours may develop in the second decade, further underlining the value of natural pigmentation as a barrier to UV damage.[26] As already discussed in Chapter 2, the lack of reports of an increased incidence of skin cancer in vitiligo is intriguing in this respect.

Two case–control studies from less sunny parts of the world are of interest. Vitaliano and Urbach,[27] reporting on squamous cell carcinoma and basal cell carcinoma patients in Philadelphia, found that cumulative lifetime solar exposure was an extremely important risk factor, and that, given the same level of cumulative lifetime solar exposure, subjects over 60 years of age were at greater risk for non-melanoma carcinoma than younger individuals. This suggests that aging per se may play a part in the development of squamous cell carcinoma, possibly related to a diminishing immune response. On the other hand, this observation could be related to the actual intensity of UV exposure rather than to a specifically age-related phenomenon. In this particular study, sensitivity to sunburn and dark or fair complexions were not shown to be risk factors for squamous cell carcinoma but only for basal cell carcinoma.

A study from the Montreal region published in 1985 controlled patients for host factors including eye and hair colour, complexion, and Celtic or Caledonian descent.[28] With these controls, it was found that significant risk factors were both occupational and non-occupational sunlight exposure, use of a long-tube sunlamp, and cigarette smoking. The exact type of long-tube sunlamp used, and details of UVB and UVA emission, are not given in this study. The association with cigarette smoking is of interest, although there was no reported association between number of cigarettes smoked and incidence of squamous cell carcinoma. There is, however, growing evidence of smoking as a risk factor for carcinoma of areas outside the lung, including the larynx and the cervix.

A number of topical treatments used for the management of intractable skin disease contain recognized carcinogens. This applies particularly to the use of topical tar, which has been recognized as a carcinogen for many years and which is used in experimental systems to induce tumours on animal skin. Despite these observations, studies over the years have not reported a significantly increased incidence of non-melanoma skin cancer or indeed of melanoma on the skin of patients with psoriasis. A large case–control study reported from Glasgow three years ago found no significant variation in the observed versus expected incidence of squamous carcinoma, melanoma, and a number of other solid tumours in patients who had used tar for psoriasis over a long period of time.[29]

Ultraviolet B has been used for many years in dermatological practice for the treatment of acne, psoriasis, and a number of other conditions. A Scandinavian study suggested that therapeutic UVB, as used in psoriasis treatment, was not associated with a greater than expected risk of squamous cell carcinoma, and further long-term studies are needed to confirm this observation.[30]

Recent interest in the possible carcinogenic potential of a number of topical agents used in acne has prompted some case–control studies. To date these do not suggest that individuals may be at increased risk of developing melanoma many years after treatment of acne.[31] No such data are yet available for squamous cell carcinoma and a case–control study

suggests that a past history of acne is a protective factor for both basal and squamous cell carcinomas.[7]

Photochemotherapy involves the use of an oral psoralen which is a photosensitizing drug in combination with exposure of the skin to long-wave UV radiation (UVA) in the 320–360 nm range of the UV spectrum. This treatment has only been available in the UK and the USA for approximately 20 years, and there is steadily accumulating evidence that patients who have received high (over 2000 J/cm^2) doses of UVA are at significantly increased risk of developing squamous cell carcinoma.[32] Even more disturbing are reports of metastases developing from these UVA-induced malignancies,[33,34] as there were early suggestions that PUVA-associated malignancies were relatively innocuous.

The more usual ratio of 3–4 basal cell carcinomas to 1 squamous cell carcinoma is reversed, indicating that the risk is of squamous cell carcinoma specifically, and not of basal cell carcinoma. At present it is therefore extremely important that all units who use photochemotherapy follow patients up even after courses of PUVA have been discontinued, and that PUVA be used for short, well-controlled courses of therapy, and never as a maintenance therapy unless there are no less-damaging alternatives.

Immunosuppression and squamous cell carcinoma

Patients who are on immunosuppressive therapy following transplantation of a kidney or other organ are also at increased risk of developing squamous cell carcinoma. As with PUVA therapy, the ratio of basal cell carcinoma to squamous cell carcinoma appears to be reversed. This observation may suggest that immunological control of early squamous cell carcinoma and precursor actinic keratoses may be of greater significance than any immunological control of the early stages of basal cell carcinoma.

Squamous cell carcinoma is also reported in sites of chronic inflammation, such as chronic ulceration or chronic sinuses.[35] This was recognized as early as 1829 with the classic Marjolin's ulcer. Squamous cell carcinoma has been reported in lesions of lupus erythematosus, and also in scars of lesions of lupus vulgaris. In the latter situation there is some doubt as to whether or not the carcinoma is the result of chronic ulceration and scarring associated with the lupus vulgaris process, or the result of treatment with intense UV lamps, or even radiotherapy, which was used in the management of this condition before the introduction of effective systemic antituberculous therapy. Exposure to X-irradiation is well established as a cause of squamous cell carcinoma, and this may develop in an area of pre-existing radiodermatitis (Chapter 6).[36,37]

The possible role of viruses in the aetiology of squamous cell carcinoma

The possible role of viruses, mainly of the human papilloma virus group, in the aetiology of squamous cell carcinoma is currently under intensive investigation. It is well known that HPV 16 and 18 are found in carcinoma of the cervix more frequently than would be expected by chance alone (see Chapter 2, page 19), and squamous cell carcinomas have been probed for a wide range of HPVs. To date HPVs have not been found in any significant numbers in patients who are not overtly immunosuppressed but develop squamous cell carcinoma. There is, however, a growing body of evidence to suggest that immuno-suppressed individuals (and once again it is the renal transplant group who have been studied most thoroughly) do have a range of HPV types in their squamous cell carcinomas. HPV 5 has been found in squamous cell carcinoma from such individuals more often than would be expected.[38]

Clinical features[39]

Squamous cell carcinoma arises on skin that is already damaged, most commonly as a result of exposure to UV radiation. The 'typical' patient is an elderly male, and the most usual sites are the back of the hand, the forearm, the face and the neck. The lesion will present as a firm, indurated, expanding nodule, which may arise on the site of a pre-existing actinic keratosis (Figures 8.1–8.5). As with actinic keratosis, the problem may be multifocal, and several primary invasive squamous cell carcinomas may develop in relatively rapid succession on sun-damaged skin. The lesion may expand rapidly on the primary site, giving rise to an ulcerated mass, and may also metastasize to local draining lymph nodes.

As discussed in Chapter 6, Bowen's disease (Figure 8.6), chondrodermatitis nodularis helicis (Figure 8.7) and cutaneous horns (Figures 8.8 and 8.9) are also recognized precursors of invasive squamous cell carcinoma, and such lesions, if not excised, must be observed for sudden growth.

Lesions developing on non-sun-exposed skin may do so adjacent to chronic ulceration (Figure 8.10). Long-standing leg ulcers should be observed with care for this change, and biopsy considered for any nodular area that shows expansion or behaviour different from that of the rest of the ulcer edge. Similarly, patients who have chronic scar tissue arising from lupus erythematosus or lupus vulgaris, or a chronic sinus, possibly as a result of previous osteomyelitis, should be warned of the possibility of the development of squamous cell carcinoma and should be instructed to report back if there is any sign of the development of a persistent raised, crusted or ulcerated nodule. Patients with chronic radiodermatitis (Figure 8.11) or old lupus vulgaris scars (Figure 8.12) should be warned to report back if a nodule develops in the scar.

Patients with chronic damage to the lower leg as a result of exposure to intense infrared radiation, for example from a coal or electric fire, will first develop an intense enhanced vascular pattern called erythema ab igne (Figure 8.13).[40] Squamous cell carcinoma may develop on this lesion (Figure 8.14), and will present as a raised, ulcerating, crusting, bleeding area. It is perhaps the European equivalent of 'Changri cancer', which develops in the skin of the thighs and genital area after long-term exposure to radiant heat under a long garment in other parts of the world. Squamous cell carcinoma of the scrotum as a result of exposure to cutting oils is very rare nowadays owing to improved working conditions and protective clothing, but is occasionally seen (Figure 8.15).

Carcinoma of the lip almost always involves the lower lip. This may relate to sun exposure, although historically clay pipes were held responsible. The first lesion seen may be a minor erosion on the lip, but frequently there is multifocal change along the entire mucocutaneous surface (Figures 8.16–8.21).

Special situations involve the development of carcinoma in the mouth, on the genitalia, and on the soles of the feet. Verrucous carcinoma of the oral mucosa may present as a persistent firm or vegetating plaque on the mucosa.[41,42] This lesion occurs most frequently in individuals who are heavy smokers and who also ingest large quantities of alcohol. The characteristic lesion will show a mixture of leukoplakia with surrounding erythroplakia (Figure 8.22) and may develop a striking verrucous pattern. Squamous cell carcinoma of the oral mucosa is most often seen in parts of the world where chewing tobacco or betel nuts is common, and it may be that there is also a synergistic effect of alcohol.

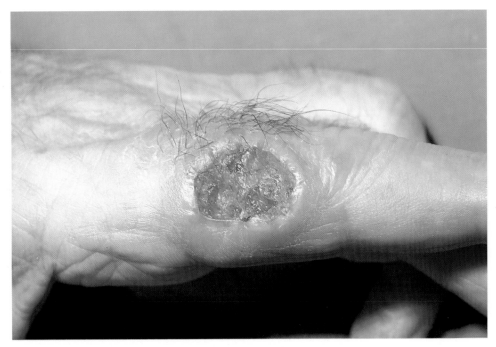

Figure 8.1 Squamous cell carcinoma on the side of the hand of a male outdoor worker. Note the obvious induration.

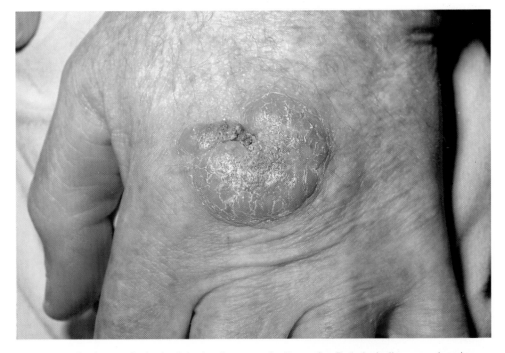

Figure 8.2 Lesion on the back of the hand, present for 7 months. Pathologically proven invasive squamous carcinoma.

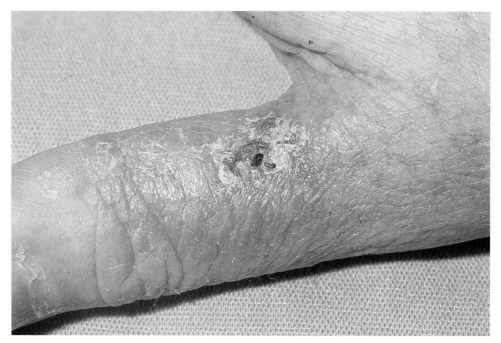

Figure 8.3   Less obvious squamous carcinoma than that in Figures 8.1 and 8.2, arising on pre-existing actinic keratosis.

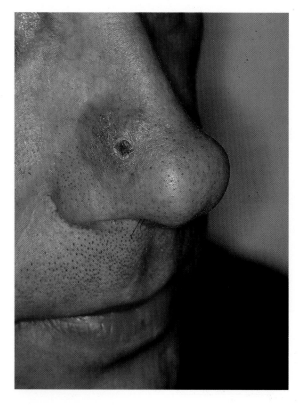

Figure 8.4   Invasive squamous carcinoma on the side of the nose. Initially this lesion was thought to be a keratoacanthoma.

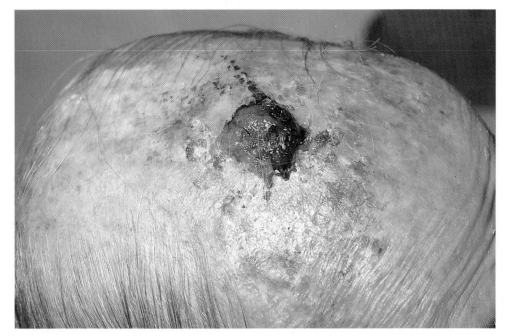

Figure 8.5   Invasive squamous cell carcinoma on sun-damaged skin of the scalp.

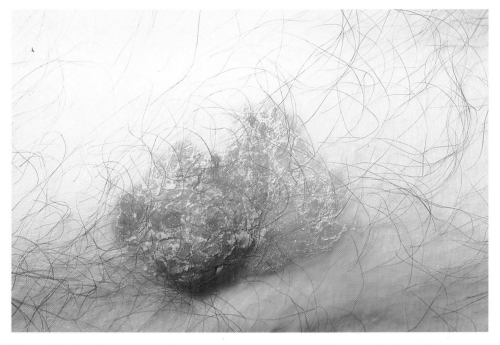

Figure 8.6   Invasive squamous cell carcinoma arising on a pre-existing Bowen's disease lesion.

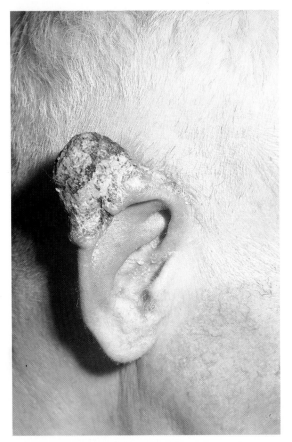

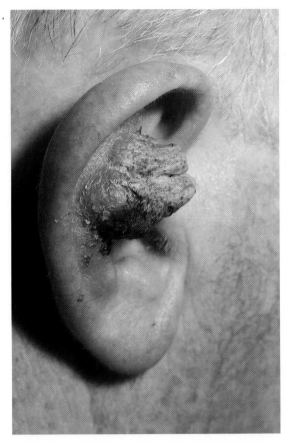

Figure 8.7   Invasive squamous cell carcinoma arising on pre-existing chondrodermatitis nodularis helicis.

Figure 8.8   Invasive squamous cell carcinoma was found at the base of this cutaneous horn on the ear of a farmer.

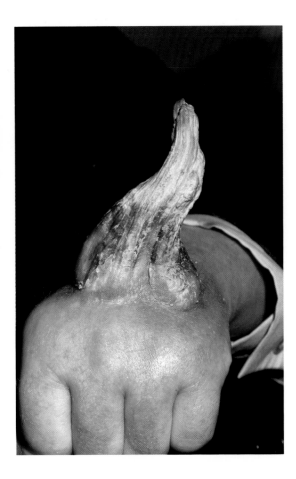

Figure 8.9   A dramatic cutaneous horn on the back of the hand of a 72-year-old male. Invasive squamous carcinoma was found at the base and the patient also had nodal metastases in the axilla. He is alive and well 10 years after surgery (patient of Dr WN Morley).

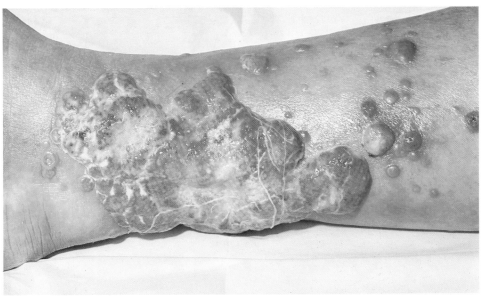

Figure 8.10   Invasive squamous carcinoma arising at site of chronic leg ulceration.

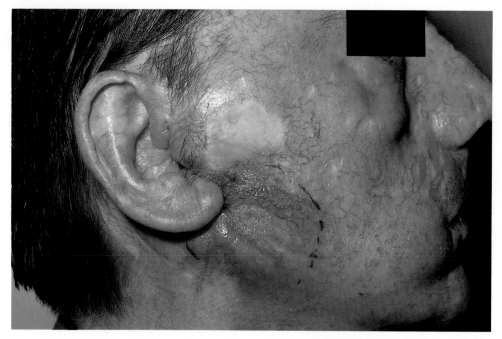

Figure 8.11   Invasive squamous carcinoma arising on radiodermatitis beneath an area of previous skin grafting.

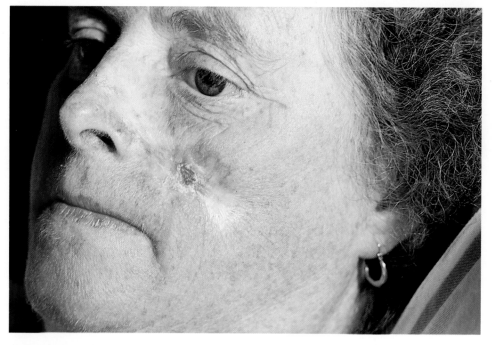

Figure 8.12   Squamous cell carcinoma arising on a site of previous lupus vulgaris.

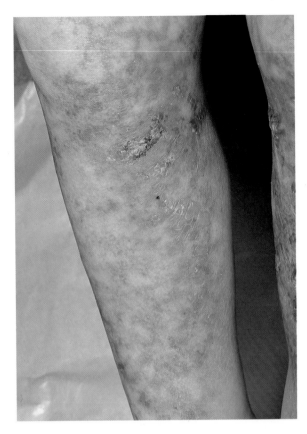

Figure 8.13 Erythema ab igne with early invasive squamous carcinoma just below the knee.

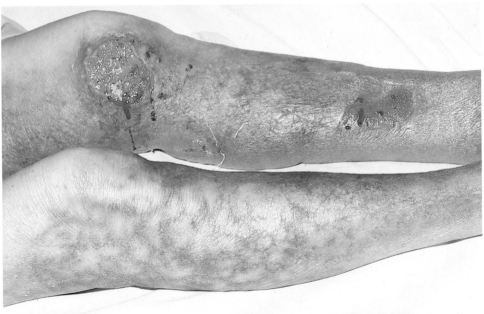

Figure 8.14 Advanced squamous cell carcinoma arising on erythema ab igne just below the left knee. This patient already had metastatic disease in the left groin.

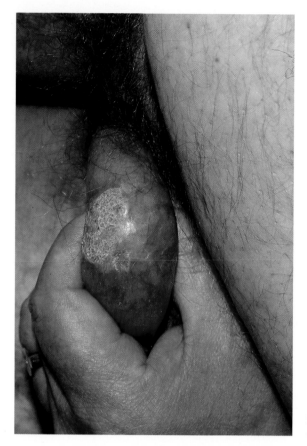

Figure 8.15 Scrotal squamous carcinoma in a male exposed to cutting oil for many years.

Squamous cell carcinoma of the genitalia (Figure 8.23) may develop in a pre-existing so-called giant condyloma of Buschke–Lowenstein (Figure 8.24).[43] This condition presents as large warty lesions, usually on the male genitalia. In the past, a viral aetiology has been postulated for this type of lesion and, recently, proof of such an association has been obtained by the use of antibodies against the human papilloma virus.[44]

Epithelioma cuniculatum usually involves the soles of the feet (Figure 8.25) and may present as a deceptively small area of ulceration with surrounding hyperkeratosis.[45,46] This lesion has a tendency to local relentless spread, and may prove extremely difficult to eradicate completely because of its tendency to burrow along the tissue spaces, causing sinus formation, and often the discharge of a cheesy, foul-smelling material.

Malignancies arising in patients receiving photochemotherapy have clinical features similar to those seen in normal individuals but these lesions may appear normally on non-exposed skin, such as the groin. Small, persistent, crusted nodules are usually the first sign of such a tumour (Figure 8.26).

Squamous cell carcinoma arising in the immunosuppressed individual is particularly difficult to detect on clinical grounds and it is a good policy to adopt an aggressive approach and to biopsy suspicious nodular or crusted lesions in these patients.

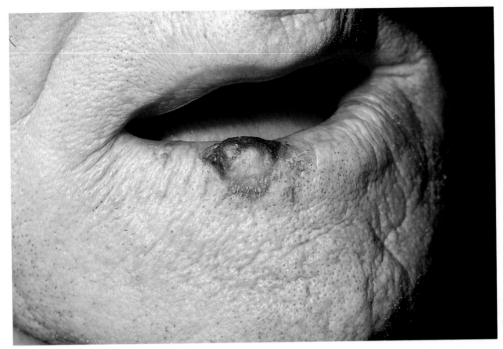

Figure 8.16   Squamous carcinoma of the lower lip. Note the involvement and induration of the entire lip margin.

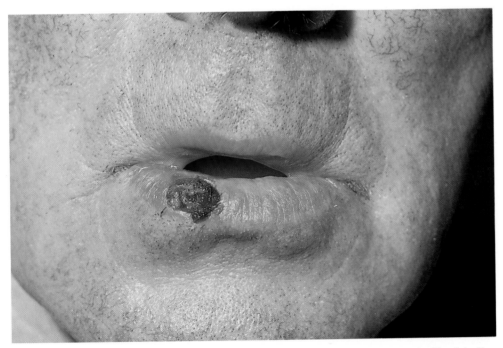

Figure 8.17   Squamous carcinoma of the lower lip. Note the two indurated areas at each side of the lip.

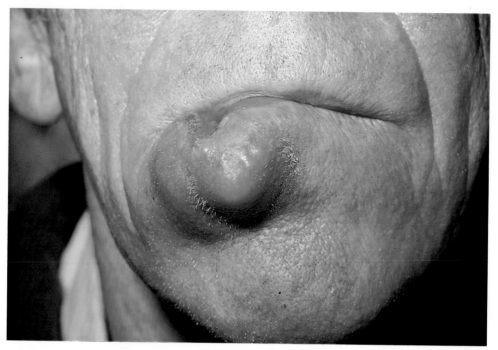

Figure 8.18 Invasive squamous cell carcinoma of the right side of the lower lip. This patient already had involved regional lymph nodes.

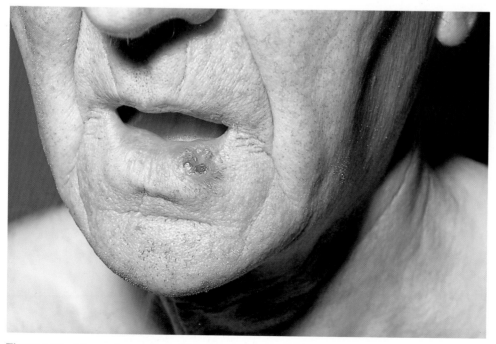

Figure 8.19 Ulcerated squamous cell carcinoma of the left side of the lower lip, also associated with spread to regional lymph nodes.

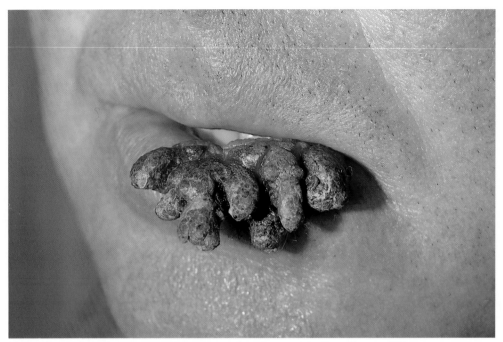

Figure 8.20 Unusual appearance of squamous cell carcinoma of the lip, with gross filiform wart appearance.

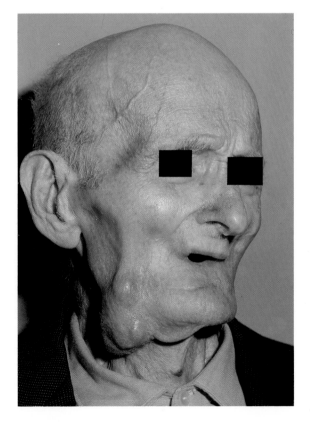

Figure 8.21 Visible metastatic spread from lower lip primary squamous cell carcinoma.

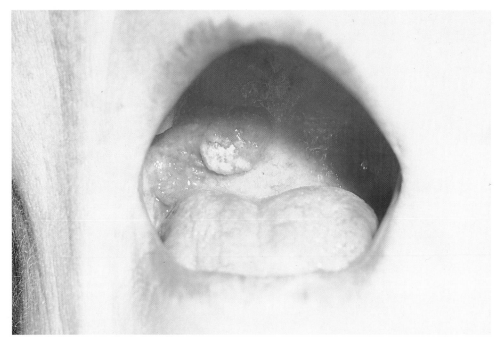

Figure 8.22   Primary squamous carcinoma of the oral mucosa.

Lesions that clinically have features of actinic keratosis or keratoacanthoma (Figure 8.27) may be found
on pathological study to be early invasive squamous
cell carcinomas.

The most common clinical differential diagnosis
will be between actinic keratosis and invasive
squamous cell carcinoma. If there is any degree of
induration of the dermis underlying the lesion,
squamous cell carcinoma should be suspected, and
the lesion biopsied. A less common problem will be
the clinical differentiation between keratoacanthoma
and squamous cell carcinoma (Figure 8.28). If the
lesion has persisted unchanged for over 6 weeks, a
diagnostic biopsy is recommended.

Pathological features

The essential feature for pathological diagnosis of
squamous cell carcinoma is evidence of a population
of cytologically malignant epidermal keratinocytes
invading the underlying dermis. The architecture is
that of an irregular downgrowth of epidermal
keratinocytes into the dermis. Large horn cysts and
individually keratinized cells will be present (Figures
8.29 and 8.30). A high proportion of squamous cell
carcinomas have a spindle cell pattern but this is not
invariably the case. Johnson and Helwig have
described an adenoid pattern, which is seen less
frequently and may include areas with an adenocystic
or pseudoglandular pattern.[47] Malignant acantholysis
with loss of normal desmosomal cohesion is seen in a
proportion of these lesions (Figures 8.31 and 8.32).

Verrucous carcinoma, giant condyloma of
Buschke–Lowenstein, and epithelioma cuniculatum
are all characterized by very florid epidermal or
mucous membrane hyperplasia with apparently little
evidence of invasion of the underlying dermis or
submucosal structure (Figures 8.33 and 8.34).[42–46]
Such invasion as is present appears to be carried out
by large, blunt tongues of epithelial or epidermal cells,

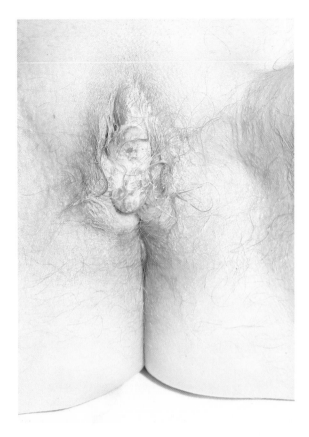

Figure 8.23 Primary squamous verrucous carcinoma of the vulva.

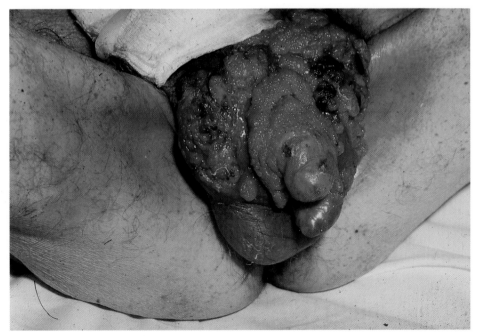

Figure 8.24 Giant condylomata of Buschke–Lowenstein of the male genitalia.

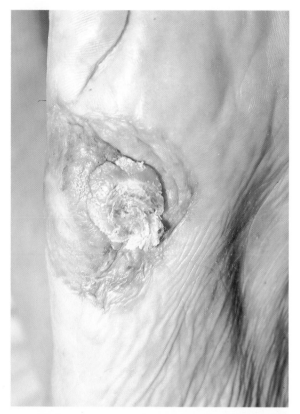

Figure 8.25 Epithelioma cuniculatum – recurrence after previous excision and grafting.

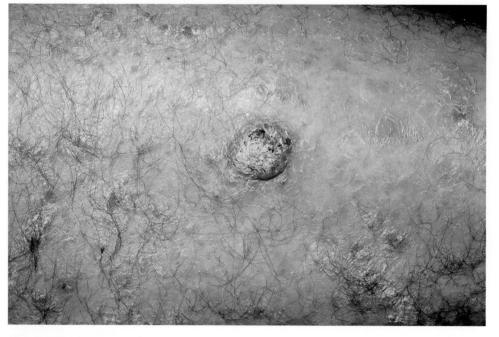

Figure 8.26 Squamous cell carcinoma on the thigh of a patient who has received 1789 J/cm² UVA in PUVA therapy and simultaneously methrotrexate.

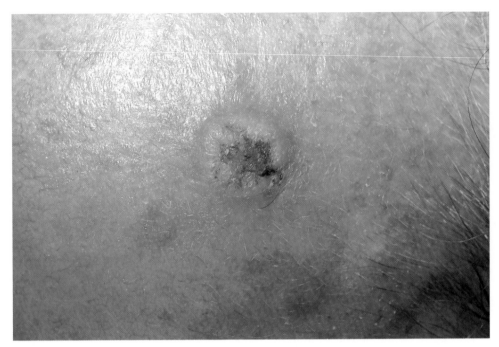

Figure 8.27   Squamous cell carcinoma with clinical appearance of keratoacanthoma in a renal transplant recipient.

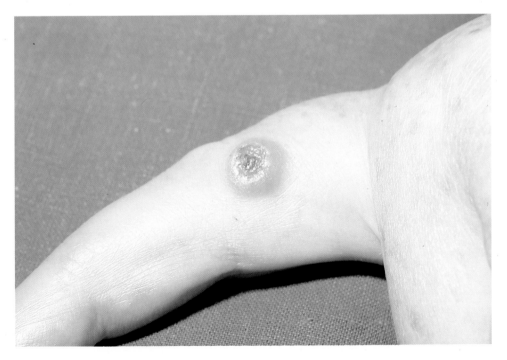

Figure 8.28   Invasive squamous cell carcinoma with clinical appearance of keratoacanthoma on a non-immunosuppressed individual. The lesion had been present unchanged for 5 months.

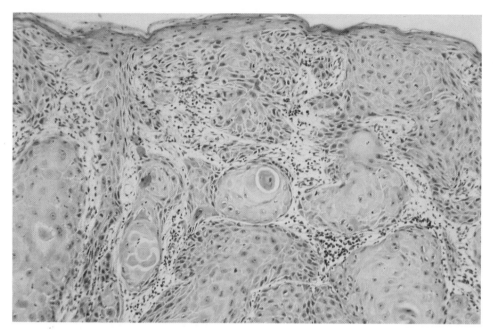

Figure 8.29 Histological features of squamous cell carcinoma, showing invasive tongues of keratinocytes with individual foci of keratinization.

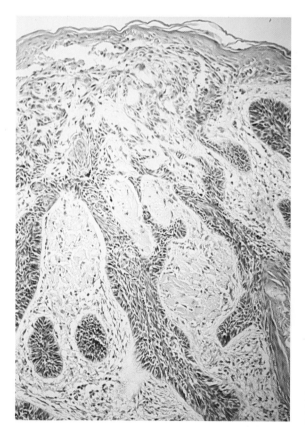

Figure 8.30 Acantholytic pattern with loss of keratinocyte cohesion seen in the adenoid type of squamous carcinoma.

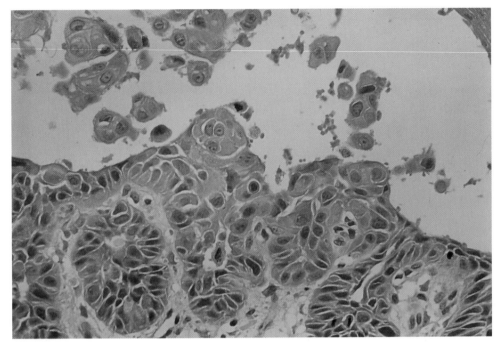

Figure 8.31 High-power view of acantholytic squamous carcinoma, showing loss of cohesion of large malignant keratinocytes.

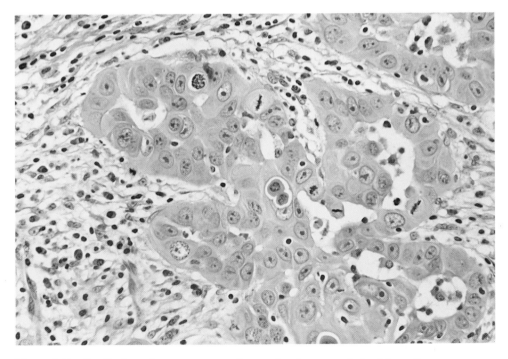

Figure 8.32 Detail of an adenosquamous carcinoma, showing a pseudoglandular pattern.

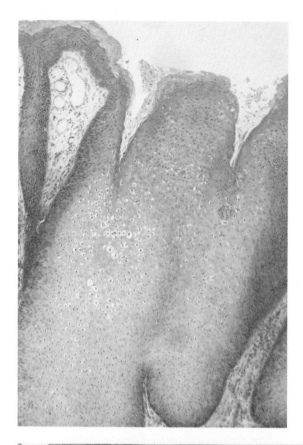

Figure 8.33 A verrucous carcinoma of the vulva, showing pale, clear keratinocytes with a blunt, invading lower border.

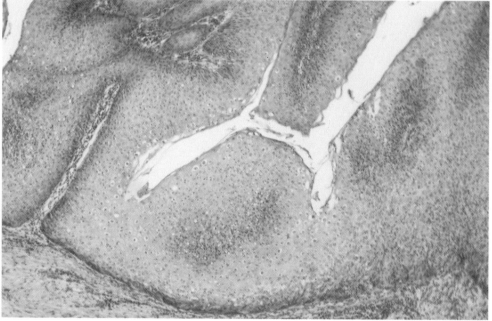

Figure 8.34 Histological features of the lesion illustrated in Figure 8.24, showing gross acanthosis and the blunt, invasive lower border.

and mitotic figures may be very infrequent. It is unwise to be lulled into a sense of false security with regard to prognosis and potential for local recurrence in this pathologically deceptively benign lesion. If complete excision is not achieved at the time of the first surgical procedure, relentless local recurrence is common, resulting in the need for further extensive surgery and possibly amputation.

There has been an attempt to relate prognosis for squamous cell carcinoma to degree of differentiation, and Broders has divided squamous cell carcinomas into grades 1–4 according to differentiation.[48] Grade 1 lesions have fewer than 25 per cent undifferentiated cells, and grade 4 lesions have more than 75 per cent undifferentiated cells. Broders' thesis was that the higher the proportion of undifferentiated cells, the poorer the prognosis. This classification is difficult to apply in that individual tumours may have some areas that could quite reasonably be classified as grade 2 and others that are grade 4, and therefore it has fallen into general disuse as a prognostic guide. Many pathologists use the eccrine sweat glands as a biologically relevant marker, and consider that tumours that have invaded below this level have declared themselves as more aggressive tumours.

The differential diagnosis of invasive squamous cell carcinoma may include a spindle cell melanoma, a keratoacanthoma, and possibly spindle cell tumours of the soft tissues and the dermis. The use of antibodies raised against the cytokeratins can be of great value in confirming that the spindle cell population is of keratinocyte origin. The great advantage of this approach is that many of these antikeratin antibodies react with material which has been fixed in formalin and processed in the conventional manner, and therefore retrospective studies are possible. Using this technique, the cytokeratin positivity will confirm that the cells are epidermal keratinocytes, whereas a positive reaction with antibodies raised against S 100 protein or NKIC 3 antibody would indicate that the tumour is likely to be a melanoma.

The problems of differentiation on pathological grounds between keratoacanthoma and early invasive squamous cell carcinoma have been discussed in Chapter 6. If there is any doubt whatever on pathological grounds that the biopsy is from squamous carcinoma rather than keratoacanthoma, complete excision of the lesion for full pathological assessment is obviously essential. If the spindle cell mass has little, if any, visible contact with the overlying epidermis, the possibility of a dermal primary origin must be considered. The lesion most likely to cause confusion is the atypical fibroxanthoma. Once again, monoclonal antibody studies will be useful, as these tumours do not stain positively with cytokeratin.

In the past, differential diagnosis of the origin of a malignant spindle cell mass in the dermis, which could be either malignant melanoma or squamous cell carcinoma, has invariably included the use of electron microscopy to identify keratohyalin granules on the one hand and melanosomes on the other. With the introduction of monoclonal antibody techniques and developments in immunochemistry, the need for electron microscopy is perhaps decreasing.

Management

In a patient with a clinical diagnosis of squamous cell carcinoma, histological confirmation is essential. In a small lesion an excision biopsy may serve for both diagnosis and treatment, but in a larger lesion an incisional biopsy to confirm the nature of the lesion is acceptable. As with basal cell carcinoma, squamous cell carcinoma is a radiosensitive tumour, and the choice for definitive therapy can therefore be made between surgery and radiotherapy. In general, there is a logical preference for surgery in that in squamous cell carcinoma the great majority of lesions have arisen on already damaged tissue, and the possibility of damaging the surrounding skin still further with radiotherapy, and perhaps stimulating the development of another primary lesion, is a very real one.

In the case of carcinoma of the lower lip, the possible multifocal nature of the lesion and greater rate of reported metastatic spread from lesions in this site should be considered. A cosmetically highly acceptable result is obtained by excising the entire lower lip area and resurfacing the deficit with mucosa from the tip of the tongue.

In the case of tumours arising on scar tissue, or in association with the epithelioma cuniculatum and Buschke–Lowenstein type of lesion, the use of Mohs' fresh tissue technique may be helpful.[49,50] The risk of metastatic spread appears to vary according to the type of damage associated with the squamous cell carcinoma. Thus it has been suggested that metastases very rarely arise in association with actinically induced squamous carcinomas. While this appears to be true in general, metastases from such lesions do occur, and patients do require follow-up. Moller et al have reported very different rates of metastases from different types of squamous carcinoma.[51] From mucocutaneous lesions of the lip in their series, the rate is 11 per cent, from actinic lesions 3 per cent, and from lesions adjacent to scars between 10 and 30 per cent.

Follow-up

Squamous cell carcinoma has the ability to metastasize and cause death. All patients who have had a pathologically proven squamous cell carcinoma should therefore be followed up, and the primary site and draining nodal basin checked at each visit. It is suggested that visits are 3-monthly in the first year and 6-monthly thereafter. In addition, however, patients who have had one primary squamous carcinoma are at increased risk of a second primary, and this, as well as secondary spread, must be sought. They should also receive appropriate advice about rationing sun exposure and the use of sunscreens.

9
Benign melanocytic lesions

A wide range of benign melanocytic lesions exists on the human skin. Benign melanocytic lesions are very much more common than malignant melanoma, and because of increasing public knowledge and concern about malignant melanoma – particularly in high-incidence areas such as Australia – it is essential that all those involved in the care of patients are aware of the clinical spectrum of presentation of these benign lesions so that prompt reassurance can be given, and where possible unnecessary biopsies avoided. A large number of individuals, particularly those who have relatives who have had malignant melanoma, develop a high degree of anxiety about benign pigmented lesions on their own or their children's skin. It is therefore extremely useful to be able to recognize the clinical features that distinguish totally benign pigmented lesions, where only reassurance is required, from those for which a biopsy is needed for histological differentiation.

The spectrum of melanocytic lesions ranges from the clinically banal simple freckle to the more difficult clinically atypical naevi, which may in a small proportion of cases be precursors of malignant melanoma.

Freckles and lentigines

Simple freckles such as those seen in the summer months on the faces of young children are merely overproduction of melanin pigment by a normal number of melanocytes for the body site involved. They are flat (macular) lesions and are usually uniformly pigmented, although they may have an irregular outline.

They may disappear almost completely in the absence of sunshine in the winter months.

The lentigo may look clinically very similar to the freckle in that it also is flat and usually regularly pigmented, but these lesions persist all year round in the absence of UV stimulation, and if biopsied it will be seen that there is a linear increase in the number of melanocytes in the basal layer. They are relatively common on areas that have been sunburned, such as the shoulders in men, and are also seen on the skin of patients who have had large doses of UVA as part of PUVA therapy. A variant which can cause clinical confusion with early small melanomas is the so-called 'ink spot lentigo', which is flat and has a small diameter, but is usually markedly irregular in outline and densely black.[1]

Acquired melanocytic naevi

Melanocytic naevi can be divided broadly into those that are acquired after birth and those that are congenital (see page 175). In the past this has been a very firm division, with acquired naevi developing mainly in the second decade and congenital naevi by definition being present at birth. There is currently a considerable degree of interest in small congenital naevi, mainly related to their malignant potential. This interest has led to a reassessment of this division between lesions present at birth and those developed between the ages of 10 and 20 years. It would appear that the division is not as clear-cut as was previously believed, and 'congenital-type' naevi – that is, those naevi that are larger than 5–10 mm in diameter, and may have terminal hair growth scattered throughout the lesion – may appear on the skin of the child up to the age of 3 or 4 years, and perhaps even later in life.

The acquired naevus is a much more common problem and the bulk of clinically visible acquired melanocytic naevi make their appearance when patients are aged between 12 and 30 years. Studies of numbers of pigmented naevi carried out in varying parts of the world show that the maximum number of acquired melanocytic naevi are present on the skin of young adults and that after the age of 35 there is a slow but steady reduction in the total numbers of visible naevi so that in geriatric practice melanocytic naevi are relatively rare lesions.[2,3]

Acquired melanocytic naevi can be divided on developmental grounds into those that are derived from the epidermal melanocyte and those that appear to be derived from dermal melanocytes. In fetal life the melanocyte migrates from the neural crest to the dermoepidermal junction, where it takes up its normal adult position in the basal layer of the epidermis. The trio of junctional, compound and intradermal melanocytic naevi is believed to be derived from the melanocytes in the basal layer.

The melanocytes are thought to transform into naevomelanocyte or naevus cells, and to slowly drop down from the basal layer into the underlying dermis. This process has been termed 'abtropfung'. At present there is no clear biological difference recognizable between melanocytes and naevomelanocytes or naevus cells in the upper layers of the dermis, although in the deeper parts of the reticular dermis naevus cells in a compound or intradermal naevus acquire a more neural morphology, and also show functional differentiation in that they lose their capacity to synthesize melanin and become cholinesterase-positive.

If naevi are biopsied on the skin of children, young adults and older adults, it will be found that the majority of naevi in children are junctional naevi, in young adults compound naevi, and in older adults intradermal naevi. This sequence has given rise to the hypothesis that junctional, compound and intradermal naevi represent a maturation process whereby the melanocytes become naevus cells and initially proliferate in continuity with the dermoepidermal junction.[4–6] At this stage the lesion would be classified as a junctional naevus. In time, groups of naevus cells become detached from contact with the dermoepidermal junction and are seen lying free in the underlying dermis. A melanocytic naevus in which cells are seen in this situation but with some cells still

present in direct contact with the overlying epidermal basal layer is referred to as a compound naevus, and a naevus in which there is no visible abnormality of the basal layer but in which naevus cells are seen lying free in the dermis is referred to as an intradermal naevus. Interesting variants of the compound naevus include the Spitz naevus, the halo naevus, and the spindle cell naevus of Reed.

There is currently a great deal of interest in both the familial and the sporadic acquired dysplastic naevus syndrome and the potential for these dysplastic naevi to transform into malignant melanoma. The familial dysplastic naevus syndrome has already been described and discussed in Chapter 4 and the sporadic variant will be considered in this chapter.

The dermally derived naevi are the blue naevi, both the commoner cell-poor type and the rarer cellular blue naevus. In normal human skin there is not an identifiable normal dermal melanocyte component, although dermal melanocytes are normal components of the dermis in many animals. It is thought that the blue naevus develops as a result of melanocytes that in fetal life have become arrested in their migration from the neural crest to their normal position at birth in the basal layer of the epidermis.

Junctional naevus

This naevus is seen clinically as a small, sandy-brown lesion present on any body site. The diameter is usually less than 1 cm, and the lateral margin of the lesion is poorly defined. It is generally macular and there is no interruption of the normal skin markings. Pathological studies suggest that junctional naevi are seen more commonly on the palms of the hands and soles of the feet (Figure 9.1) than on other body sites, but a detailed investigation of the relationship of numbers of such naevi to surface area has not, to the author's knowledge, been conducted. These naevi are usually present on the skin of younger individuals under the age of 30. The most common clinical differential diagnosis would be from a simple lentigo, and this may not be possible without biopsy and pathological examination.

Pathology

A proliferation of naevomelanocytes with the biochemical capacity to produce melanin pigment will be seen in contact with the basal layer of the epidermis. The proliferating melanocytic cells usually form 'theques' or clusters of four or more naevus cells, which may be slightly larger than the surrounding keratinocytes. Upward proliferation of these clear cells through the epidermis is not seen in the benign junctional naevus. It has been stated in the past that only melanocytic naevi showing this so-called junctional activity have the potential for malignant change, but occasionally acquired naevi appear to undergo malignant change in a deep intradermal component, and malignant change in a congenital naevus appears to arise more frequently in this intradermal component than in the more superficial areas (see below).

Compound naevus

This lesion is seen in large numbers on the skin of young adults and may affect any body site (Figure 9.2). The acquired compound naevi are usually between 3 and 5 mm in diameter and are raised papular lesions. The shade of pigment varies from a light tan to a relatively dark brown, but tends to be uniform throughout the lesion. The pigmentation tends to stop fairly abruptly, and is only seen on the area of elevation. There is not usually a flat, macular halo of pigment around the palpable naevus.

Pathology

The compound naevus shows the presence of naevomelanocytes both in contact with the overlying basal cells and also lying free within the papillary dermis in clusters. As with the junctional naevus, there is no evidence of upward movement of naevus cells through the epidermis, and the naevus cells are small, regular packeted cells with relatively small quantities of cytoplasm and a small nucleus with regular chromatin.

Unusual, but not worrying, pathological features seen in some compound and intradermal naevi are balloon cells, granuloma formation, bone formation and amyloid.[7,8] These are not usually apparent clinically.

Intradermal naevi

These lesions very often present as small, fleshy skin tags with little, if any, visible melanin pigment (Figure 9.3). It is not uncommon to see one or two dilated vessels, and terminal hair growth may be seen from the lesion. These lesions appear most often on the face. The average patient is in his or her third decade or older. It is relatively common for a small granuloma to develop in the dermis in association with the naevus cells, and this may give rise to rapid growth, inflammation, pain, and anxiety about possible malignant change.

Pathology

The essential features of an intradermal naevus include the presence of a normal epidermal basal layer with no evidence of an increase or decrease in melanocyte population. Lying free in the dermis, and often extending deeply into the reticular dermis, is a population of small, compact, polygonal naevus cells. These cells may be packeted and have a relatively epithelioid appearance in the more superficial areas of the lesion, but may undergo a slow transformation so that in deeper parts of the lesion a smaller, more neural-looking naevus cell predominates. This morphological change is accompanied by functional change in that appropriate biochemical tests using the dopa reaction indicate that the superficial cells have retained their biochemical ability to produce melanin pigment while the deeper cells have lost this ability, and indeed many are cholinesterase-positive. This functional change is in keeping with the neural appearance of these more deeply situated naevus cells.

In older individuals, loose, pendulous skin tags may be removed, mainly from the face and neck, and reveal simply a skin tag with fibrous stroma and one or two residual naevus cells. This observation has given rise to the speculation – which obviously cannot be proved absolutely – that this is the final stage in the maturation and disappearance of the junctional, compound and intradermal naevi.

The Spitz naevus, or juvenile melanoma

The Spitz naevus is a variant of the compound naevus and is important for the pathologist in that it may, on histological examination, be confused with malignant melanoma. Clinically there is rarely any confusion, and if good clinicopathological communication exists,

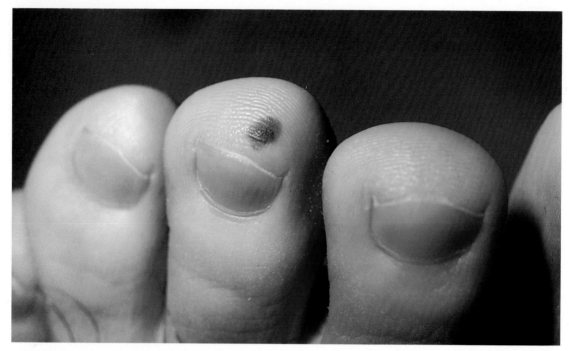

Figure 9.1 Junctional naevus on the toe of a 28-year-old. Histological examination proved this to be a pure junctional naevus. At this age, the majority of naevi on other body sites will be compound.

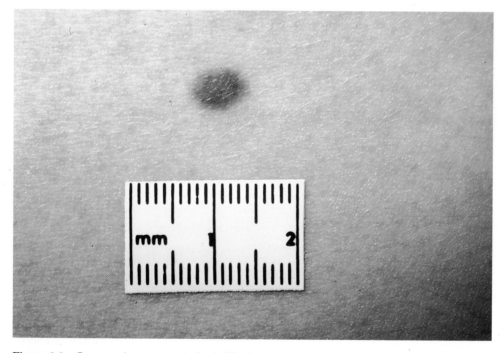

Figure 9.2 Compound naevus on the back. The lesion measures 6 mm in diameter and is uniform in shape and pigmentation.

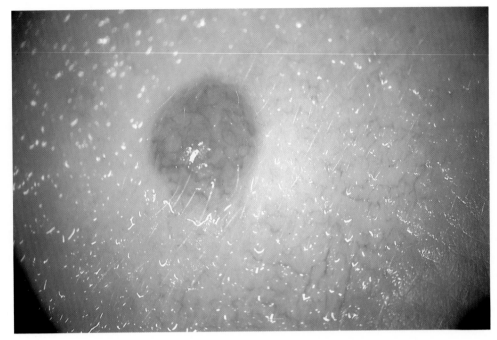

Figure 9.3   Magnified view of an intradermal naevus on the chin. This lesion is 5 mm in diameter and virtually no pigment is seen.

this lesion should be less of a problem in practical management than it would sometimes appear to be.

Until 1948 the Spitz naevus was inappropriately classified as a malignant melanoma. Its eponymous name was given because the late Sophie Spitz recognized that there appeared to be a subclass of 'melanomas' in children that never metastasized and did not cause death.[9] From this observation the subset of benign Spitz naevi has been identified. The term Spitz naevus is preferred to juvenile melanoma, to avoid confusion with a truly malignant lesion.

Clinical features

Spitz naevi are most common in children and young adults but a number of studies have indicated that they may be seen at almost any stage in life. Pathologists should, however, become steadily more cautious about making the diagnosis with increasing age of the patient.

In children these lesions present as raised, red, papular lesions, most commonly on the face (Figures 9.4–9.6). They may grow rapidly over a period of months to reach approximately 1 cm in diameter and then remain unchanged for several years as firm, red, papular lesions. In older patients there may be more pigment present and the lesions will appear as uniform black or brown lesions. Facial lesions are less common in older individuals, and the back of the hand is a more common site (Figure 9.7).

A rare situation is that in which the patient, usually a child, develops over a short period of time large numbers of Spitz naevi on one body site (Figure 9.8). This phenomenon of multiple, or agminate, Spitz naevi is not understood but strongly suggests a local blood-borne spread of naevus cells with the ability to proliferate in the immediate area of the original lesion but not beyond this area.[10–12]

Pathology[13,14]

Pathological examination will show a pattern in which naevus cells are seen in contact with the basal layer and also lying free in the underlying dermis. However,

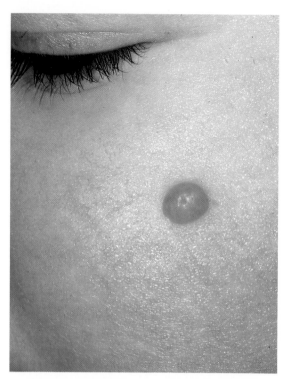

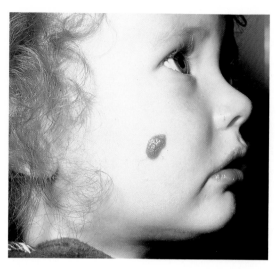

Figure 9.5   Larger Spitz naevus on the cheek of a 2-year-old.

Figure 9.4   Typical Spitz naevus on the cheek of a 4-year-old. This lesion had not been present 5 months before the photograph was taken.

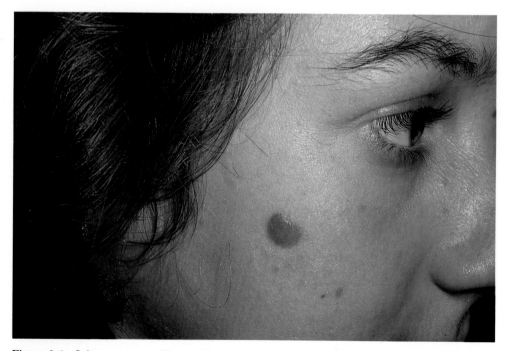

Figure 9.6   Spitz naevus on a 12-year-old.

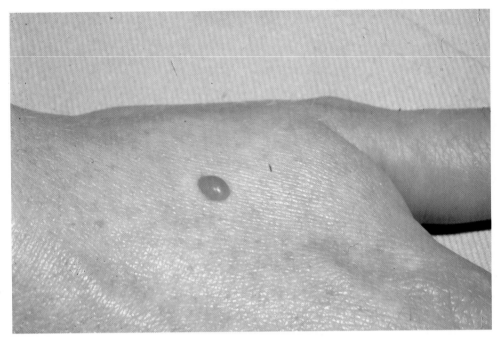

Figure 9.7   Spitz naevus on the back of the hand of a 22-year-old.

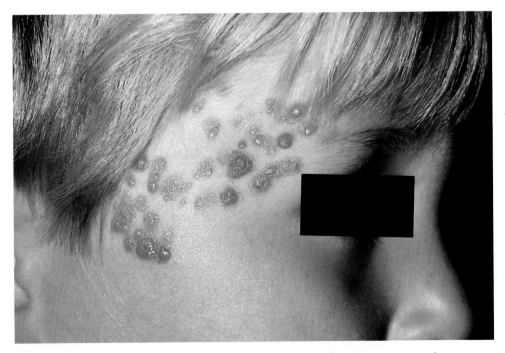

Figure 9.8   Multiple, or agminate, Spitz naevi on the face of a 5-year-old boy (patient of Dr DT Roberts).

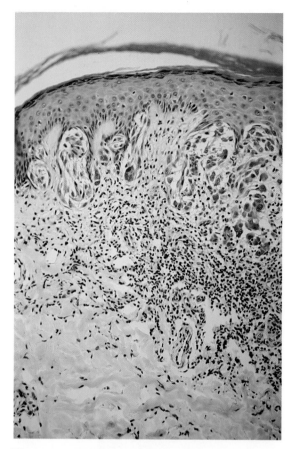

Figure 9.9 Pathology of the lesion illustrated in Figure 9.6. Note the acanthosis, vascular dilatation, and lymphocytic infiltrate.

4. occasional mitotic figures in the naevus cell population; and
5. the presence of a mild lymphocytic infiltrate around the intradermal naevus cells.

The naevus cells themselves may be either spindle or epithelioid in type, giving rise to the alternative names spindle and epithelioid cell naevus. The architecture of the lesion is that of a small, well-circumscribed naevus and the epidermis on either side of the lesion shows no abnormalities. In addition there is an absence of any upward movement of cells of the melanocyte series through the epidermis.

A less common sclerotic naevus is occasionally seen with very little or no abnormality at the dermoepidermal junction. This sclerotic or desmoplastic naevus has many features of a purely intradermal Spitz naevus.[15] For many dermatopathologists the differentiation between a true Spitz compound naevus and a malignant melanoma with some Spitzoid features is one of the most difficult to make. When faced with a lesion of this type, it is most important to know the age of the patient and the site of the lesion. Even with this information, however, there will be a small proportion of such lesions in which accurate differentiation between benign Spitz naevus and Spitzoid malignant melanoma cannot be made on simple morphological examination and conventional haematoxylin and eosin staining with absolute confidence. It is hoped that some of the newer monoclonal antibodies raised against cells of the melanocyte series may be of value in this most difficult differential diagnosis.

in addition to this pattern of a compound naevus, certain more specific features are seen (Figure 9.9). These are:

1. a degree of acanthosis or thickening of the epidermis;
2. the presence of homogeneous pink globules or Kamino bodies in the region of the dermoepidermal junction;
3. the presence of large numbers of thin-walled dilated capillaries admixed with the naevus cells, possibly explaining the bright red colour of the lesions in young people;

The desmoplastic naevus

Two series of these naevi have been reported,[16,17] and there is a view that they may be variants of Spitz naevi. They are most commonly seen on the upper limbs of young adults, and clinically are raised, red, firm lesions. A likely clinical differential diagnosis is dermatofibroma (see page 285). The pathology, however, is that of an intradermal naevus which appears to have elicited a very vigorous desmoplastic response in the surrounding collagen. Individual naevus cells may be relatively large, usually epithelioid, cells, and they may have large intranuclear inclusions, but mitotic figures are rare. These naevi are benign, and are not precursors of, desmoplastic malignant melanoma (see page 188).

The halo naevus[18]

This interesting variant of a compound naevus is found most frequently on the trunk skin of young adults. On Caucasian skin the lesions are frequently recognized during the summer months, and are seen as brown, pigmented naevi surrounded by a depigmented halo of otherwise normal skin. These lesions are not obvious on Caucasian skin during the winter months, but become apparent in the summer because the surrounding normal skin tans in response to sunlight, whereas the halo area does not (Figures 9.10–9.12). Multiple lesions are frequent, and the natural history of this lesion, if not surgically excised, is that over a period of months the central naevus will disappear spontaneously, leaving the depigmented area, which may persist for several years before natural repigmentation takes place.[19]

This model of a naturally destroyed melanocytic lesion is obviously of great interest, and the mechanism, if understood, might be of practical value in the management of malignant melanoma. Patients with halo naevi have in their serum an antibody that is cytotoxic to melanocytes.[20]

Pathology

The pathology is that of a compound naevus with a dense lymphocytic infiltrate throughout the dermal component of the lesion. The density of the infiltrate and the close contact of the lymphocytes actually in the body of the lesion is important, as in a number of other situations naevus cells may be associated with a lymphocytic infiltrate at the edge of the lesion. On initial pathological examination, it may be difficult to identify the dermal naevus cell component because of the intensity of the lymphocytic infiltrate. In this case the use of one of the monoclonal antibodies, such as S 100, which stains both benign and malignant cells of the melanocyte series, may be of value in identifying naevus cells. This antibody reacts on conventionally processed material and therefore can be used retrospectively.

Pigmented spindle cell naevus of Reed

This interesting variant of a compound or occasionally a junctional naevus was identified by Richard Reed et al in 1975.[21] Before this time it may well have been confused with early malignant melanoma, as were Spitz naevi before 1948. The bulk of lesions reported to date have been seen on females, most commonly on the thigh area. They present as densely pigmented blue-black palpable lesions between 5 mm and 1 cm in diameter (Figures 9.13 and 9.14).

Pathology[22]

As the name implies, the lesion is a spindle cell naevus with large quantities of melanin pigment within both the naevus cells that are situated in the basal layer of the epidermis and those in the papillary dermis. Large quantities of melanin pigment are also seen lying free in the dermis and in melanophages. An important point common to all benign naevi is the absence of any cells of the melanocyte series percolating through the epidermis above the basal layer. This feature is one that may be particularly valuable in differentiating benign naevi from early malignant melanoma, as involvement of the suprabasal layers of the epidermis is seen in the malignant lesions.

Naevus 'en cocarde'

This term is occasionally used to describe the striking clinical appearance of concentric rings of darker and lighter pigmentation, which looks rather like a rosette (Figure 9.15).[23,24] There is no particular prognostic significance, and the pathology is that of an ordinary compound naevus.

Clinically atypical naevi (previously sporadic dysplastic naevi)

This condition was first described by Elder et al in 1980,[25] and followed on the earlier descriptions by Clark and Lynch of the association between familial atypical naevi and malignant melanoma. Elder reported that in a series of patients with non-familial melanoma, a large number of the patients studied had pigmented melanocytic naevi that were larger than 5 mm and had an ill-defined border (Figures 9.16–9.19), irregular pigmentation, erythema and accentuated skin markings. Since this time large numbers of studies have been carried out on naevus patterns both in patients with malignant melanoma

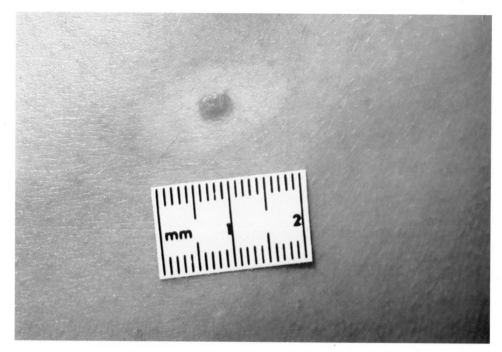

Figure 9.10   Halo naevus on a 15-year-old boy's back.

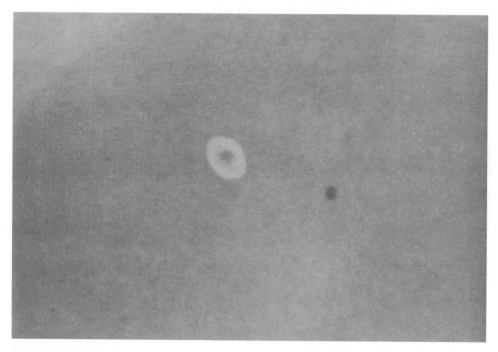

Figure 9.11   Halo naevus on the shoulder of a 12-year-old.

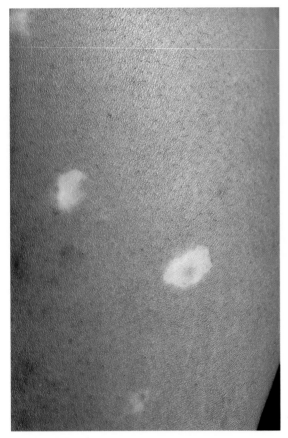

Figure 9.12   Halo naevi on genetically dark skin can be very striking.

and in their families.[26–29] The majority of studies to date comprise patients referred to centres with a particular interest in pigmented lesions and are not epidemiological studies of an unselected population. The bulk of studies do, however, confirm that patients with large numbers of such atypical naevi appear to be at increased risk of malignant melanoma. The exact magnitude of this increased risk in the non-familial situation varies according to reports from individual centres and may reflect heterogeneity. A consensus conference hosted by the American National Institutes of Health[30] recommended that the term clinically atypical naevi be used to describe the clinical features of these lesions and that the term dysplasia be reserved for pathological use.

Pathology[31,32]

The pathological features of clinically atypical naevi can be divided into architectural abnormalities, cytological abnormalities, and abnormalities indicating a host response to the naevus.[33] The great majority of these naevi are compound naevi, although a few are junctional in type. The architectural features seen are the large size of the lesion, with its irregular lateral margins, the presence of atypical lentiginous hyperplasia of melanocytes in the basal layer of the epidermis, and the fusion of epidermal ridges and horizontal orientation of melanocytes (Figure 9.20). The cytological abnormality is that of a melanocytic naevus cell population with large nuclei, intense hyperchromatic staining, and occasional mitotic figures. The host response features recognized are the presence of collagen fibroplasia within and around the dermal naevus cell population, the presence of a lymphocytic infiltrate in and around the dermal naevus cells, and apparent neovascularization, most commonly at the base of the naevus.

Blue naevus

The blue naevus is a naevus derived from melanocytes in the dermis that are thought to have become arrested in fetal life during migration from the neural crest to the dermis to the epidermal junction. Thus the 'abtropfung', postulated as the method of development of the acquired compound and intradermal naevi, has not occurred.

Clinical features

Blue naevi are often recognized in older children and young adults. The majority present, as their name suggests, as dense, blue-black regular lesions, commonly on the face (Figure 9.21).[34] The cellular blue naevus is said to occur more frequently on the wrist and buttock areas and is also a densely pigmented, often papular, blue-black lesion.[35] These lesions often give rise to concern about malignant melanoma because of the intensity of the pigmentation, but this pigmentation is uniform, whereas blue-black pigmentation in malignant melanoma is usually admixed with varying shades of brown and also with red because of the inflammatory response.

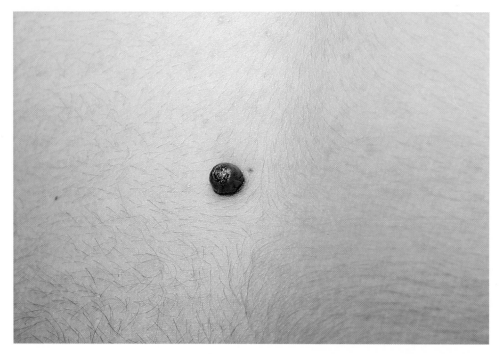

Figure 9.13 Pigmented spindle cell naevus on the small of the back.

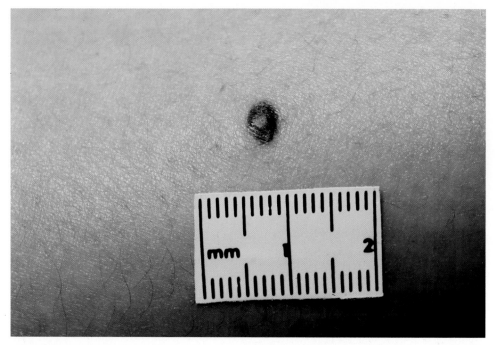

Figure 9.14 Pigmented spindle cell naevus on the thigh of a 20-year-old female.

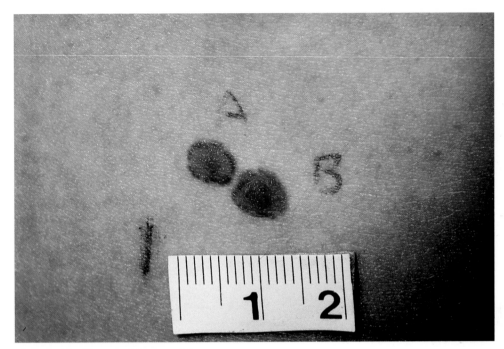

Figure 9.15 Two naevi 'en cocarde'.

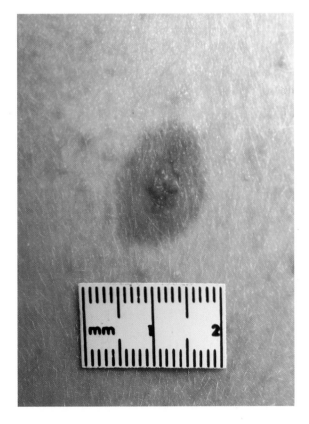

Figure 9.16 A clinically atypical naevus showing the pinkish hue, irregular and indistinct lateral border, and 'poached egg' appearance of a central nodule with a surrounding macular area.

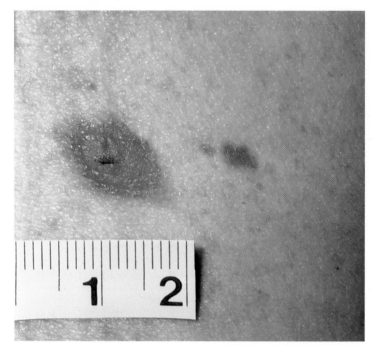

Figure 9.17   A clinically atypical naevus with a diffuse, indistinct lateral edge.

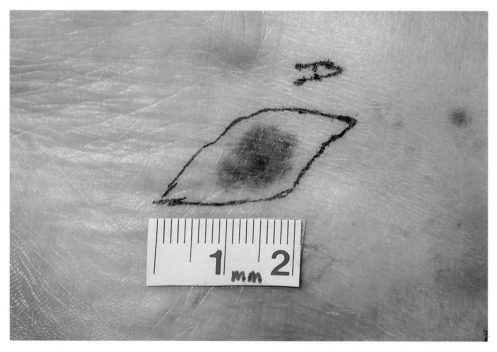

Figure 9.18   A large clinically atypical naevus with irregular central pigmentation.

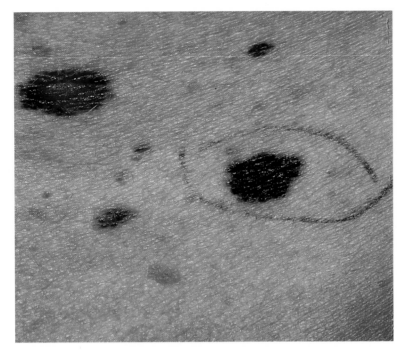

Figure 9.19   Two clinically atypical naevi on the back of a 38-year-old male who already had had four primary melanomas excised.

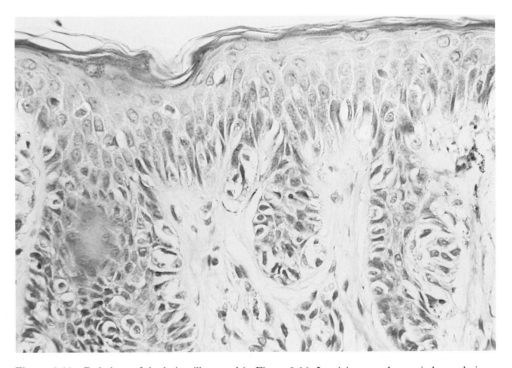

Figure 9.20   Pathology of the lesion illustrated in Figure 9.16. Lentiginous melanocytic hyperplasia, fibrosis of dermal collagen, and cytologic atypia of melanocytes are all seen.

Two rare variants of the blue naevus are the naevus of Ota (Figure 9.22) and naevus of Ito (Figure 9.23).[36–38] These are seen on the face and shoulder area respectively and are unusual in a Caucasian population, although they are seen more frequently in the Japanese.

Pathology

The pathology of the blue naevus is that of a spindle cell population of melanocytic naevus cells in the dermis. The cells tend to be large and bipolar, and are interwoven between collagen bundles. They do not form the regular packets of naevus cells seen in the intradermal naevus described on page 159.

A more densely populated dermis is seen in the cellular variant of the blue naevus, and the cytology of individual cells may be masked by large quantities of melanin pigment (Figure 9.24). This can be removed easily using a melanin bleach, so that the cells comprising the lesion can be seen more clearly. The overlying epidermis is normal.

Combined naevus (Figure 9.25)

A combined naevus is a naevus that shows features of a junctional naevus in that there is proliferation of melanocytic naevus cells adjacent to and in contact with the dermoepidermal junction, and also a component of naevus cells, which are considered to be derived from the blue naevus. The two cell populations are usually quite distinct, having a band of normal dermis between them. Without this band distinguishing such a lesion from a normal compound naevus would be extremely difficult. Clinically these lesions may simulate malignant melanoma.

Management of acquired melanocytic naevi

Melanocytic naevi may be removed for a variety of reasons. The most usual medical reason is concern that a malignant melanoma has developed in a pre-existing, melanocytic naevus. The second most

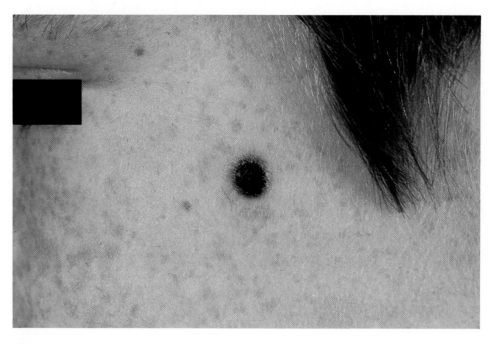

Figure 9.21 Blue naevus on the cheek of a 9-year-old boy.

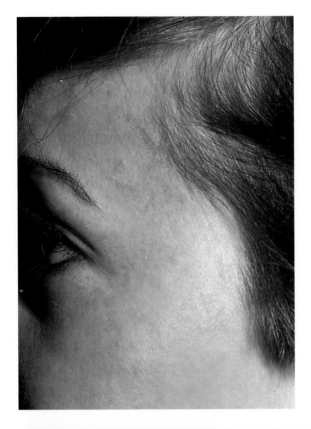

Figure 9.22   Diffuse facial pigmentation of naevus of Ota.

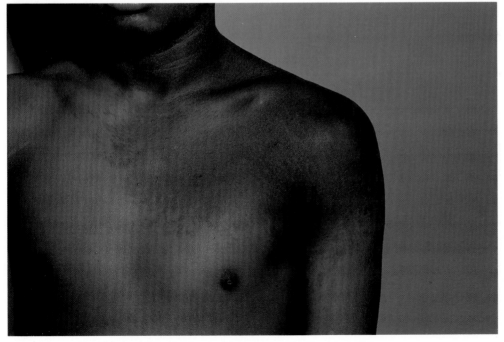

Figure 9.23   Naevus of Ito.

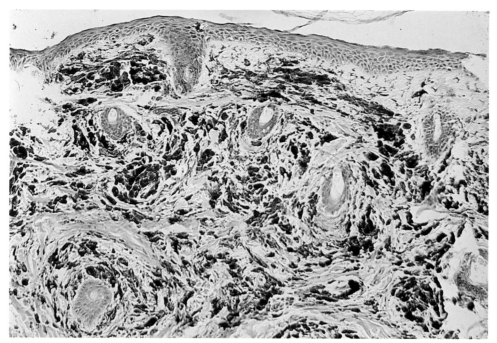

Figure 9.24 Pathology of a blue naevus.

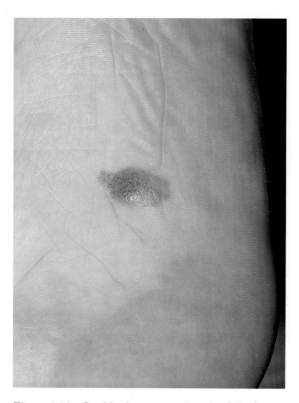

Figure 9.25 Combined naevus on the sole of the foot.

common reason for removal of melanocytic naevi is cosmetic, and the third is prophylactic, in that it has been widely believed in the past that melanocytic naevi on sites of regular minor trauma, such as the waist and shoulder areas, are more likely to undergo malignant change. Older textbooks have suggested that naevi on the palms of the hands, soles of the feet and genitalia are more likely to undergo malignant change and therefore should be prophylactically excised. There is no good statistical evidence to support this policy, but early palmoplantar melanomas (see Chapter 10) may look deceptively benign on clinical examination, and the policy of a rather more aggressive approach to local removal of naevi in these sites may be justified for this reason.

In the case of lesions that, on clinical examination, appear to fall into the spectrum of junctional, compound and intradermal naevi, excision is rarely necessary on medical grounds, although it may be considered appropriate if the patient is extremely concerned about the possibility of malignant change. Although on pathological examination between 20 and 50 per cent of all melanomas are said to have arisen in association with a melanocytic naevus, banal melanocytic naevi are so common that it has been calculated that the risk of malignant change in an individual acquired naevus is very low indeed.

Total excision, with a narrow margin of 1–2 mm of normal skin around the lesion, is all that is required. It is, however, essential that all pigmented naevi that are excised are sent for histological confirmation that the lesion is indeed a benign melanocytic naevus and does not show any features whatever of malignant change. For this reason, scalpel excision is recommended as a more appropriate method of therapy than a shave biopsy or a punch biopsy. A further reason for this policy is the problem of the traumatically activated naevus, sometimes called a pseudomelanoma.[39] This is a naevus that has been excised only partially, and the remaining tissue is stimulated into mitotic activity, producing a histological picture very like that of an early malignant melanoma.

Spitz naevi are frequently excised because of their history of relatively rapid growth, and, before pathological examination, are often thought to be vascular lesions rather than lesions derived from melanocytes. Once again, a scalpel excision with a narrow margin is the most appropriate procedure.

Halo naevi do not require excision and it is suggested that reassurance and possibly re-examination 3–4 months after the first referral is appropriate management of such lesions.

In the case of pigmented spindle cell naevi, there is frequently concern that the lesion in question is a malignant melanoma and excision biopsy is often essential to confirm the benign diagnosis.

The same problem frequently arises with blue naevi because of the intensity of the pigmentation, and once again an excisional biopsy of a small lesion is recommended. While a proportion of clinically atypical naevi may be precursors of melanoma, current evidence suggests that this proportion is very small in those with no family history of melanoma, but much greater if there is such a history. In most centres at the present time atypical naevi are monitored at 3-monthly intervals, and excised only if there is evidence of growth or change. A policy of 'preventive excision' is not logical because of the apparent rarity of malignant progression. As a general policy it is recommended that excision be considered in the case of any apparently benign pigmented naevus in an adult that is showing growth, inflammation, or change. Children develop new naevi and existing naevi may grow and therefore this policy is not so appropriate in the first decade of life. At present there is experimental work in progress assessing the safety, efficacy and cosmetic results of laser treatment for pigmented lesions which are cosmetically undesirable but in which the risk of malignant change is low, such as the naevus of Ota.[40]

Labial melanotic macules[41]

These lesions are relatively common, and patients referred are frequently young women concerned about their appearance.

They are usually solitary (Figure 9.26), and multiple lesions should alert the physician to the possibility of the Peutz–Jeghers syndrome (Chapter 4). The lesions are usually seen on the lower lip, suggesting that they arise in response to UV stimulation.

Solitary lesions are usually found to be simple ephelides on pathological examination. This term is used to describe a focal increase in melanin pigment in keratinocytes with no evidence of an increase in the number of melanocytes.

Excision is therefore only required on cosmetic grounds.

Congenital melanocytic naevi

Congenital melanocytic naevi can be divided into giant, intermediate and small congenital naevi on the basis of either widest diameter or total surface area. A popular division is to consider as small lesions those with a diameter of less than 1.5 cm, intermediate lesions those with a diameter of less than 20 cm, and large or giant lesions those with a diameter of greater than 20 cm. An alternative, and perhaps more practical, working definition is to define as giant all large naevi that cannot be excised completely.

Until 1980 the bulk of interest in the congenital naevus centred around the giant, garment or bathing trunk naevus and its potential for malignant change. In the past five years there has been a considerable degree of interest in smaller congenital naevi and their potential for malignant change.[42]

Incidence

In a number of studies small congenital naevi have been found to be present on the skin of around 1 per cent of newborn infants. One of the largest studies was that carried out by Walton et al who, in a study of 1058 infants, identified 41 lesions that were initially thought on clinical grounds to be congenital melanocytic naevi;[43] however, histological examination reduced this number to only 11. A recent Danish study[44] of 314 babies confirmed this 1 per cent

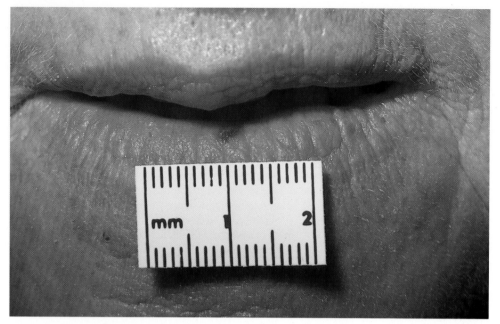

Figure 9.26   Solitary labial melanotic macule. No naevus cell population was seen on pathological examination of this lesion.

incidence, and a study carried out at about the same time in Oklahoma[45] on 830 newborn infants identified congenital naevi in 5 of 500 white babies but 17 of 228 black babies.

No satisfactory incidence figures exist for intermediate-size congenital naevi, and the incidence of giant garment or hairy pigmented naevi is reported as being very low, possibly 0.002 per cent of all newborn infants.

Clinical features

Congenital pigmented naevi are by definition present at birth. In the case of the intermediate or giant congenital naevi, the diagnosis will be apparent at birth, with a pigmented lesion covering a large part of the body surface (Figure 9.27). In early infancy the colour may be a pale coffee or tan, but it tends to darken with age. Hair follicles are often involved in this malformation, and the lesion shows excessive growth of terminal hair even in early neonatal life. Many of these unfortunate children have large numbers of small congenital naevi in addition to the

giant lesion (Figures 9.28 and 9.29), and the children with lesions covering any part of the spine may have bony defects, such as an occult spina bifida. Infants with giant naevi on the head and neck area may also have involvement of the underlying component of the central nervous system, and pigmentation of the leptomeninges.[46]

In the case of isolated small congenital naevi, care must be taken in making the clinical diagnosis, as the published studies referred to above, which have carried out biopsies to confirm clinical suspicion, suggest that in newborn infants as many as 50 per cent of pigmented lesions thought to be congenital naevi are other lesions (Figures 9.30 and 9.31).[43] Vascular abnormalities are a common cause of clinical confusion.

Pathology[47]

The pathology of the 'classic' congenital naevus is that of a naevus in which the bulk of the melanocytic cells are situated in the deeper two-thirds of the reticular dermis and involve the appendages. The presence of naevus cells within eccrine sweat glands, hair follicles and sebaceous glands is a relatively specific sign that the lesion in question has been present since birth. The overall architecture of the typical congenital naevus shows a diffuse naevus pattern scattered through a large area of the dermis in contrast to the usual focal packeted nature of naevus cells in the acquired intradermal naevus. There may be some lentiginous change and junctional activity in the overlying epidermis.

With the recent interest in the possible malignant potential of small congenital naevi, a larger number of pathological studies have been carried out on these previously neglected lesions. Studies to date suggest that the pathology described above is not invariably found in all pigmented naevi that have been present since birth or early life, and that some congenital naevi biopsied during the first year of life may show a pattern indistinguishable from that seen in a compound naevus found on adult skin. Care must be taken therefore in interpreting the pathological

features of melanocytic naevus to be those of acquired or congenital lesions without good clinicopathological correlation.

A feature seen relatively frequently if naevi are biopsied in the first year of life is the phenomenon of transepidermal elimination of naevus cells.[48] This feature is not seen in adults with acquired naevi, and can, on scanning-power microscopy, give the architectural appearance suggestive of a superficial spreading type of malignant melanoma. Closer examination of the lesion will show that the naevus cells within the epidermis are in packets rather than being individually distributed, and that they do not have the cytological appearance of malignant cells.

Recognizing malignant change within a pre-existing congenital naevus can be extremely difficult. The most common pattern is that of the development of an apparent clone of malignant cells in the dermal component of the lesion.[49] In these lesions there is rarely a connection between the dermoepidermal junction and the malignant focus within the pre-existing naevus.

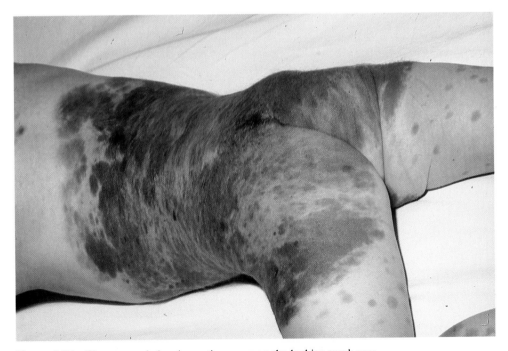

Figure 9.27   Giant congenital melanocytic naevus on the bathing-trunk area.

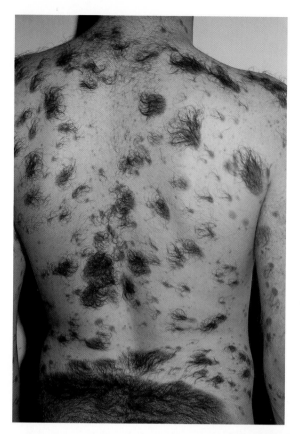

An additional feature that is occasionally seen, and that may give rise to pathological concern, is the presence of naevus cells in vascular channels. This does not automatically imply that the lesion has undergone malignant change, and 'benign metastases' to lymph nodes of cytologically non-malignant cells are occasionally seen.

Speckled lentiginous naevus (naevus spilus)[50]

This rare variant of a melanocytic naevus has in the past been confused in the literature with Becker's naevus (Chapter 5). In the author's opinion, Becker's naevus is primarily an epidermal disorder with coincidental hyperpigmentation, whereas the speckled lentiginous naevus does contain naevus cells derived from

Figure 9.28 This 24-year-old male has a giant congenital melanocytic naevus on the bathing-trunk area and multiple smaller congenital naevi on the upper back.

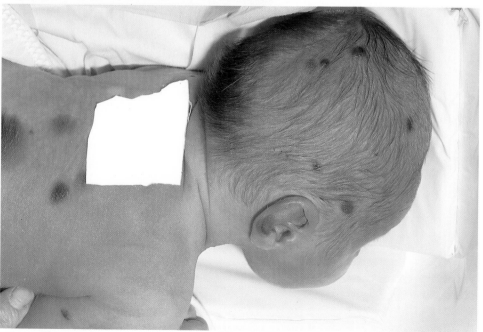

Figure 9.29 Neonate with multiple small and intermediate-sized congenital naevi.

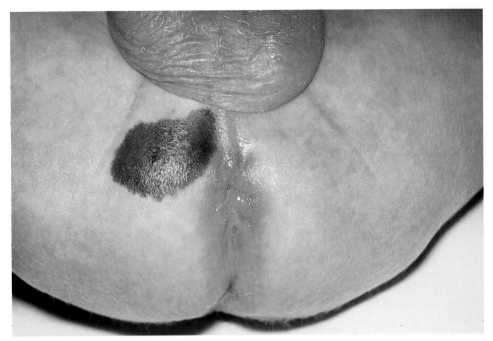

Figure 9.30   Congenital melanocytic naevus on the buttock area. All such lesions should be photographed routinely in the neonatal period.

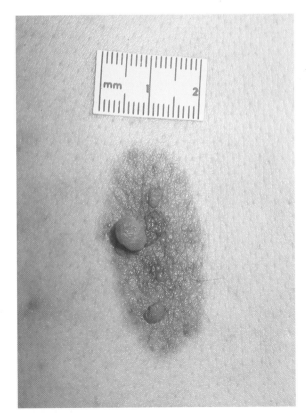

melanocytes. The term 'naevus spilus' appears to be responsible for part of this confusion, and it is therefore suggested that the term should be abandoned.

The clinical appearance is that of a large macular area of increased pigmentation with darker naevoid lesions within this area (Figure 9.32). These darker lesions are frequently elevated and papular.

Pathology

The pathology of this lesion is that of small compound naevi set within an area in which there is an increased number of melanocytes in the basal layer of the epidermis. Thus a lentiginous pattern is seen throughout the lesion with focal areas of compound naevus contained within it.

Figure 9.31   Benign papillomatous change in a congenital naevus on the back of a 4-year-old.

There have been a number of recent individual case reports of melanoma developing within these speckled naevi, but as the incidence of the naevi in the population is not established it is not yet clear whether or not 'preventive' excision should be recommended. The fact that malignant change can occur in these lesions does, however, mean that patients should be warned to seek advice if they notice change in such lesions.[51–53]

Management of congenital naevi

The two problems involved in the management of congenital naevi are the currently believed potential for malignant change of such lesions, and the cosmetic appearance of the lesions. In the case of the giant pigmented naevus, it is established that there is a risk of malignant change. A number of published studies are unsatisfactory in terms of the total numbers of patients studied, and are really a series of case reports. One of the more useful studies comes from Scandinavia.[54] A cohort of patients who had giant naevi were monitored over a period of several years, and although the exact number of patient years of observation is not stated in the text, the lifetime risk of malignant change was calculated to be 4.6 per cent. Given this figure, prophylactic excision of the naevus would seem entirely justified. Frequently, however, this is not feasible in terms of the size of the lesion and the availability of normal skin for grafting. The simultaneous presence of both giant and smaller lesions can reduce very greatly the area of skin available for grafting. The use of tissue expanders may in the future make prophylactic excision of even very large lesions a practical proposition.

A relatively new approach to the problem is shaving of the naevus within the first 48 hours of life. The theory is that at this time a large number of naevo-melanocytes will be in the superficial dermis and epidermis, and so a large proportion, but not all, of the naevus cells will be removed. Thus the risk of malignant change may be reduced by reducing the number of potentially malignant cells, and the cosmetic appearance may be improved by a reduction

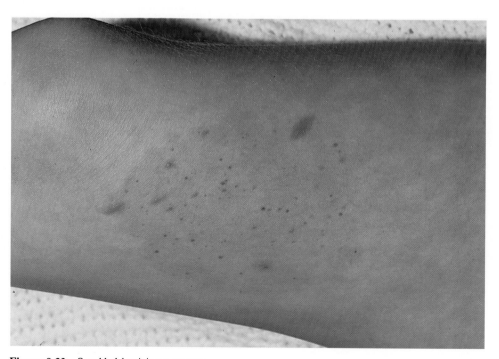

Figure 9.32 Speckled lentiginous naevus.

in pigmentation. Few centres have as yet carried out this technique for longer than 5 years, and thus the benefit to the patient in terms of reduced malignant change is not yet established.

Cosmetic cover of the lesions is generally unsatisfactory, because of the combination of pigment and terminal hair.

Management of the small congenital naevus is at present a subject of active investigation. A number of workers have evidence to suggest that these naevi do transform on occasion into malignant melanoma, but the exact rate of transformation is not established.[55-57] The great rarity of malignant melanoma before puberty suggests that patients are not at great risk in the first decade of life, and that if excision is considered necessary on cosmetic or prophylactic grounds, it can be delayed until the child is aged 10–12 years. In the author's opinion, evidence that small congenital naevi can transform into malignant melanoma is not at present so great that a positive campaign to seek out and remove all such naevi is justified, and the surgical workload involved would be considerable.

10
Malignant melanoma

Of all cutaneous malignancies, malignant melanoma attracts the most attention. This is not because it is at present the commonest type of skin cancer, but because it causes the greatest number of deaths. A high proportion of these deaths are in relatively young people, and therefore knowledge of the early clinical features of malignant melanoma – at a point when complete surgery is likely to be curative – is necessary for all those involved in examining the skin of patients or the public. Thus, community nurses, chiropodists and beauticians as well as doctors should all have some knowledge of the features of early curable melanoma.

Incidence

Cutaneous malignant melanoma is a particularly interesting tumour for epidemiological studies. The current rate of increase in the incidence of melanoma is 5–7 per cent per year, faster than for any other malignancy except lung cancer in women. Studies from many parts of Europe,[1-3] Australia[4] and North America[5] all document a virtual doubling in the incidence of melanoma each decade for the past three or four decades, and at present the trends in incidence continue upwards for all countries in which accurate records are kept. The steepest increases are currently recorded from Australia, which already has the highest incidence rates, and mainly affect older males, in whom the incidence has doubled in only seven years.[4] A similar steep rise in the incidence of melanoma (including thick lesions) is seen in Scotland.[3] At present the bulk of this increase is in thinner tumours (less than 1.5 mm thick). This has given rise to suggestions that changes in pathological criteria for the diagnosis of malignant melanoma are partly responsible for this rapidly increasing incidence. However, multinational pathological reviews have not confirmed this suggestion,[6] and at present one of the explanations for this rapidly increasing incidence is that the time of diagnosis has been brought forward by greater public awareness arising in part from improved health education about pigmented lesions.

Mortality

Melanoma-associated mortality is also rising steadily, but the curve is less steep than for incidence. The reason for this is thought to be that a higher proportion of current newly diagnosed melanomas are relatively thin and therefore potentially curable. An interesting observation with regard to melanoma mortality is that there does appear to be at present a slight flattening of the curve. It has been suggested that the highest melanoma mortality is being seen at present in cohorts of men born around 1930 and women born in the 1940s.[5,7,8] Several studies looking at melanoma and mortality in relation to migration indicate that the earlier in life a person arrives in a country with long hours of sunshine, the greater the risk of melanoma.[9] It is not yet established whether the reason for this is greater vulnerability of young melanocytes to malignant change, or merely greater opportunity in childhood for long hours of outdoor sun exposure. In younger people mortality appears to be levelling, but at present a falling mortality trend has only been seen in the United Kingdom, and there only in females following a public education campaign aimed at promoting earlier diagnosis.[10]

Aetiology (Table 10.1)

Case–control studies[11,12] indicate that the major risk factors for apparently sporadic melanoma are the presence of large numbers of naevi of any type, the presence of freckles, a history of severe sunburn, and fair or red hair and blue eyes.

Over the past decade much has been written on the subject of so-called dysplastic naevi, now termed

Table 10.1 Risk factors for melanoma.

- Family history of melanoma in two or more first-degree relatives
- Large numbers of banal melanocytic naevi
- Freckles
- Presence of clinically atypical naevi
- History of severe sunburn
- Born in tropical climate
- First few years of life in tropical environment

atypical naevi, with the recommendation that the term dysplasia be restricted to pathological use.[13] A number of studies have indicated that large numbers of clinically atypical naevi are a risk factor for melanoma, and that this risk is greatly increased in the setting of familial melanoma where patients may have not only a family history of melanoma in one or more first-degree relatives but also large numbers of these clinically atypical naevi.[14,15]

Case–control studies carried in out in North America, Australia and Europe[11,16–19] all incriminate excessive exposure to natural sunlight as a major factor in the aetiology of cutaneous malignant melanoma. The relationship, however, is complex and there appears to be a subtle interaction between the nature of sun exposure and skin type. It is possible that those who can and do develop a suntan with relative ease – so-called skin types 3 and 4 – might reduce their risk of melanoma with a year-round tan, but those who do not tan easily – skin types 1 and 2, who form the bulk of the melanoma population – appear to increase their risk with any type of sun exposure, whether year-round, intermittent or burning. This contrasts with non-melanoma skin cancer, where there is a clear relationship between cumulative lifetime sun exposure and skin cancer risk. In the case of melanoma, current studies suggest that short episodes of acute exposure to ultraviolet (UV) radiation, leading to severe sunburn, are more important than the number of hours of exposure in a lifetime. Thus the type of sun exposure experienced by those living in a Northern European climate who enjoy two or more holidays each year in a tropical, sub-tropical or even Mediterranean environment does appear to be a risk factor for melanoma.

A recent paper[20] has suggested that two-thirds of all melanomas worldwide can be attributed to excess UV exposure and that the remaining third, which are mainly found in non-Caucasians, appear to be due to other factors. Work on these other factors continues, and at present the roles of occupation, diet and alcohol intake have all been investigated.[21] No clear relationship

emerges from occupation and melanoma risk and, although there are some complex interactions between dietary unsaturated fatty acids and melanoma risk, once again these studies have not been fully confirmed. There is an association between melanoma and excess alcohol intake.[21] Patients receiving L dopa have a higher than expected incidence of melanoma, but this mainly relates to individual case reports,[22] and the increased risk is not therefore quantitated.

Individuals who use artificial sources of UV exposure such as sun lamps or sunbeds do appear to increase their risk of melanoma, but in these individuals it is always difficult to control for exposure to natural sunlight.[23–25] Nevertheless, there are now studies from several parts of Europe and also from Canada indicating that regular use of a sunbed does add to melanoma risk.

A number of papers have studied the possible role of exposure to unshielded fluorescent lighting as a melanoma risk and there are contradictory reports on this, with some studies reporting a positive finding and others failing to confirm this observation.[26]

Patients with xeroderma pigmentosum (Chapter 4, page 30) have an increased risk of malignant melanoma, indicating that faulty DNA repair may also be a risk factor for melanoma. Interestingly, patients who are albinos do not have an increased risk of melanoma, although they have a greatly increased risk of squamous cell carcinoma. This suggests that it is possible that some of the intermediates in the melanin synthesis pathway are carcinogenic and important in normally pigmented individuals. In albinos these intermediates will be absent, and this may explain the lack of increased melanoma risk in comparison with risk for other cutaneous malignancies.

The role of female hormones in melanoma has been thoroughly investigated.[27] One of the reasons for this interest has been that in certain parts of the world, including the United Kingdom, the incidence of melanoma is higher in females than males, but the prognosis is better. It has been suggested that this may be due to minor hormonal influences which are overridden in areas of high solar intensity such as Australia, where the incidence of melanoma is the same between the sexes. These studies have led to intensive investigation of the possible role of oral contraception in the aetiology of melanoma. Careful studies have not shown any significant risk associated with taking the oral contraceptive, even over long periods of time, provided the new lower-dose hormonal preparations are used.

A significant proportion of melanomas occur on body sites not easily or regularly exposed to UV radiation.

This has lead to the suggestion that exposure of the skin on other sites may stimulate production of what has been termed a solar circulating factor,[28] and that this factor may activate melanocytes at points distant from the area of direct sun exposure – giving rise, for example, to melanoma in the axillae or the soles of the feet. While this is an attractive hypothesis, 25 years on there is still no solid evidence to support it.

In summary, current evidence strongly incriminates UV radiation as the major cause of melanoma. Animal models of melanoma are relatively poorly developed, but those that are available at present include the opossum, a fish model and a new transgenic mouse model.[29] In all of these models UV radiation delivered in the first few days of life increases melanoma risk. Further work is needed, however, to link these observations to molecular events leading to malignant transformation of the melanocyte.

General clinical features of malignant melanoma

The most likely patient to present with malignant melanoma is a Caucasian female aged 30–50 years with a growing pigmented lesion on her leg. Females are more commonly affected than males, and the leg is the commonest site in women. In males, the back is the commoner site. Melanoma is extremely rare in children.

General pathological features

The essential feature of all invasive malignant melanomas is the presence of melanoma cells invading the dermis and deeper tissues. The cells may be of spindle, epithelioid or mixed type, and there may be variation in the type of cells seen in different parts of the tumour – so-called intralesional differentiation. Occasionally, balloon cells may compose a proportion of the tumour cell population. Melanin pigment may be present, in varying quantities, in tumour cells, lying free in the dermis and in macrophages. Fine intracytoplasmic melanin pigment seen deep in the lesion is a useful aid to diagnosis, as this is not seen in the deeper cells of a benign naevus.

Occasionally, a malignant melanoma may have a cell population that is predominantly composed of small naevus-like cells, so that on scanning-power microscopy the lesion looks deceptively benign. Careful examination at higher magnifications will reveal that this population has a large number of atypical mitoses and other features of malignancy.

The terms borderline melanoma and minimal deviation melanoma have been suggested to describe level 3 and level 4 lesions of this type (see below). These terms tend to cause confusion and it is suggested that the term malignant melanoma of small naevoid cell type is a more appropriate and safer term.

Some melanomas, particularly those arising in skin that shows other signs of serious actinic damage, may be associated with a very dense desmoplastic stroma and may have a relatively scanty cell population. This pattern may be associated with neurotropic spread, and causes particular difficulties for the pathologist in determining completeness of primary excision. Microscopic control of excision margins using the fresh tissue technique is recommended for such cases.

Possible pitfalls in pathological reporting of malignant melanoma

Pathological reporting of malignant melanoma is not always straightforward, as there are problems associated with both overdiagnosis and underdiagnosis.

Overdiagnosis may arise when congenital naevi are biopsied early in life, when vulvar lesions are biopsied, with dysplastic naevi, and when examining naevi that have recurred after incomplete excision. Congenital naevi in infants may show upward movement of large pigment-containing cells through the epidermis, usually a sign of melanoma. However, these usually occur in clusters rather than as single cells, and the phenomenon of transepidermal elimination of naevus cells in early infancy in these lesions has been discussed in Chapter 9. Vulvar lesions in young women may have a pathological appearance very similar to that of a severely dysplastic naevus or an early superficial spreading melanoma, and careful clinicopathological collaboration is needed to avoid unnecessary and inappropriate surgery. In both these lesions and in dysplastic naevi the absence of single cell invasion of the overlying epidermis may be helpful, as this is a feature found in early melanoma rather than in benign lesions. In the case of the recurrent naevus after incomplete excision, a good clinical history will prevent problems. Without this, the pathological features of a traumatically irritated naevus can be very similar indeed to a severely dysplastic naevus, or even to early superficial spreading melanoma.

The risk of underdiagnosis arises with a melanoma having features of a Spitz naevus, and with a melanoma of the small naevoid cell type described above. It is wise to be increasingly cautious about diagnosing Spitz naevus with advancing age, although, as stated in Chapter 9, true Spitz naevi may be seen in the elderly. Pointers, but not absolute markers, towards melanoma rather than Spitz naevus include a ragged lateral margin with spread of abnormal epidermal melanocyte activity beyond the invasive or intradermal area, a lack of overall symmetry, upward movement of melanocytic cells through the epidermis, and large numbers of melanocytic cells in mitosis.

Epidermotropically metastatic melanoma

Occasionally, secondary melanoma may mimic melanoma. This usually occurs with multiple tumour deposits on a limb, and the cells lie in small nests immediately beneath the epidermis.

Clinical subsets of malignant melanoma

Many years ago Wallace Clark and his colleagues suggested that malignant melanoma could be divided on clinical pathological grounds into 3 main types.[30] These were the superficial spreading melanoma, nodular melanoma and lentigo maligna melanoma. A fourth variant, the acral or acral lentiginous melanoma, was added later. Some workers prefer not to use these subdivisions and consider all cutaneous malignant melanoma of the skin as forming part of a spectrum. In the author's opinion, the Clark subclassification is of clinical value, as lesions that might be included in the differential diagnosis of, for example, a lentigo maligna melanoma would not be included in the differential diagnosis of a nodular melanoma. Similarly, the aetiological factors discussed above appear to differ slightly in that the profile of UV exposure of the lentigo maligna melanoma patient is different from that of the superficial spreading and nodular melanoma patient.

Lentigo maligna melanoma

These lesions are found predominantly on the light-exposed skin of older individuals. In a recent large Scottish series,[31] 90 per cent were found on the head and neck area and 10 per cent on other sites, mainly on the backs of the hands and the lower legs. The bulk of affected patients are in the seventh or eighth decade at the time of presentation, but the age range is lowering and a small number of individuals with this type of lesion are now seen in the fourth and fifth decades, even in temperate climates. In Australia and New Zealand larger numbers present at a younger age.

Clinical features

The initial clinical feature of the lentigo maligna type of melanoma is a slowly expanding in situ or radial growth phase. This is seen as a macular area of increased pigmentation, frequently on the temple or cheek area (Figures 10.1–10.3). If biopsied at this

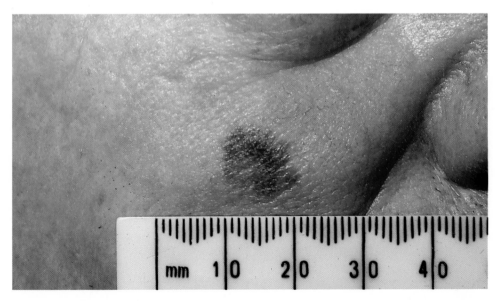

Figure 10.1   Early lentigo maligna on the cheek.

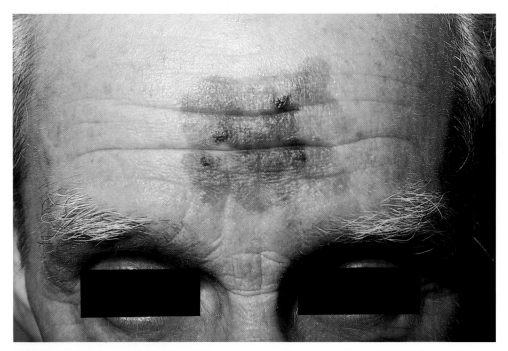

Figure 10.2 More extensive lentigo maligna on the forehead.

Figure 10.3 Extensive lentigo maligna on the nose.

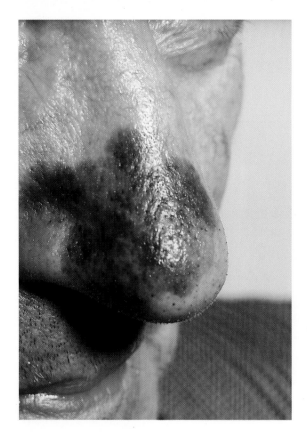

stage the lesion will show neoplastic melanocytes confined within the epidermis. The terms precancerous melanosis of Dubreuilh, or preinvasive lentigo maligna, or Hutchinson's melanotic freckle, are all appropriate for this lesion, which would be classified as a level 1 or intraepidermal lesion and would not be recorded in the majority of cancer registries as invasive malignant melanoma.

If left untreated, this lesion will slowly expand laterally across the skin surface, and central regression may be seen at the same time as lateral spread continues. Thus the lesion may take on quite a different shape over a period of years, and this may be apparent from a study of family photographs. Involvement of the pinna and the conjunctiva may occur.

After a very variable period of time, an invasive phase may develop within this pre-existing lentigo maligna (Figures 10.4–10.6). Once melanoma cells are seen in the dermis the term lentigo maligna melanoma is appropriate, and at this stage the tumour has developed the capacity for metastatic spread. The

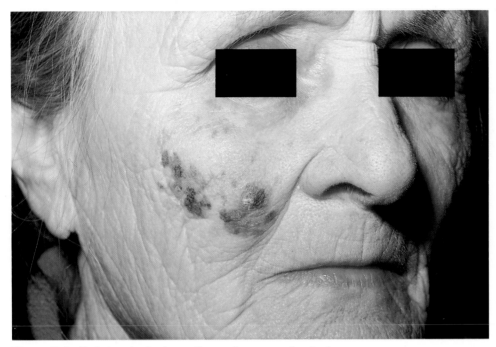

Figure 10.4   Early invasive lentigo maligna melanoma on the cheek.

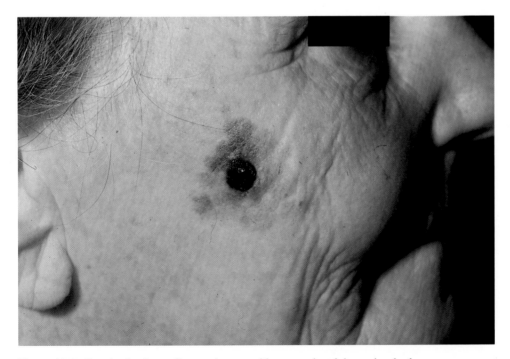

Figure 10.5   Invasive lentigo maligna melanoma with a central nodule on the cheek.

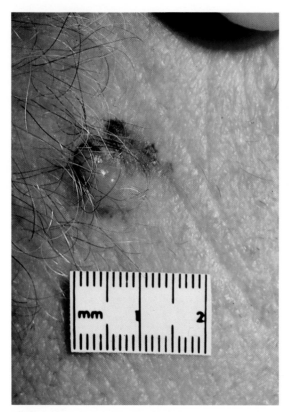

Figure 10.6   Invasive lentigo maligna melanoma with a non-pigmented central nodule on the cheek.

development of the vertical or invasive growth phase is usually seen clinically as the development of a more densely pigmented raised nodule within the pre-existing paler macular area. The rate of growth of these nodules can be relatively rapid.

Pathology

In the preinvasive or lateral growth phase, the lentigo maligna is an intraepidermal proliferation of usually spindle-shaped malignant melanocytes replacing the basal layer of the epidermis. The epidermis is usually thin, and the underlying dermis shows striking evidence of solar elastosis. At the time of the development of vertical growth phase, a lymphocytic inflammatory response may be seen around a few early invasive malignant melanocytes in the underlying dermis (Figure 10.7). As the numbers of invading melanoma cells become greater, this lymphocytic infiltrate is no longer seen.

A small proportion of invasive lentigo maligna melanomas develop a desmoplastic pattern.[32] Desmoplastic melanoma is a term used to describe malignant melanoma cells associated with a particularly dense and sclerotic fibrous stroma. This is

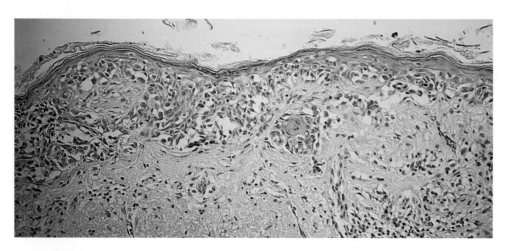

Figure 10.7   Pathology of early invasive lentigo maligna melanoma, showing malignant melanoma cells starting to invade a dermis that shows striking actinic damage.

sometimes seen in association with metastatic spread of the neoplastic melanocytes along nerves; hence the term neurotropic melanoma.[33] This type of malignant melanoma is particularly difficult to treat because of the great difficulty in determining, on pathological examination, that excision of the lesion is complete along the nerve trunks.

Superficial spreading malignant melanoma

Clinical features

This type of melanoma comprises the great majority of all melanomas seen in Europe, Australia and the USA, and the relative proportions appear to rise as the incidence of melanoma rises. Superficial spreading melanomas are seen most often on the female calf and the male back and clinically present as irregularly shaped pigmented areas. As clinical skill at early diagnosis improves, the diameter of these early melanomas at the time of diagnosis falls, and they may now be only 0.5–0.6 cm in diameter. The lateral outline of the melanoma is usually rather irregular, frequently with a notch, and the pigmentation tends to be variable, with areas of brown, black and even blue due to deeply situated melanin pigment and red due to inflammation (Figures 10.8–10.12). At a relatively early stage in its development, superficial spreading melanoma may ooze or crust at a time when obvious ulceration is not visible.

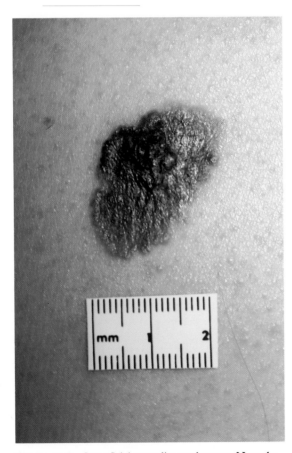

Figure 10.8 Superficial spreading melanoma. Note the size and the irregular edge.

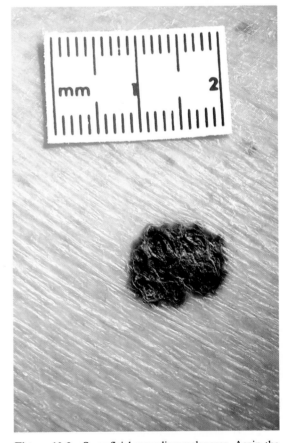

Figure 10.9 Superficial spreading melanoma. Again the edge is irregular. This lesion caused clinical confusion with a basal cell papilloma.

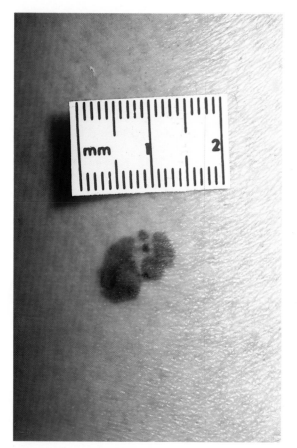

Figure 10.10 A small but easily recognized superficial spreading melanoma. Note the irregular edge and colour.

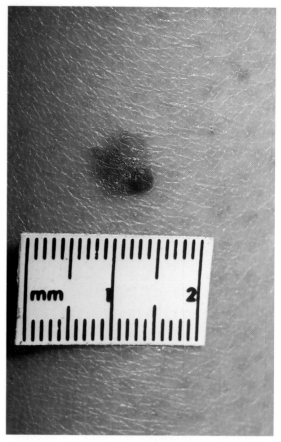

Figure 10.11 Early superficial spreading melanoma recognized by the patient after a public education campaign.

The natural history of the early superficial spreading malignant melanoma is that it may expand both laterally and into the superficial papillary dermis over a period of months or perhaps even years. In time, central nodules may develop within the lesion (Figures 10.13 and 10.14).

Approximately 50 per cent of patients with superficial spreading melanoma will give a history of a pre-existing apparently benign pigmented naevus on the site of development of the malignant melanoma. This clinical history does not always correlate with the pathological appearance, and there may be both false-positive and false-negative observations. This may be due, on the one hand, to destruction of all visible naevus cells by the malignant process, and on the other, to the fact that the patient may mistakenly consider an in situ radial growth phase of the melanoma as a benign naevus.

Patients with multiple primary melanomas usually have superficial spreading lesions. Approximately 2–5 per cent of melanoma patients have more than one primary tumour,[34] and these patients should be screened carefully for the presence of either the familial or the so-called sporadic dysplastic naevus syndrome, now better termed atypical mole syndrome.

epidermal involvement there is downward vertical invasion of malignant melanocytes through the papillary and reticular dermis.

Nodular malignant melanoma

The term nodular malignant melanoma should be used only for those lesions that appear to develop with a nodule as the earliest clinically recognizable growth phase. It is assumed that there must be a phase during which malignant cells are confined to the epidermis, but this is not clinically visible and the first visible sign of a lesion is a raised, usually blue-black nodule with normal skin surrounding (Figures 10.16 and 10.17). These lesions may grow rapidly, and this rapid growth may be associated with breakdown of the overlying epidermis and ulceration. The average age at presentation with nodular melanoma is a few years younger in most series than the age at presentation with superficial spreading melanoma, and considerably younger than the average age of presentation with lentigo maligna melanoma. Any body site may be involved, but the trunk appears to be more frequently involved than is the case with other types of melanoma.

The clinical differential diagnosis of nodular melanoma frequently includes both benign and malignant vascular tumours, and it may be impossible to differentiate clinically between this type of lesion and a rapidly growing nodular melanoma (see Figures 10.24 and 10.25). Histology is essential in this situation.

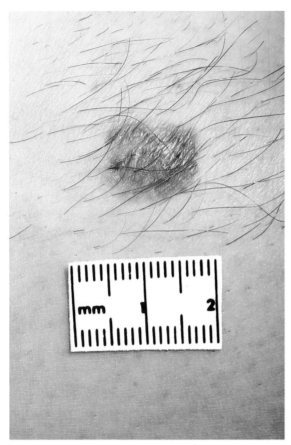

Figure 10.12 Early superficial spreading melanoma developing in a congenital naevus.

Pathological features

Superficial spreading malignant melanoma shows upward invasion of individual melanoma cells both singly and in nests through the epidermis in a pattern similar to that seen in Paget's disease (Figure 10.15). For this reason, an alternative name for superficial spreading melanoma is Pagetoid melanoma. This involvement of the epidermis is seen throughout the lesion and is often marked at the lateral margins, which extend some distance beyond the area overlying the vertically invasive component. In addition to this

Pathology

The essential pathological feature of a nodular malignant melanoma is a very sharp transition (within an area of 3 rete pegs) from normal epidermis to an area of invasive malignant melanoma with downgrowth of malignant melanoma cells into the dermis. Thus an impression is obtained of a rapidly expanding clone of cells with a particularly malignant and invasive phenotype.

Nodular melanomas tend to invade deeply relatively rapidly, and in this type of lesion it is particularly important to examine all parts of the pathological specimen carefully for signs of vascular invasion in the deeper component of the lesion.

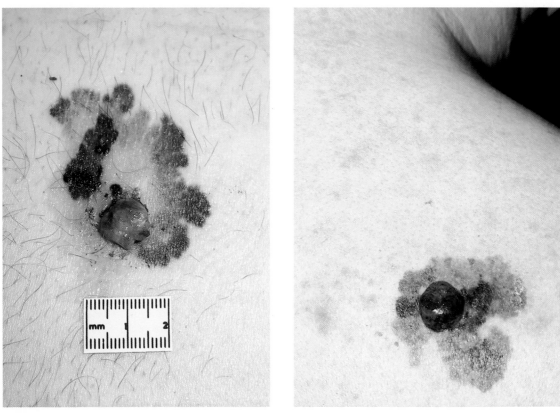

Figures 10.13 and 10.14   Large superficial spreading melanomas with central raised nodules.

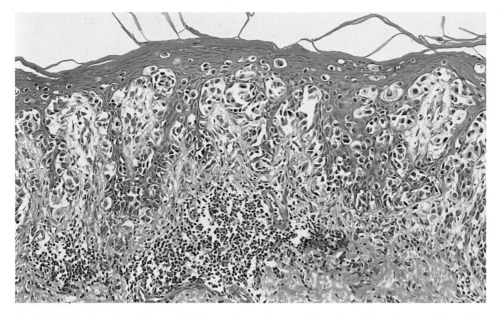

Figure 10.15   Pathology of a superficial spreading melanoma. Note the epidermal permeation with melanoma cells in a Pagetoid fashion.

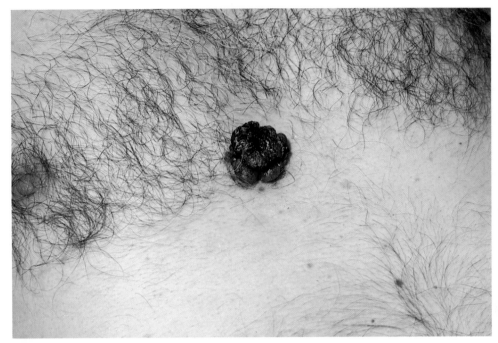

Figure 10.16 Nodular melanomas on the anterior chest.

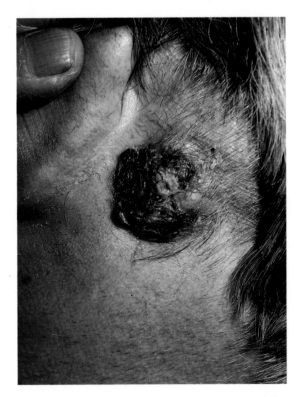

Figure 10.17 Large nodular melanoma behind the left ear. The lymph nodes were already involved.

Acral lentiginous melanoma

Acral lentiginous melanomas are, by definition, found mainly on the palms of the hands and soles of the feet, although a small number of lesions with this type of clinicopathological presentation are found on the non-hair-bearing areas of the upper wrists and ankles. These lesions are seen much more often on the feet than on the hands, with, in Scotland,[2] a ratio of 8 lesions on the feet to 1 on the hand. Initially, the lesion may present as a deceptively banal-looking pigmented macular area, hence the term lentiginous. In time, however, raised, densely black nodular areas will develop within this macular area of pigmentation (Figures 10.18–10.20). The timescale over which these lesions grow is not well established.

Subungual malignant melanoma

Subungual or periungual malignant melanoma may be regarded as a variant of the acral lentiginous malignant melanoma. This is a subset of melanomas in which there is some evidence that there may be delay in making appropriate diagnosis on the part of the medical profession, and it is therefore particularly

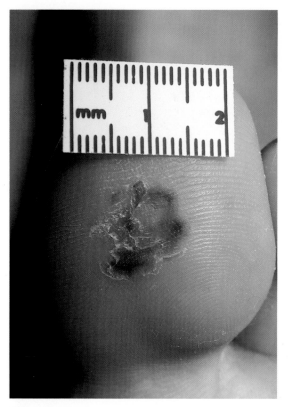

Figure 10.18   An early acral lentiginous melanoma on the first toe.

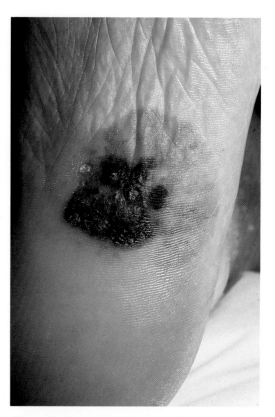

Figure 10.19   A typical large acral lentiginous melanoma on the heel.

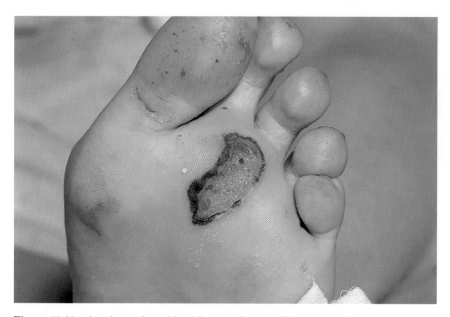

Figure 10.20   An ulcerated acral lentiginous melanoma. This pattern of peripheral pigmentation with central loss is fairly common.

Pathology

The pathology of acral lentiginous melanoma is similar to that of superficial spreading melanoma. Large numbers of malignant melanoma cells are seen both singly and in clusters, percolating through the epidermis and also invading the underlying dermis. A feature that is relatively common in acral lentiginous melanoma is the presence of an unusually dense lymphocytic infiltrate in and around the melanoma cells in the dermis and in the basal layer of the epidermis. The pathologist examining an acral lentiginous melanoma should be particularly careful to examine all parts of the specimen, as areas of focal lentiginous proliferation separated by areas of relatively normal epidermis are fairly common.

Differential diagnosis

From the descriptions above it will be seen that, while malignant melanomas of all four main types have certain features in common, there are features that are relatively specific to, for example, the nodular versus the lentigo maligna melanoma type of lesion.

In the early growth stages of all types of melanoma, the most important feature suggesting the diagnosis is change in a pigmented lesion in an adult. The change may relate to size of the lesion, to colour variation with different shades of brown or black, or to the development of a more irregular shape. Some individuals with what is subsequently shown pathologically to be early melanoma give a graphic description of irritation and minor itch developing in the lesion.

The clinical differential diagnosis will include, in the case of lentigo maligna melanoma, the preinvasive lentigo maligna phase, the flat type of seborrhoeic keratosis or basal cell papilloma, and the pigmented actinic keratosis (Figure 10.22). In the case of superficial spreading melanoma, the differential diagnosis will include dysplastic naevus (Figure 10.23), occasionally a congenital naevus, and rarely a basal cell papilloma. Nodular melanomas may be impossible to distinguish clinically from vascular lesions (Figures 10.24 and 10.25), and acral lentiginous melanomas may be clinically similar to benign naevi, plantar warts with thrombosed capillaries (Figures 10.26–10.28) and so-called 'talons noirs', which are haemorrhages into the epidermis from trauma, often seen on the heels of joggers. Large surveys of preoperative accuracy of clinical diagnosis have suggested

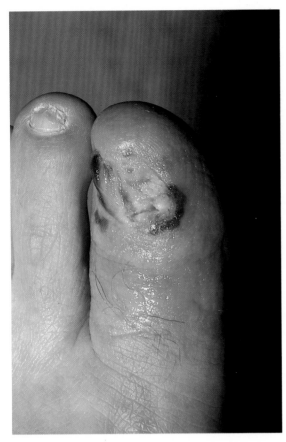

Figure 10.21   An advanced subungual melanoma also showing pigment on the nail-fold (Hutchinson's sign).

important to examine carefully any persisting area of periungual pigmentation or of nail destruction accompanied by pigmentation. On occasion, such lesions are initially misdiagnosed as fungal infection with associated nail pigmentation, or as simple traumatic injury. It is essential that a diagnostic biopsy be taken from this type of lesion if there is any clinical doubt whatever.

A feature of value in examining a pigmented nail is the presence or absence of pigment on the nail-fold proximal to the actual nail. The presence of pigment in this site is known as Hutchinson's sign and is an important diagnostic marker. Pigmentation in this area is not seen in association with a traumatic subungual haemorrhage, nor with fungal infection. Its presence is strongly suggestive of subungual malignant melanoma (Figure 10.21).

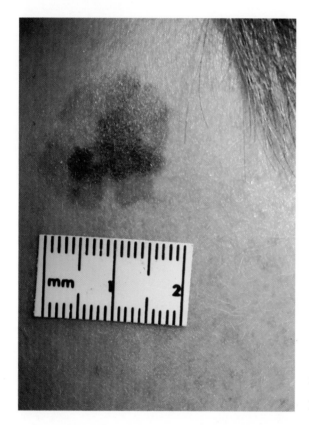

Figure 10.22 Flat type of basal cell papilloma (seborrhoeic keratosis) mimicking lentigo maligna. Histology is essential in such cases.

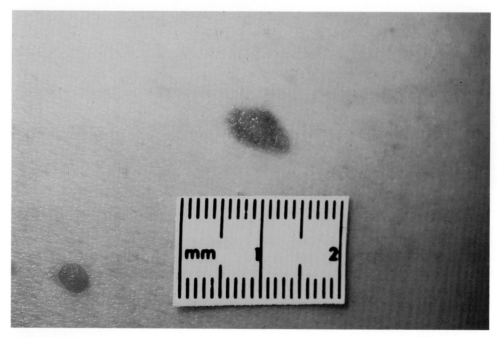

Figure 10.23 A clinically atypical naevus with some clinical features of early superficial spreading melanoma.

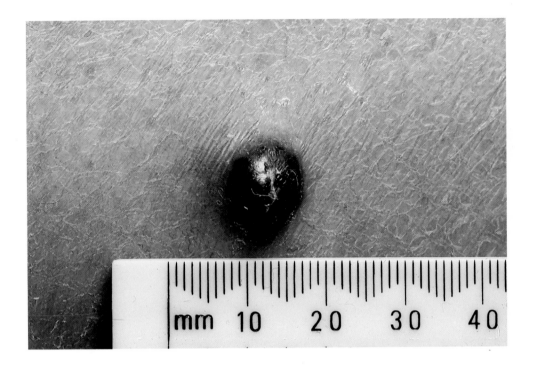

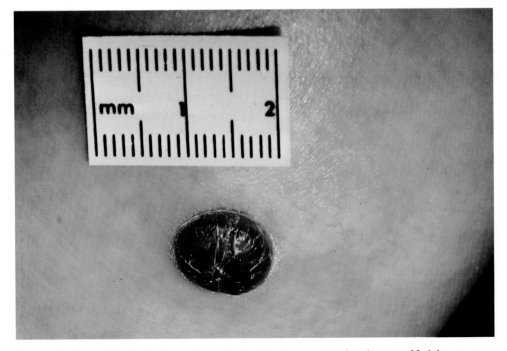

Figures 10.24 and 10.25 Benign angiomas both referred as suspected melanomas. Nodular melanoma can look very similar, and pathological confirmation of a clinical impression is essential.

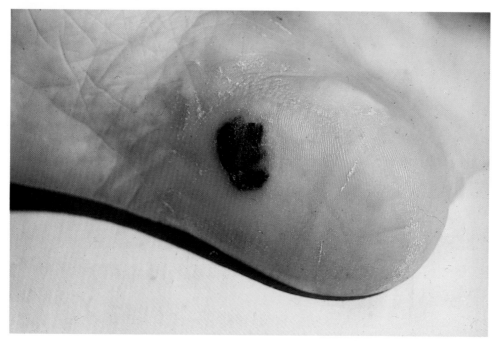

Figure 10.26 Acral melanoma or plantar wart? This is actually a melanoma, but had been treated as a plantar wart before referral.

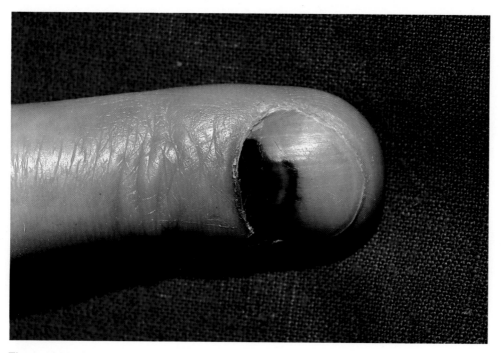

Figure 10.27 Subungual haemorrhage mimicking melanoma. Note the lack of pigment on the nail-fold. Compare with Figure 10.21.

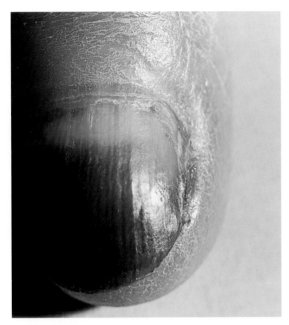

Figure 10.28 A pigmented nail due to fungal infection mimicking subungual melanoma. Note the lack of pigment on the nail-fold.

Skin surface microscopy and imaging as aids to melanoma diagnosis

There is currently great interest in increasing the accuracy of preoperative diagnosis of melanoma by using both simple magnification in vivo and also image analysis of captured surface features of pigmented lesions. Skin surface microscopy has been developed over the past 25 years[35-37] and the latest equipment is simple, inexpensive and portable. The dermatoscope is a small illuminated hand-held magnifier similar in size to an auriscope. With magnifications of × 10 in vivo, features highly suggestive of but not as yet totally specific or sensitive for melanoma can be identified, and other features that are found very much more frequently on non-melanocytic lesions can be seen. The melanin pigment network associated with lesions arising from melanocytes is seen as a fine reticulate network which in benign melanocytic lesions, such as naevi, streams out towards the lateral margin, and in malignant lesions tends to be more interrupted and clumped. Non-melanocytic pigmented lesions such as pigmented basal cell carcinomas and angiomas can be relatively easily identified in vivo by this technique, but reliable distinction between benign and malignant melanocytic lesions is not yet routinely available.

The use of image analysis is also at present at the experimental stage. The principle of the technique is to capture the surface features of the pigmented lesion on computer and analyse accurately such features as the degree of pigment variation, the irregularity of the perimeter of the lesion, and the quantity of red pigment contributing to the overall colour of the lesion. To obtain an algorithm which separates melanoma from all other non-melanoma pigmented lesions requires accurate analysis of large numbers of all types of lesions which may come into the differential diagnosis, and at present this work is in progress. Preliminary analysis suggests that, as with use of the dermatoscope, identifying non-melanoma pigmented lesions may be relatively easy, but that separating early melanoma from atypical naevi will be much more difficult.

that an accuracy rate of no more than 50 per cent is common, emphasizing the absolute necessity of a diagnostic biopsy in the majority of lesions. Guides such as the American ABCDs and the British seven-point checklist (Table 10.2) are helpful in discriminating at the clinical level those lesions that are likely to be melanoma from those that are not.

Table 10.2 Seven-point checklist to aid clinical distinction between melanoma and non-melanoma pigmented lesions.

Major features
- Change in shape of a previous pigmented lesion
- Change in size of a previous pigmented lesion
- Change in colour of a previous pigmented lesion

Minor features
- Size > 6 mm in diameter
- Inflammation
- Oozing or crusting
- Mild itch

Urgent specialist referral is recommended if any one of the major features or two or more of the minor features are present

Prognostic features of importance (Table 10.3)

Both clinical and pathological features of the primary tumour are of prognostic significance.

Table 10.3 Prognostic factors for melanoma.

Tumour thickness	Consistently, the most important prognostic feature
Growth phase – radial/horizontal or vertical	Radial growth phase tumours may not yet have acquired the capacity to metastasize
Clark levels	Deeper levels associated with poorer prognosis
Angioinvasion	
Ulceration	Significant even if only microscopic
Mitotic count	
Pathological evidence of regression	Conflicting reports here

1. By far the most important feature is the tumour thickness measured from the granular layer to the deepest invasive melanoma cell in the manner advocated by the late Alexander Breslow[38] (Figure 10.29) – hence the term Breslow thickness. All studies show that there is a direct linear relationship between tumour thickness and survival. Any study looking at other putative prognostic factors should always control for Breslow thickness, to ensure that they are truly independent variables. There have in the past been suggestions that there were specific 'breakpoints' in tumour thickness at which there was a stepwise deterioration in prognosis, but a survey of a very large number of patients has not confirmed this suggestion,[39] and at present tumour thickness is considered a continuous variable.

2. An additional important pathological prognostic sign is the division of melanomas into those in the radial or horizontal growth phase and those in the vertical growth phase.[40] The term radial or horizontal growth phase describes a melanoma in which there is invasion into the dermis (Clark level 2, see below) but the malignant cells in the dermis do not yet form a coherent tumour mass 25 or more cells across. Vertical growth phase melanoma describes the situation in which there is a clearly demarcated larger cluster of cells invading the dermis. Long-term follow-up of patients with tumours only in the radial or horizontal growth phase shows 100 per cent survival and it is suggested that these tumours have not yet developed metastatic capacity.[41]

3. The Clark levels of invasion are also important prognostic factors. These relate the deepest invasive tumour cells to surrounding structures. The Clark level system uses five levels of invasion. These are: level 1, intraepidermal or in situ melanoma; level 2, invasion of the papillary dermis; level 3, invasion of the papillary dermis down to the reticular dermis and expansion of the papillary dermis; level 4, invasion of the reticular dermis; and level 5, invasion of fat. Many centres use both the Breslow thickness and Clark level measurements, as it has been shown that a thin melanoma measured by the Breslow technique may have a poorer prognosis when it is a lesion classified as level 4 rather than level 3. This seems biologically logical, as, clearly, the lesion that has invaded to level 4 has exhibited a greater degree of destructive and possibly metastatic potential.

4. The presence of tumour cells in vessels is also confirmed in most series as a very poor prognostic sign.

5. Several large studies also indicate that visible ulceration and even microscopic ulceration are poor prognostic signs independent of tumour thickness.

6. Mitotic count in melanomas is also found in most series to be a significant prognostic feature, with high mototic counts associated with a poor prognosis.

7. Pathological evidence of regression, defined as dermal sclerosis amounting to scar tissue formation with associated streaks of melanin pigment and necrotic melanoma cells, has in the majority of studies been associated with a poor prognosis in melanomas less than 1.5 mm thick, and here the assumption is that the tumours were originally thicker and still carry the prognosis associated with their original thickness.[42–44]

Clinical features said in some series to affect prognosis include sex of patient, body site, and age at diagnosis. All of these features may be related to tumour thickness, and it is therefore once again essential to control for tumour thickness in trying to establish if any or all of these features are independent prognostic features in their own right.

Current work on prognosis in melanoma patients is concentrating on trying to integrate all features of known or suspected prognostic significance and relate these to survival prospects over time in an appropriate model.[45,46] Such models should enable more accurate counselling of patients and relatives at the time of diagnosis.

Management

The cornerstone of successful treatment of melanoma is early diagnosis and prompt appropriate surgical therapy. Patients who have melanomas removed when they are less than 1.5 mm thick have over 90 per cent disease-free five-year survival prospects, but those whose tumours are removed when only 2 mm thicker, at 3.5 mm or greater, have a less than 50 per cent chance of surviving disease-free to five years.

If melanoma is clinically suspected, biopsy should be performed. With small melanomas, this will usually be an excision biopsy with a narrow margin – 2–5 mm – of surrounding clinically normal skin.

Biopsy technique for suspected melanoma

In the author's opinion, biopsies of lesions in which the suspicion of melanoma is strong are best carried out by those who will perform definitive surgery if melanoma is confirmed. This will allow for optimal planning of the excision, and will minimize doubts about orientation of specimens, exact excision margins and other problems.

In the case of pigmented lesions in which the suspicion of melanoma is low, but diagnostic histology is still required to confirm that the lesion is, for example, a basal cell papilloma or benign naevus, the biopsy can quite reasonably be carried out by the primary care practitioner.

There are possible dangers of an incisional rather than an excisional biopsy in suspected melanomas, because of theoretical risks of disseminating tumour cells into vessels. Papers can be cited to either support or refute this hypothesis, but as the public becomes more aware of the potential dangers of pigmented lesions and comes for medical advice with smaller lesions, this problem is becoming much less common in practice; the lesions requiring biopsy are small, and an excision biopsy with a narrow margin of 1–2 mm of normal skin around the lesion is appropriate and has the added advantage that the entire sample is available for histological examination. There is no evidence to suggest that this type of excisional diagnostic biopsy followed 1–2 weeks later by definitive melanoma surgery, if required, alters the patient's prognosis in any way. A punch biopsy should never be made into a possible melanoma because of the possibility of pushing tumour cells deeper into the dermis.

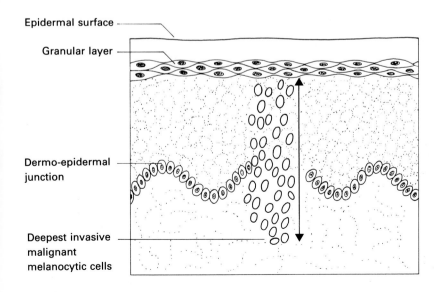

Figure 10.29   Measurement of Breslow thickness.

Frozen section diagnosis of melanoma is not recommended for routine use. This is because artefacts may be introduced which could cause problems in distinguishing, for example, between melanoma and Spitz naevus. With modern pathology techniques, a specimen can be conventionally processed in 24 hours.

It has been suggested that injecting large quantities of local anaesthetic close to a primary melanoma could force acantholytic tumour cells into vascular channels. This complication has not been proven, but it would seem prudent to use local, or even regional, anaesthesia inserted at a reasonable distance from the lesion.

Once the diagnosis of primary cutaneous melanoma is histologically confirmed, the extent of surgical treatment of the primary lesion will depend on the thickness of the tumour. The current trend is to reduce the margin of normal skin excised around the tumour, and trials are in progress to establish just how far this can be reduced without increasing the risk of local or distant recurrence. In practical terms, this means that many patients who in the past might have had skin grafts will nowadays have direct closure. This in turn means that a much higher proportion of melanoma surgery is now carried out on a day-patient basis.

Until the results of these trials are available, a reasonable working practice advocated by Taylor and Hughes[47] is to excise 1 cm of normal skin around the tumour for every millimetre of tumour thickness up to 3 mm. Thus, a primary tumour up to 1 mm thick will only require 1 cm clearance in all directions. Despite these suggestions for a reduction in lateral clearance in comparison with previous routine practice, it is still important that an adequate clearance in depth is achieved, and the depth of excision should at least be down to subcutaneous fat.

In the past, many arguments have been advanced for and against removal of the deep fascia. Current evidence would suggest that this should depend on the body site, and removal or retention does not by itself affect the prognosis.

Proof that a narrower lateral margin of excision for thinner tumours will not lead to an increase in either local or distant recurrences is emerging from the World Health Organization (WHO) Melanoma Group Trial.[10] This study has compared the disease-free interval and survival in patients with limb melanomas less than 2 mm thick which have been randomized to receive either 1 or 3 cm clearance of normal skin around the primary tumour. At median follow-up of 5 years there is no significant difference in survival rates between the two groups, but there is a higher incidence of local recurrence in the group with a narrower excision margin.

Lymph node dissection and sentinel node biopsy

For many years there have been arguments over the value to the patient of adjuvant or prophylactic lymph node dissection for patients with primary tumours in the intermediate and thicker groups. The logic of this approach is that if nodes from these groups are removed and pathologically examined at the time of primary surgery and before there is any clinical evidence of node involvement, up to one-third of patients will have microscopic nodal metastases. However, long-term follow-up, comparing disease-free interval and survival in patients who have had prophylactic node dissection with matched patients who had node dissection only when the nodes became clinically palpable, has shown a survival benefit for only around 15 per cent. The group who appear to benefit most are those with intermediate-thickness tumours, but even here the proportion apparently benefiting is small, and the procedure may be associated with post-operative morbidity of persistent limb oedema.

To try to overcome these problems and identify the section of this population who do require nodal excision at the time of removal of the primary tumour, Morton[48] has introduced the concept of selective lymph node biopsy of the so-called sentinel draining lymph node. This node is identified by injecting blue dye around the site of the primary melanoma, exposing the draining lymph nodes, and biopsying the node into which the dye first drains. Extensive studies have indicated that if this node is free of tumour cells, the chances of malignant cells in other nodes in the draining node basin is very slim indeed. Thus a positive node identified by this technique would be an indication that a full node dissection was justified, but a negative result would indicate that this was not required. At present trials are in progress to confirm this hypothesis.

Arterial limb perfusion

The use of intra-arterial limb perfusion with high concentrations of melphalan and associated hyperthermia has been used in both a therapeutic and an adjuvant setting.[49] It is of value therapeutically in controlling locally recurrent disease confined to a limb, but a large controlled trial of the value of adjuvant limb perfusion in thick, poor-prognosis primaries on limbs has not shown any survival benefit. Dramatic clearance of locally recurrent disease is seen after perfusion with tumour necrosis factor alpha, but this approach is also associated with significant toxicity and is at present only available in highly specialized centres.

Interferon adjuvant therapy

Large numbers of studies have been carried out using interferon in both an adjuvant and a therapeutic setting. Results to date suggest that, in the therapeutic setting, a small number of patients do benefit and obtain a worthwhile extension of survival. Controlled trials are in progress looking at the possible benefits of adjuvant interferon both after excision of a thick poor-prognosis primary, and also after excision of pathologically-involved lymph nodes when the patient has been rendered tumour-free. The bulk of the studies in progress relate to recombinant alpha interferon, but gamma interferon is also under investigation.

Other adjuvant therapy

At present there is no standard adjuvant chemotherapy or immunotherapy regime which has been shown in controlled trials to improve the poor prognosis associated with a thick primary tumour. A large number of melanoma vaccines are at present in controlled trials and the results are awaited with interest.

Follow-up

After primary surgery, melanoma patients should be followed up for local or distant recurrence. The value of extensive staging procedures is debatable, as most patients who develop secondary spread show involvement of regional lymph nodes first. A full clinical examination, chest X-ray and full blood count are minimal requirements, and in some centres patients with thick primary tumours receive a routine computerized tomography (CT) scan. There is no established follow-up routine, but a common practice is to follow patients monthly for the first 3 months while the wound is healing, 3-monthly thereafter for up to 2 years, 6-monthly to 5 years, and then annually.

Patients with thick primary tumours will most often have problems with recurrence in the first 2 years, and patients with thin primaries who develop recurrence may not do so until 5–10 years after primary surgery.

If a patient develops local recurrence in a limb after removal of a primary melanoma on that limb (stage 2a disease), further surgery and possibly arterial limb perfusion is the recommended therapy. CO_2 laser ablation may also offer useful control of this type of recurrence. When palpable lymph nodes develop (stage 2b disease), a full node dissection is appropriate. At present there is no proven chemotherapeutic regime that prolongs survival after a therapeutic node dissection, but as stated above a number of studies are in progress, run by such groups as the melanoma sections of the WHO and the European Organization for Research and Treatment of Cancer (EORTC), looking at the possible value of both interferons and chemotherapy. If possible, patients should be entered into structured studies run by such groups rather than offered chemotherapy on a random and ad hoc basis, as only in this way will useful information on the value of adjuvant therapy be obtained.

Female patients: pregnancy and hormonal supplements

Many women who have had melanoma may wish to start or continue the oral contraceptive, to embark on a first or subsequent pregnancy or to take hormone replacement therapy. Provided the melanoma did not develop explosively during a period of intense hormonal stimulation as in pregnancy, there is no evidence to suggest that any of these will have an effect on subsequent prognosis. A large study of the possible effect of pregnancy on melanoma conducted by the WHO Melanoma Program has reported no deterioration in prognosis for patients who embark on a pregnancy after melanoma.[50] It must be borne in mind, however, that for women with thicker tumours the prospects of survival without any additional problem of pregnancy are poor, and the possibility of a motherless child is very real.

Management of disseminated disease

Once a patient has disseminated disease, the prospects for cure are very poor. A large number of trials have reported a response rate of around 20 per cent with DTIC as a single agent but responses are usually

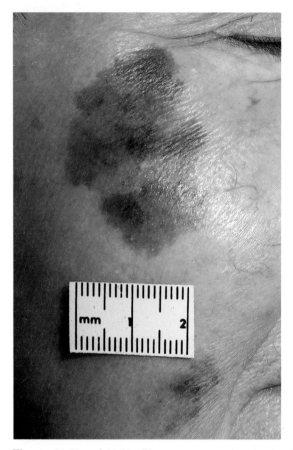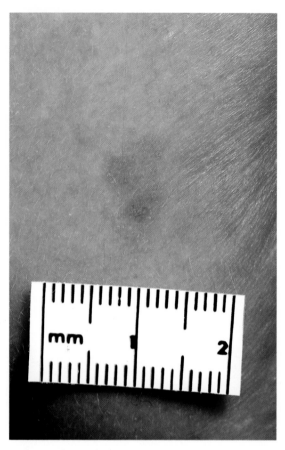

Figures 10.30 and 10.31   Biopsy-proven non-invasive lentigo maligna before and after cryotherapy.

short-lived. The nausea associated with DTIC can now be controlled with ondansetron, and multiple drug regimes such as BELD (Bleomycin Eldesine Lomustine and DTIC) may offer a higher response rate, of up to 45 per cent, but again these are usually of relatively short duration.[51]

Early encouraging results with interleukin 2 have not been confirmed. It is thus very important to consider quality of life before embarking on chemotherapy which is likely to be toxic and unlikely to be curative.

Radiotherapy

Radiotherapy has little to offer in primary melanoma as, in general, melanoma is not radiosensitive, but palliative radiotherapy can be of great value in the management of cerebral metastases and in the relief of pain from bony secondaries.

In some centres lentigo maligna is treated with radiotherapy (see below).

Management of lentigo maligna

In the preinvasive lentigo maligna stage, this lesion is treated in some centres with cryotherapy with good cosmetic results (Figures 10.30 and 10.31). If this approach is contemplated, it is essential to carry out a pretreatment biopsy to confirm that that lesion is not invasive, and the patient should be followed up regularly as local recurrence is possible.

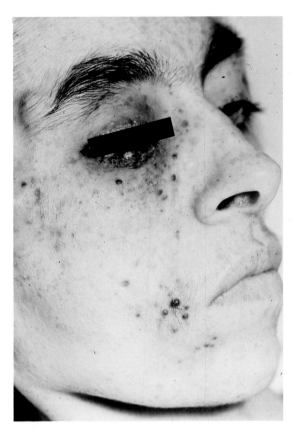

Figure 10.32   Malignant blue naevus.

Conclusion

The incidence of melanoma is increasing at a rate very much faster than our ability to treat advanced disease. Until we understand the exact aetiological sequence involved in UV exposure and can mount a logical preventive campaign, it is essential that both the medical profession and the public are taught to recognize melanoma at an early growth stage while the prospects for cure by limited surgery are good.

In the case of both lentigo maligna and invasive lentigo maligna melanoma, radiotherapy is a valid treatment alternative, as this lesion is relatively radiosensitive. In the case of frail elderly patients, this may well be the most appropriate therapy.[52,53]

Malignant blue naevus

This is an extremely rare tumour, and is most easily recognized if it develops in a naevus of Ota or Ito (Figure 10.32). Patients may present with multiple nodules and, on pathological examination, a spindle cell neoplastic lesion will be seen, having no connection with the overlying dermis. Necrosis within the lesion is a useful diagnostic sign.[54]

11

Cutaneous lymphomas, pseudolymphomas and histiocytosis X

The following clinical presentations will be described and discussed in this chapter:

Mycosis fungoides
The Sézary syndrome
Pagetoid reticulosis
CD30 lymphomas:
   Lymphomatoid papulosis
   Primary CD30 cutaneous T-cell lymphoma
   Actinic reticuloid
   Lymphomatoid pityriasis lichenoides
Lymphomatoid granulomatosis
B-cell cutaneous lymphoma
Malignant angioendotheliomatosis
Hodgkin's disease
Crosti's lymphoma
Angiolymphoid hyperplasia with eosinophils
Follicular mucinosis
Histiocytosis X

Terminology

In the USA the term cutaneous T-cell lymphoma (CTCL) has been used for the past 15 years in many centres as an inclusive term to describe the bulk of lymphomas presenting in the skin. In Europe there is less enthusiasm for this term, and in the UK and elsewhere a number of centres use the term mycosis fungoides to describe the most common T-cell lymphoproliferative disorder of the skin, and the terms Sézary syndrome, Pagetoid reticulosis, and so on, as appropriate. If the term cutaneous T-cell lymphoma is preferred, it is suggested that the clinical type of cutaneous T-cell lymphoma be added to the description.

A very small number of lymphomas presenting in the skin are of B-cell origin and they will be considered briefly at the end of the chapter.

Incidence

Cutaneous T-cell lymphoma of all types is still a rare entity, although this apparent rarity may in part reflect under-registration of cases managed in private practice or on an outpatient basis, as in many parts of the world incidence figures are collated from inpatient data. Very few countries have incidence figures for cutaneous T-cell lymphoma as a separate entity, but figures from the USA would suggest that the incidence rate is of the order of two new cases per million of the population annually. Thus the rate of development of new cases is low, very much lower than that of, for example, malignant melanoma in most parts of the world. However, it should be remembered that cutaneous T-cell lymphoma is frequently diagnosed in the fifth or sixth decade, and is a disorder with which many patients live for 20 or 30 years. Thus, the overall prevalence of cutaneous T-cell lymphoma in the community may be considerably higher than that of more aggressive types of malignancy, which have a higher incidence but shorter survival period.

Historical background

The name mycosis fungoides was first used by the French dermatologist Alibert in 1806.[1] Alibert saw only one case in his lifetime, and used the term mycosis fungoides because the unfortunate patient had mushroom-like cutaneous nodules. Several years after this first description, the French dermatologist Bazin, after observing a number of patients, suggested that a discernible progression of disease could be traced from a premycotic stage to a mycotic and finally to a tumour stage.[2] Shortly after this it was suggested that this orderly pattern of disease progression did not always occur, and that the tumorous or 'd'emblée' stage could develop without a prior premycotic plaque stage. At the end of the nineteenth century the erythrodermic variant of mycosis fungoides was also identified.

The Sézary syndrome, considered by some to be the leukaemic variant of mycosis fungoides, was first reported in 1938 by Sézary and Bouvrain.[3] They described the presence of the triad of erythroderma, a leukaemic blood picture with atypical mononuclear cells, and peripheral lymphadenopathy.

Since this time the term Sézary syndrome has been used rather more loosely, and is now used by some to describe any cutaneous T-cell lymphoma in which more than 5 per cent of the peripheral blood mononuclear cells are atypical. This can give rise to problems in comparing results of therapy in different series.

Thirty years later, in 1968, Lutzner et al[4] used electron microscopy to identify the typical hyperconvoluted nucleus of the T-cell involved in cutaneous T-cell lymphoma. In the 1970s Edelson and his collaborators[5] used the immunological and ultrastructural techniques then available to identify the atypical circulating mononuclear cells as T-lymphocytes.

Since 1980, and the advent of commercially available monoclonal antibodies recognizing T-lymphocytes and subsets, there have been a large number of publications confirming that the great majority of patients with cutaneous T-cell lymphoma have a proliferation of T-helper lymphocytes, which locate preferentially in the skin.[6,7]

Studies of cutaneous T-cell lymphoma have been carried out with the aim of establishing whether or not it is a malignant disorder from the very earliest stages, or whether it is initially a reactive process which, in some patients, later transforms to a malignant proliferation. The results, in those cases in which a large enough number of lymphocytes can be extracted from the cutaneous lesions for T-cell receptor beta-chain DNA analysis to be performed, suggest that the disorder is monoclonal, implying a malignant proliferation,[8] and more recent studies,

looking at gene rearrangement in cells extracted from both epidermis and dermis separately, suggest that the first signs of gene rearrangement are seen in the epidermis.[9]

Aetiology

At present the reason for the T-helper proliferation resulting in cutaneous T-cell lymphoma is not understood. A number of case–control studies have been carried out in both the USA and the UK. Studies in the USA suggested that mycosis fungoides patients were exposed to air pollution, pesticides, solvents and detergents more frequently and more intensely than were appropriate control patients.[10–12] A case–control study in Scotland has not confirmed these observations, but has observed that in the mycosis fungoides patients there was a higher incidence of atopy than in the control group.[13]

A number of workers have postulated that mycosis fungoides is a disease of antigen persistence in which an initially reactive process is stimulated by inadequate handling and clearance of unidentified antigen or antigens, and that in a proportion of cases this initially reactive dermatitis process is transformed into a malignant proliferation.[14–16] The observation that atopics are over-represented in those suffering from mycosis fungoides could be interpreted as supportive evidence for this view, as it is well established that they over-react to a wide range of ingested and inhaled antigens.

Retroviruses and mycosis fungoides

The identification of adult T-cell leukaemia lymphoma and the presence of antibodies to HTLV-1 in the serum of affected patients in Japan has stimulated a search for similar antibodies in patients with all types of cutaneous T-cell lymphoma in various parts of the world. Outside Japan, antibodies to HTLV-1 are found almost exclusively in negro patients of Caribbean extraction with cutaneous T-cell lymphoma and in coloured patients from the south-eastern part of the USA. Patients with adult T-cell leukaemia lymphoma usually have a rather more aggressive type of disease than cutaneous T-cell lymphoma of the mycosis fungoides type, with hypercalcaemia, a persistent leukaemic phase, and a rapid downhill course. Studies suggesting that antibodies to HTLV were present in a proportion of European patients have not been confirmed in more recent studies using more sensitive tests.[17]

Cutaneous T-cell lymphoma of the mycosis fungoides type

Clinical features[18]

The common age range at presentation with cutaneous T-cell lymphoma of the mycosis fungoides type is in the sixth and seventh decade, although rare childhood cases are reported.[19] In the majority of

reported series, males are affected more frequently than females. The characteristic clinical progression of patients with mycosis fungoides is an initial phase during which the patient complains of small pruritic plaques, covering less than 10 per cent of the body surface (Figures 11.1 and 11.2).[20] Some of these resolve spontaneously, while new lesions appear elsewhere. These lesions appear most frequently on the trunk, particularly on the breast and buttocks. Biopsies taken at this point in time are not usually diagnostic of cutaneous T-cell lymphoma, and although the clinical suspicion is high, there are at present no ancillary diagnostic tests of value at this stage.

After a variable period of time, frequently 2–3 years, the erythematous elevated pruritic plaques become

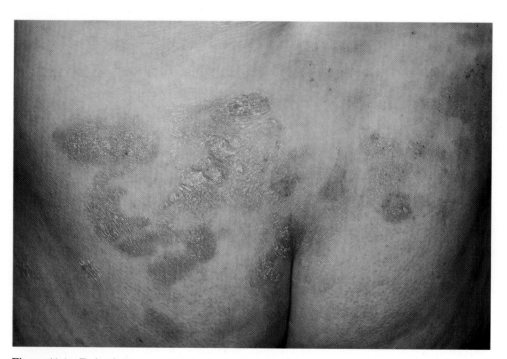

Figure 11.1   Early plaque-stage mycosis fungoides, buttock lesions.

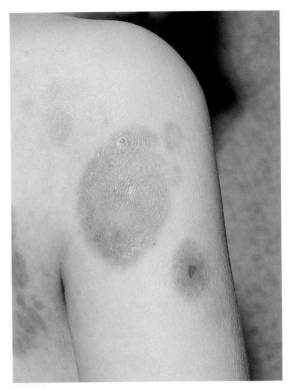

Figure 11.2 Early plaque mycosis fungoides on the upper arm.

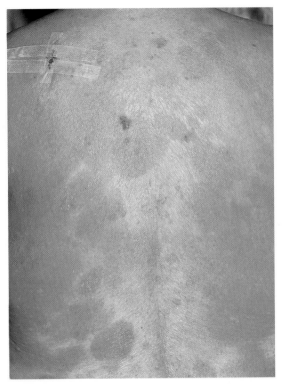

Figure 11.3 Extensive plaque mycosis fungoides on the back.

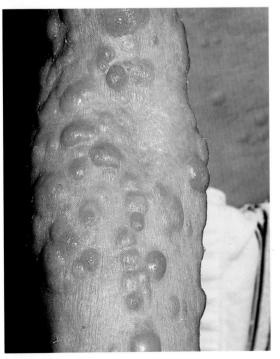

Figure 11.4 Nodular mycosis fungoides on the forearm.

more numerous (Figure 11.3), and additional nodules may develop (Figure 11.4). More than 10 per cent of the body surface may now be involved, and the pattern of spontaneous resolution of individual plaques seen in the earlier phase becomes less frequent.

Biopsies of plaques at this stage should show confirmatory signs of cutaneous T-cell lymphoma, and a study in the USA has reported an interval of nearly 4 years between clinical suspicion of mycosis fungoides and pathological confirmation. The essential feature for this diagnosis is the presence of atypical T-helper lymphocytes with convoluted nuclei in the epidermis. These cells appear to have a particular affinity for the epidermis, in that they will be seen colonizing the epidermis even when the total infiltrate

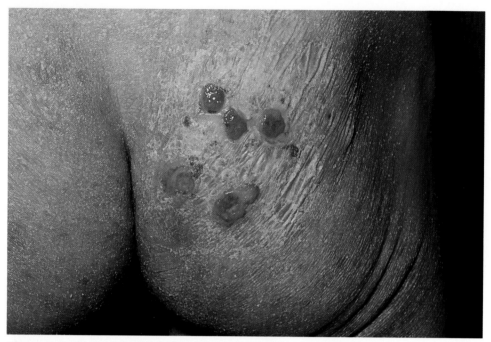

Figure 11.5   'Tumeur d'emblée' variant of mycosis fungoides, buttock lesions.

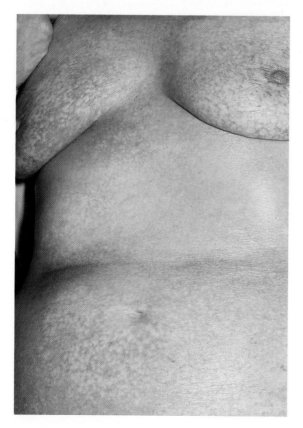

in the dermis is fairly sparse. There is little, if any, spongiosis, and this will help in distinguishing the condition from a dermatitis reaction.

Once large plaques develop on the cutaneous surface, there is a tendency for them to show partial central resolution with peripheral extension. This can give rise to very striking and bizarre annular and polycyclic shapes, commonly seen on the trunk. The peripheral margin of the polycyclic rings may break down to give annular ulceration, and nodules may develop in and around these large plaques. These nodules rapidly break down and ulcerate.

A proportion of patients with mycosis fungoides present with raised nodules as the first clinical sign. This is the so-called 'tumeur d'emblée' type (Figure 11.5). Others may present with either poikiloderma (literally dappled skin, Figure 11.6) or erythroderma (Figure 11.7). The patients with the poikiloderma

Figure 11.6   Poikilodermatous mycosis fungoides lesions on abdominal and breast skin.

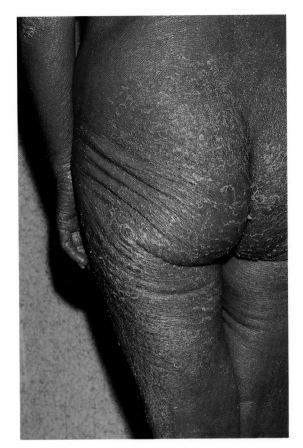

Figure 11.7 Erythrodermic mycosis fungoides.

type of presentation show colour changes on the skin of the breast and buttock area, which may be atrophic, painful and pruritic. This initial type of presentation tends to be associated with a slow extension of similar lesions over the rest of the body surface rather than the progression reported above from small plaques, to larger plaques covering a large part of the body surface, to nodules.

Patients with erythrodermic mycosis fungoides tend to present with a rather more acute disorder, and the interval between clinical presentation and the ability to make a definitive pathological diagnosis is shorter than for patients presenting with plaque-type disease. These patients frequently have a total body erythroderma with profuse fine scaling, and at an early stage may show evidence of damage to the skin appendages with hair loss and nail dystrophy.

Many patients with cutaneous T-cell lymphoma have exclusively cutaneous problems for many years. The majority of patients do not, in the early stages, have palpable lymphadenopathy or evidence of involvement of other organs. Because of the advanced age of many patients at first presentation, a number may die of causes unrelated to their cutaneous T-cell lymphoma, and at autopsy will be found to have no involvement of organs other than the skin.

A proportion of patients with cutaneous T-cell lymphoma will, however, develop palpable lymphadenopathy. This proportion varies in reported series, but appears to be larger in the USA than in Europe. Node biopsy of these lesions may reveal either what is interpreted as a reactive dermatopathic lymphadenopathy, or evidence of frank involvement with malignant T-helper cells.[21] It has been suggested that the barrier to the spreading of cutaneous T-cell lymphoma from the skin to other organs lies between the skin and the lymph nodes, as once clinical lymphadenopathy, which is due to histologically proven infiltration with malignant T-cells, is present, the disease frequently progresses much more rapidly, with involvement of other organs and death. The proportion of patients who develop cutaneous T-cell lymphoma outwith the skin and who die from it varies in series reported from various parts of the world. Series reported from the USA[22,23] in the period 1960–75 suggested that cutaneous T-cell lymphoma was frequently a fatal disease, whereas series from other parts of the world, particularly Europe, suggested that it tended to follow a more chronic benign course. Retrospective analysis of clinical, pathological and therapeutic variables in these series is difficult. It may be that the American series have a higher mortality because of the concentration of patients with more aggressive disease in specialized centres, whereas series from other parts of the world may have included patients with relatively benign simulants of cutaneous T-cell lymphoma. Careful prospective studies using modern pathological techniques with monoclonal antibodies and T-cell receptor probes will allow long-term follow-up and comparisons of clearly defined cohorts.

Pathology

The essential histological feature of cutaneous T-cell lymphoma of the mycosis fungoides type is the identification of atypical lymphocytes in the epidermis and

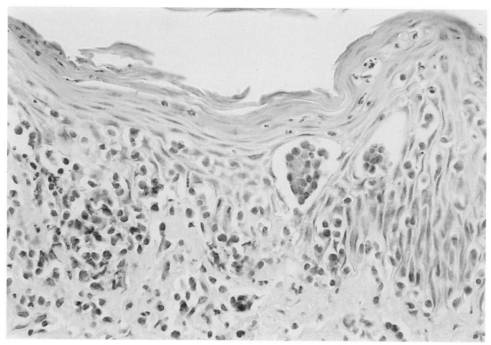

Figure 11.8 Low-power view of mycosis fungoides stained with haematoxylin and eosin, showing two large, Pautrier-like abscesses.

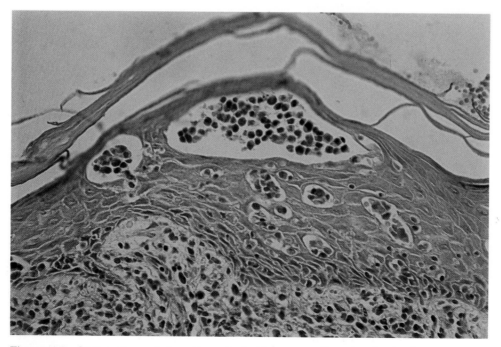

Figure 11.9 Section of mycosis fungoides stained with haematoxylin and eosin, showing several Pautrier microabscesses.

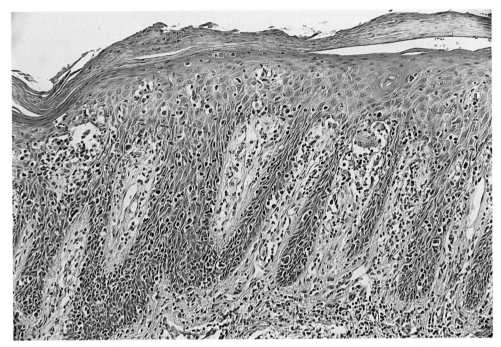

Figure 11.10 Histology of the patient illustrated in Figure 11.7. Note the rather psoriasiform epidermis but also the presence of Pautrier abscesses.

in the papillary dermis (Figures 11.8–11.10). The lymphocytic infiltrate is characterized by the use of monoclonal antibodies as being predominantly T-helper lymphocytes. It should, however, be borne in mind that the great majority of cutaneous lymphocytic infiltrates of all types, both benign and malignant, are of the T-helper subclass, and therefore the presence of T-helper cells in the epidermis and papillary dermis is not specific for cutaneous T-cell lymphoma. The pattern of distribution of this T-helper infiltrate in mycosis fungoides is epidermotropic, and epidermal spongiosis is minimal. In the early stages, there may be small numbers of other cell types, particularly eosinophils, present, but the infiltrate becomes more monomorphic with advancing disease.

Careful examination under the high-power objective of the microscope will reveal that the T-cells in the epidermis are frequently present in clusters forming the so-called Pautrier microabscesses, and examination of thin sections cut at 1–2 μm under oil immersion, or ultrastructural studies, will reveal that these T-cells are atypical, having large hyperconvoluted nuclei. These are the T-cells identified by Lutzner, and morphologically they are very similar to the circulating atypical mononuclear cells seen in the Sézary syndrome.[3,4]

If cutaneous T-cell lymphoma is untreated, and progressive disease develops, the volume of the cutaneous T-cell infiltrate tends to increase, and very large numbers of atypical T-lymphocytes may be found in cutaneous nodules. In some patients with advanced disease there appears to be a relative loss of the epidermotropic quality of the T-lymphocytes, but this is not an invariable finding.

In the early stages of cutaneous T-cell lymphoma, a small proportion of T-suppressor lymphocytes will be found with the predominant T-helper lymphocyte population, but as the disease progresses, sequential studies suggest that the ratio of T-helper to T-suppressor lymphocytes in the skin rises.

If peripheral blood smears are examined from patients with cutaneous T-cell lymphoma of the mycosis fungoides type, a large number of patients will be found to have a small proportion (1–2 per cent) of circulating atypical lymphocytes. The presence of small numbers of such cells should not automatically lead to a diagnosis of the Sézary syndrome, which should be reserved for patients who have 5 per cent or more of such large atypical cells present. Purists would also advocate that erythroderma and lymphadenopathy are required for this diagnosis.

Examination of the bone marrow, 'blind' lymph node biopsy of clinically impalpable nodes, and liver and spleen biopsy in early mycosis fungoides generally yield negative results, and such procedures are not considered necessary for routine staging of cutaneous T-cell lymphoma although they have in the past been regarded as necessary in investigative and research studies.[23]

Staging of cutaneous T-cell lymphoma

Table 11.1 gives the Tumour Nodes Metastases (TNM) classification of cutaneous T-cell lymphoma currently used with an additional B classification for the peripheral blood. Slightly different staging classifications are in use in certain parts of the world.

The use of one or other of the currently defined staging systems is recommended as part of the initial investigations of a patient with suspected cutaneous T-cell lymphoma so that therapeutic studies may be reported on a well-defined group of patients and valid comparisons can be made between series from different centres.

At present there is some interest in the use of radio-labelled monoclonal antibodies raised against T-lymphocytes in imaging clinically unidentified deposits of mycosis fungoides cells. Reports are divided on the value of this technique, which is still in the early stages of development.[24,25]

Other investigations

Workers in Europe have advocated the use of DNA cytophotometry and the nuclear contour index

Table 11.1 TNM B classification of cutaneous T-cell lymphoma.

T0	Clinically suspicious plaques, pathologically non-diagnostic
T1	Limited plaques covering less than 10 per cent of the body surface. Pathology diagnostic
T2	Generalized plaques covering 10 per cent or more of the body surface. Pathology diagnostic
T3	One or more cutaneous nodules. Pathology diagnostic
N0	No clinical lymphadenopathy
N1	Lymph nodes clinically palpable. Pathology shows only reactive lymphadenopathy
N2	No clinically palpable lymph nodes but pathology shows CTCL in nodes
N3	Clinically palpable lymph nodes. Pathology confirms CTCL
M0	No involvement of internal organs
M1	Visceral organs involved (organs should be specified)
B0	Atypical lymphocytes, if present, comprise less than 5 per cent of white count
B1	More than 5 per cent of total white count composed of atypical lymphocytes

measurement as useful assessments of patients whose histology is not confirmatory of mycosis fungoides.[26]

DNA cytophotometry is a method of quantifying the total DNA in the cell nucleus, and high levels are in general associated with a malignant phenotype. Measurement of the nuclear contour index involves taking a representative selection of cells seen on ultrastructural examination, and relating the perimeter of the nucleus, which is an index of the degree of nuclear convolution, to the nuclear diameter. Clearly, this is a time-consuming technique, and there is a degree of bias possible in selecting the cells to be measured. It has, however, been suggested that using these tests it may be possible to assign patients either to a benign reactive or early mycosis fungoides group earlier than is possible by conventional haematoxylin and eosin examination. Few centres carry out these tests at the present time and confirmation of their value from other centres would clearly be of value. A comparison of these tests with analysis of DNA from the T-cell receptor would also be a useful contribution. It may be that these sophisticated aids to earlier diagnosis will become more widely used when we have curative therapy available for early disease.

Management[27]

The management of mycosis fungoides varies greatly in different centres and in different continents. This reflects the fact that at present there is no proven curative method of managing this condition. In general there is a tendency in Europe to approach treatment in terms of disease control rather than cure, and to aim for symptom relief rather than to offer early and aggressive chemotherapy. In the USA a large study has recently been carried out with the aim of identifying and treating mycosis fungoides in a more aggressive manner in the early stages of the disease, aiming at cure rather than at palliation. This approach was based on the observations of the improved prognosis in the leukaemias and in Hodgkin's disease with an early and aggressive approach to therapy. Preliminary reports of the results of this study do not suggest that this is a major therapeutic advance.

Once the pathological diagnosis is confirmed, the patient's symptoms and need for therapy should be assessed. Mild pruritus and the presence of a few plaques in an elderly patient may be quite adequately controlled with a topical steroid. In some cases this may need to be augmented with UVB therapy, particularly in the winter months. This regime may be all that is required to keep a patient completely symptom-free and is a perfectly acceptable approach to management in an elderly individual who is not in great discomfort.

If plaque lesions are more extensive and severe pruritus has not responded to topical steroids and/or UVB, alternative therapies to be considered are photochemotherapy (PUVA), topical nitrogen mustard, and radiotherapy in the form either of electron beam or local tumour dose radiotherapy to individual plaques and nodules. The choice of treatment will depend on the type of disease present, the patient's age and general condition, local availability, and the physician's experience.

Photochemotherapy

Photochemotherapy has now been used for the management of mycosis fungoides for two decades.[28-31] The majority of centres that have used photochemotherapy report good results with PUVA, provided maintenance treatment is used. A large number of treatment schedules have been established and studies comparing regimes which treat to clearance of lesions and then discontinue PUVA with treatment regimes which treat to clearance and then reduce the UVA dose for maintenance therapy show that the latter approach is more satisfactory.

Most centres using PUVA for routine treatment of mycosis fungoides carry out skin biopsies at 3–6 month intervals. A comparison of histology before and during PUVA therapy will show that the cutaneous T-helper cell infiltrate is grossly reduced, but has not disappeared completely, and, in comparison with the pretreatment appearance, there is a clearance of lymphocytes from the epidermis and a relative aggregation of mycosis fungoides cells in the deeper parts of the dermis (Figures 11.11–11.14).[32] The Langerhans cell population is greatly reduced during PUVA therapy, but it has not been established whether or not this reduction is in any way related to the good response to PUVA seen in patients with mycosis fungoides. PUVA is particularly useful therapy for patients who complain of extensive and severe pruritus, as relief of pruritus may be achieved within 3–4 days of starting PUVA therapy.

As with other conditions requiring long-term PUVA therapy, patients with mycosis fungoides do require regular supervision and examination in case of development of non-melanoma skin cancer or preceding actinic keratosis. Reports of these events in mycosis fungoides patients to date are very few.[33]

Most patients on PUVA therapy will need to use emollient therapy, as PUVA tends to dry the skin, but few will require other topical treatments, and in general it is possible to withdraw potent topical steroid therapy.

Topical nitrogen mustard and BCNU therapy

The use of topical nitrogen mustard for the control of mycosis fungoides was first introduced by Van Scott and Kalmanson and is a popular method of managing patients in many centres.[34] It is of particular value for

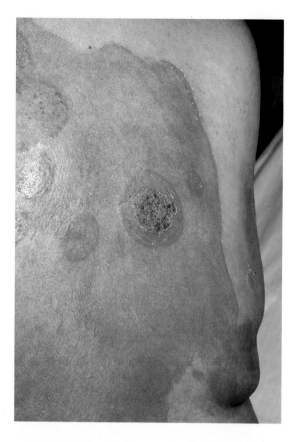

patients who live at a distance from a PUVA centre and who cannot readily attend for maintenance therapy. Early reports used an aqueous solution which had to be made up immediately before application to the skin because of instability. This was expensive and inconvenient. More recently many centres have advocated the use of an aqueous cream containing nitrogen mustard which has a shelf-life of some 3 months.[35]

Patients using topical nitrogen mustard should be instructed to apply the preparation to the affected skin lesions using protective gloves for the hands. Initially, the treatment may need to be used daily, but with response this can be cut down to twice or even once

Figures 11.11 and 11.12   Clinical and histological features of advanced plaque mycosis fungoides with early tumours before therapy.

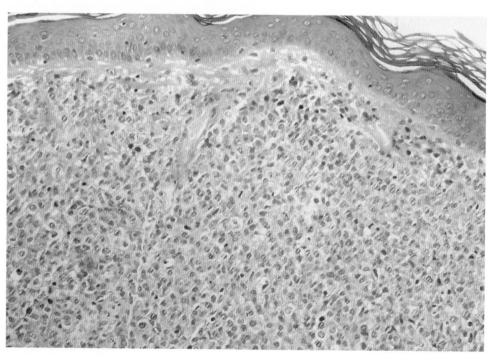

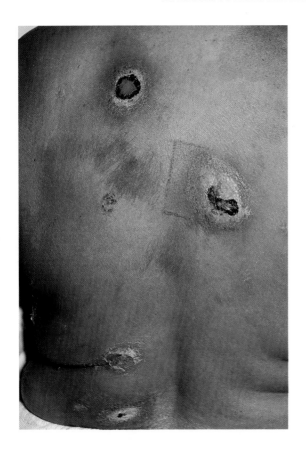

per week. A number of patients develop an allergic contact dermatitis to nitrogen mustard which appears to be relatively common in fair-skinned Caucasians. A desensitization regime can be used but personal experience would suggest that patients find this regime difficult to follow.

There are reports of non-melanoma skin cancer developing on the skin of patients who have used nitrogen mustard in this way, and therefore careful follow-up is needed.[36]

Topical BCNU therapy has been used in the same way, and a recent review of 15 years' experience suggests 5-year survival rates of around 77 per cent.[37]

Figures 11.13 and 11.14 The same patient as in Figures 11.11 and 11.12 after 4 weeks' PUVA therapy given three times per week.

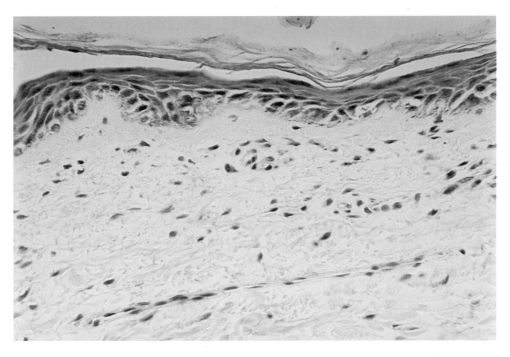

Electron beam therapy

The pioneering work by Fuks[38] using electron beam therapy as a form of superficial radiation treatment for mycosis fungoides has been developed in many centres. This treatment is based on the principle that electrons will only penetrate a few millimetres into the dermis and epidermis, and thus the dose of radiation will be maximal where it is most needed. In the 1970s, and before the introduction of photochemotherapy, electron beam therapy was used widely in many centres. It was suggested that, if used early and aggressively, electron beam therapy could result in cure rather than control of mycosis fungoides. In the event, it has been found that long-term remissions lasting 5 or even 10 years have been achieved with doses of 3000 cGy of radiation given over varying treatment schedules, but a great number of patients who had electron beam therapy many years ago have now experienced recurrence of the disease so once again this treatment should be regarded as palliative rather than curative. A relatively common treatment schedule in the UK is a total dose of 3000 cGy, divided into 10 doses of 300 cGy given twice weekly for 5 weeks.[39] Temporary alopecia will occur, and nails may be shed if they are not protected. The eyes must be protected, and use of internal eyeshields will prevent persistence of periorbital lesions. The electrons are generated in a linear accelerator, from which patients stand several metres away. Different radiation fields may need to be designed according to the locally available machine to allow uniform treatment of all body sites.

Short-term side-effects of this therapy include temporary increase in pruritus, nausea, limb oedema, and, occasionally, marrow suppression. Longer-term problems include telangiectasis and a persistent dry skin.

Many of the individual treatment modalities advocated for mycosis fungoides can be used in combination, and the combined use of electron beam and chemotherapy is reported to be beneficial.[40]

Chemotherapy

At present there are no systemic chemotherapeutic regimes of confirmed proven value in mycosis fungoides. In the early stage of the disease, treatment logically should be aimed at the epidermis rather than the peripheral blood, and in later disease stages many patients appear to respond poorly, if at all, and rapidly develop opportunistic infections, which frequently are the cause of death. There are in the literature a few reports of short-term benefit following use of the specific anti-T-cell cytotoxic drug, deoxycoformycin. This drug is specific for T-cells, but is toxic to both normal and malignant T-cells, so severe immunosuppression is a recognized side-effect. The place of this drug in the therapy of mycosis fungoides is not yet established.

Retinoids, interferons and photopheresis

Both retinoids and interferons have been used with benefit in patients with T-cell lymphoma. Etretinate and also isotretinoin have been reported to be of benefit, using relatively high doses, in the order of 1.5–2.0 mg/kg of retinoid per day. Remissions, even of lymph node disease, are reported.[41–44]

A second experimental approach to the management of mycosis fungoides is the use of interferons,[45–48] which have been used both singly and in combination with either retinoids or PUVA, with additional benefit.[49] Controlled trials are needed, but the diversity of presentation and subsequent disease progression in mycosis fungoides makes this a particularly difficult area for accurate assessment of response.

A further experimental approach to therapy for mycosis fungoides and the Sézary syndrome (see below) is the use of photopheresis, pioneered by Edelson et al.[50–52] This involves connecting the patient to a leucopheresis machine, and, after giving oral psoralen, irradiating the patient's white cells ex vivo with UVA while they are passing through a thin-walled polythene filter before returning them to the patient. Some long-term remissions have been reported in a small number of patients treated by this method but to date there are no comparative trials. This approach implies that treating cells in the peripheral blood rather than in the skin may be of value, and it is of interest that this approach currently looks much more promising than systemic chemotherapy. The mechanisms involved in the observed beneficial effect are not yet understood, but an increasing number of centres now have access to photopheresis technology.

The therapeutic use of monoclonal antibodies in mycosis fungoides appears to have some temporary benefit in a small number of patients.[53]

The Sézary syndrome[3]

The clinical presentation with the Sézary syndrome is usually that of an elderly male with erythroderma (Figures 11.15 and 11.16), lymphadenopathy, and a high total white count with a high proportion, frequently over 50 per cent, of atypical lymphocytes. It is, however, possible for patients to have the Sézary syndrome with a normal total white count, but an abnormal subpopulation.

Examination of a peripheral blood film will show the presence of cerebriform mononuclear cells. These large Sézary cells have a very large nucleus with scanty cytoplasm and even on light microscopy the hyperconvoluted shape of the nucleus will be apparent.

Diagnosis of the fully established Sézary syndrome is relatively straightforward, based on clinical observation, skin biopsy, and peripheral blood examination. However, as with classic mycosis fungoides, the early stages of the Sézary syndrome may be difficult to diagnose as patients may have erythroderma associated with atopic dermatitis, psoriasis, or a persistent unidentified contact allergy. In all of these situations there may be reactive benign dermatopathic lymphadenopathy, and a small proportion (1–3 per cent) of atypical circulating mononuclear cells may be seen. Recent work from the Netherlands has suggested that in this situation useful aids to earlier diagnosis are the presence of an expanded T-helper subset in the peripheral blood with a ratio of helper to suppressor T-cells greater than 10 and a nuclear contour index greater than 5.5.[54,55]

Pathology

Biopsy of the skin in the Sézary syndrome will show the presence of large numbers of T-lymphocytes.[56] Marker studies will show that the majority of these cells are of the T-helper subset.

The epidermotropic distribution of the lymphocytes seen in classic mycosis fungoides is not always present in the Sézary syndrome, and a more dense infiltrate may be seen in the papillary dermis. Biopsy of palpable lymph nodes in the early stages may show only a reactive pattern, but later will show the presence of Sézary cells. Examination of the bone marrow will frequently reveal the presence of Sézary cells. The total circulating leucocyte count may be very high indeed in leukaemic phases of the Sézary syndrome, and in severe cases 90 per cent or more of the circulating mononuclear cells may be Sézary cells.

Management

Patients with erythroderma due to the Sézary syndrome respond well to photochemotherapy, provided a low initial dose of UVA is used. However, it is often necessary to combine this with a cytotoxic drug such as low-dose oral chlorambucil. This combination can provide useful long-term maintenance therapy.

Some patients with the Sézary syndrome have relatively few cutaneous lesions but have large numbers of atypical circulating mononuclear cells. These patients respond well to low-dose chlorambucil and prednisolone therapy.[57] There are reports of treatment of the Sézary syndrome with combination therapy such as CHOP, but, as with mycosis fungoides, patients with the Sézary syndrome tend rapidly to become immunosuppressed and develop opportunistic infections.

There is currently considerable interest in the use of photopheresis as described in the section on mycosis fungoides for the Sézary syndrome.[52] Photopheresis should be particularly successful in this condition, as the peripheral blood cells are treated directly.

Pagetoid reticulosis (localized epidermotropic reticulosis, or Woringer–Kolopp disease)

In 1939 a description was given of a 13-year-old boy having a single polycyclic plaque on the left forearm that had been present since he was aged 7. Woringer and Kolopp reported that biopsy of this lesion showed atypical mycosis-like cells invading the epidermis.[58] Since this time, a small number of patients have been described with this entity and its exact relationship to the more aggressive types of cutaneous T-cell lymphoma is still debated.

Clinical features[59]

The majority of cases reported to date are in men, and the lesions present as isolated, slowly expanding

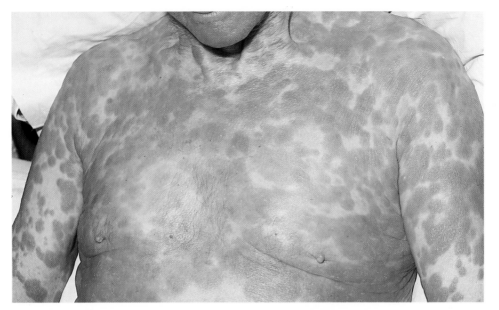

Figure 11.15   Extensive lesions on the trunk in the Sézary syndrome.

plaques, most often on the lower limb (Figure 11.17). There is frequently a history of the lesion being present in isolation for 2–3 years and slowly expanding peripherally. Some patients give a history of trauma before the appearance of the lesion, and the clinical differential diagnosis may well include a cutaneous fungal infection. The great majority of cases reported to date are Caucasian.

Pathology

A skin biopsy will show a dense lymphocytic infiltrate in the papillary dermis and epidermis. In comparison with classic mycosis fungoides, the infiltrate in Woringer–Kolopp disease is more epidermotropic (Figure 11.18). The alternative name, Pagetoid reticulosis, describes well the dense infiltration of the epidermis with T-lymphocytes in a pattern similar to the epidermal colonization of Paget's disease. Marker studies have been carried out in only a small number of patients. These report that the lymphocytes bear the T-subset marker, but some reported cases are predominantly T-suppressor cells in contrast to the T-helper cells more common in other types of cutaneous lymphoma.[60] In addition to the T-lymphocyte population, histiocytes have been reported in association with the lymphocytic infiltrate.[61]

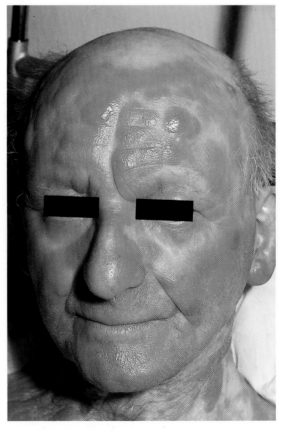

Figure 11.16   The Sézary syndrome – facial appearance.

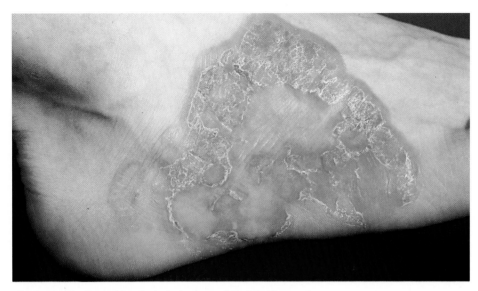

Figure 11.17   Pagetoid reticulosis (patient of Dr RS Chapman).

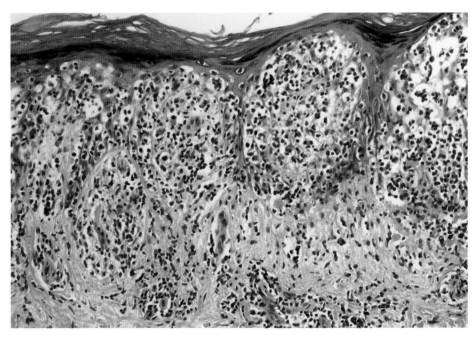

Figure 11.18   Histological features of Pagetoid reticulosis, showing striking epidermotropism.

Management

This condition frequently affects young people and may persist with relatively little change for many years. There is not, in contrast to mycosis fungoides, a tendency for new lesions to appear in other sites. The bulk of reported cases have been treated successfully with local low-dose radiotherapy, and follow-up studies suggest that the lesion does not occur on the original site, nor do new lesions appear in other sites.

CD30 lymphomas[62]

The Ki 1 or CD30 antigen is seen on Reed–Sternberg cells in Hodgkin's disease, and also on the cells of some large-cell lymphomas, of both B- and T-cell origin, on isolated large cells in lymphomatoid papulosis, and in a miscellaneous group of conditions, including so-called regressing atypical histiocytosis.

Primary CD30 cutaneous T-cell lymphoma

Clinical features

This condition is seen in adults, who usually present with one large isolated nodule on the trunk.

Pathology

The diagnostic features are the absence of epidermotropism, and the presence in the dermis of dense infiltrate (usually T-cell) which contains multinucleate giant cells and numerous mitotic figures. T-cell markers and gene rearrangement studies both confirm the T-cell nature of these cells.

Treatment

Many of the nodules regress spontaneously, but radiotherapy is effective for persistent lesions. The prognosis is excellent with over 90 per cent of patients alive and disease-free at 5 years.

Lymphomatoid papulosis

This condition was described by Macaulay[63] in 1968, who reported a clinically benign self-healing 'rhythmical paradoxical' skin eruption that had many clinical features similar to the acute form of pityriasis lichenoides but a histology suggesting a malignant lymphoma.

Clinical features

Patients with lymphomatoid papulosis may present at any time in adult life. In a recent Danish study, the mean age at presentation was 43 years.[64] Patients give a history of the development of recurrent crops of erythematous papules, mainly on the trunk, which rapidly break down to form necrotic ulcerated lesions. These lesions heal slowly, with scarring, and after a variable period of time a fresh crop appears (Figures 11.19 and 11.20). The clinical appearance of these lesions may be confusing. In the erythematous and papular stage, a vasculitis may be suspected, and the scarring may even suggest self-inflicted dermatitis artefacta.

Pathology

The pathological features of lymphomatoid papulosis are those of a dense T-lymphocyte infiltrate involving the epidermis and the papillary dermis. In comparison with the lymphocytes in mycosis fungoides, the lymphocytes involved in lymphomatoid papulosis may be even more cytologically atypical and disturbing, strongly suggesting a rapidly progressive malignant lymphocytic proliferation (Figures 11.21 and 11.22).

In 1982 Willemze and colleagues suggested that two types of lymphomatoid papulosis could be identified.[65] Type A showed predominantly atypical cerebriform T-lymphocytes, and type B showed large numbers of cells that were apparently non-lymphocytic and possibly related to the Langerhans cell series. No other group has as yet related these pathological varieties to prognosis or to response to treatment. Cell marker studies on lymphomatoid papulosis have confirmed that the majority of lymphocytes in this condition are of the T-helper subset. A proportion of the cells are very large, with a morphology

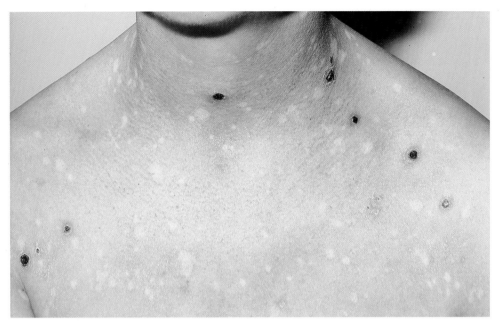

Figure 11.19   Clinical features of lymphomatoid papulosis.

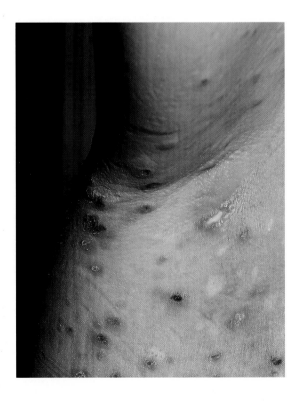

Figure 11.20   Lymphomatoid papulosis, showing numerous active lesions in the axilla.

similar to the Reed–Sternberg cells of Hodgkin's disease, and these cells are also CD30 positive.

Management

The original description of lymphomatoid papulosis suggested that patients might continue for many years with recurrent crops of these lesions, which did not progress. This has been confirmed in a number of series, but in addition there are individual case reports of patients with apparently classic lymphomatoid papulosis developing mycosis fungoides, or Hodgkin's disease, either before or after the diagnosis of lymphomatoid papulosis is made.[66]

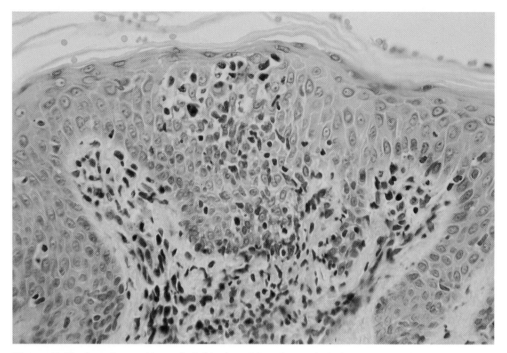

Figure 11.21 Lymphomatoid papulosis histology. Note the cytological appearance of atypical lymphocytes in the epidermis.

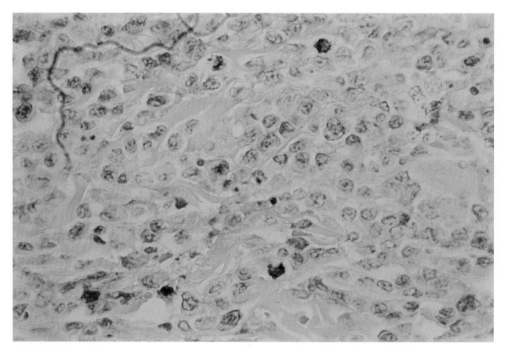

Figure 11.22 High-power view of the histology of dermal infiltrate in lymphomatoid papulosis. Note numerous atypical mitoses.

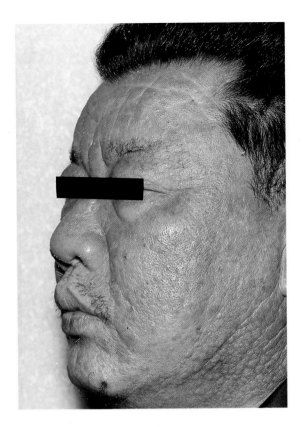

In some individuals new crops of lymphomatoid papulosis lesions can be averted by potent topical steroids or by injection of intralesional steroid. Other individuals find that low-dose maintenance photochemotherapy prevents the development of lesions, and the use of single agent cytotoxic drugs such as methotrexate has been reported to be effective.[67] Individual choice of treatment will depend on local availability and the degree of discomfort. Long-term follow-up is clearly necessary.

Actinic reticuloid

This condition was first recognized by Ive et al[68] in 1969, who described a group of individuals, mainly males, who developed very severe and persistent photosensitivity and who were found on phototesting to be sensitive to UV radiation of all wavelengths, and even to light in all the visible part of the spectrum.

Figure 11.23 Actinic reticuloid. Note the thickened facial skin.

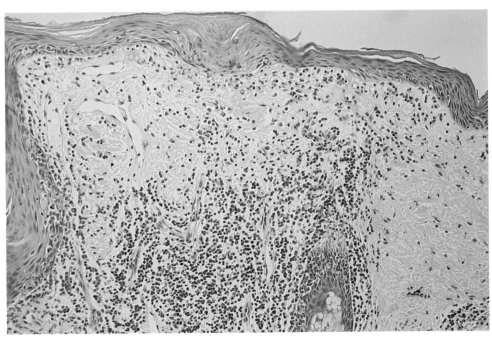

Figure 11.24 Histological features of actinic reticuloid. Note the deep lymphocytic infiltrate and surrounding solar elastosis.

These patients had a dense and deep lymphocytic infiltrate with atypical cells present in their skin. The original paper suggested that treatment was difficult and unrewarding.

Clinical features

Since the original publication a number of workers have confirmed the existence of this severe and persistent photodermatitis. Some groups prefer the term chronic photodermatitis/actinic reticuloid, but others use the term actinic reticuloid to describe an acute and persisting photodermatitis with sensitivity to wavelengths right through the UV spectrum and into longer-wave visible light.

The clinical appearance is usually that of an elderly male with erythematous thickened indurated skin on the face and neck (Figure 11.23). There is usually a very sharp transition between thickened exposed and normal unexposed skin on the back of the neck, and the facial appearance may be coarsened and leonine. Other exposed sites, such as the hands, are involved in a similar fashion. The patient may give a history of slight improvement in the winter months but of rapid and severe deterioration on exposure to any sunlight. These patients may also react to sunlight through window-glass.

Pathology

The pathology of actinic reticuloid is that of a dense infiltrate of T-lymphocytes involving the epidermis and dermis (Figure 11.24). In contrast to cutaneous lymphoma of the mycosis fungoides type, this lymphocytic infiltrate extends deeply throughout the entire dermis. There may be some non-lymphoid cells present, notably eosinophils.

Management

Once the diagnosis is confirmed, a search should be made for evidence of coexistent mycosis fungoides or other lymphoma, as this may be present initially, or may develop some years after actinic reticuloid is diagnosed. If no such problem is found, the patient should use broad-band UVA and UVB sunscreens. In practice, it is often found that physical titanium dioxide-containing sunscreen barrier preparations are required to control

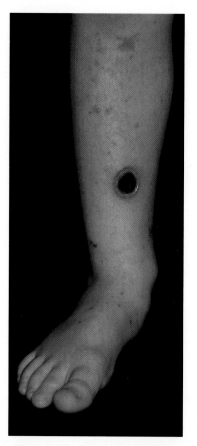

Figure 11.25   Deep vasculitis lesions in a patient with lymphomatoid pityriasis lichenoides.

this condition. Patients must be advised to avoid exposure to all sunlight. The windows of their homes can be screened with an appropriate UV-screening film. Some patients respond well to systemic azathioprine.

These measures may greatly improve the patient's condition, but low-dose systemic steroids and/or azathioprine may also be required to maintain the skin in a comfortable condition.[69] Topical steroids are of variable value. Once again, long-term follow-up is essential.

Lymphomatoid pityriasis lichenoides

This entity was described by Black and Wilson Jones[70] shortly after the description by Macaulay of lymphomatoid papulosis. There are many similarities between the two conditions.

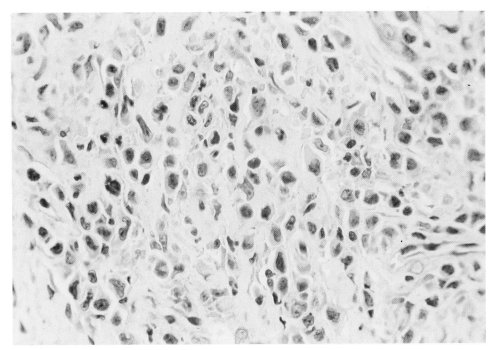

Figure 11.26 High-power view of dermal infiltrate in lymphomatoid pityriasis lichenoides, showing striking lymphocytic nuclear atypia. This biopsy was taken 20 years ago from a 3-year-old boy who is now a fit and healthy 23-year-old.

Clinical features

The patients with lymphomatoid pityriasis lichenoides may be of any age and children have been reported with this condition. Patients present with scaling plaques and small crops of elevated papules. In contrast to lymphomatoid papulosis, most of the individual lesions are slightly smaller but a small number break down to form such large necrotic ulcerating areas (Figure 11.25). The condition may persist with seasonal remissions and recurrences for many years.

Pathology

The pathology is that of a lymphocytic vasculitis. As with the other conditions in this group, individual lymphocytes show cytologically disturbing features suggestive of a malignant phenotype. Despite these cytological features in an individual patient, the condition may persist as a chronic problem with little change for many years (Figure 11.26).

Management

The patient should be screened for evidence of mycosis fungoides or other lymphoma, and if the results of this screening are negative, it may be possible to control but not completely clear the condition with potent topical steroid applications or with UVB therapy. PUVA has been reported to be used successfully in this condition, and there are individual case reports suggesting that a wide range of oral preparations, such as dapsone and tetracycline, may be of value.

Lymphomatoid granulomatosis

Lymphomatoid granulomatosis was first described in 1972.[71] Initially this was a problem that mainly involved the pulmonary system, but over the past decade cutaneous involvement with lymphomatoid granulomatosis has been described. A study in 1979 reported that cutaneous lesions were present in 40 per cent of 152 cases.[72] These may be either an erythematous rash or cutaneous nodules.[73,74]

Clinical features

The clinical features of lymphomatoid granulomatosis are very variable, but the general pattern is that of extensive indurated violaceous plaques, reddish or blue nodules, ulceration, dry skin or acquired ichthyosis and follicular hyperkeratosis. The loss of body hair and absence of sweating reflects the striking damage seen to the skin appendages on pathological examination.

Pathology

The pathology of cutaneous involvement with lymphomatoid granulomatosis is that of a deep-seated granulomatous mixed lymphohistiocytic infiltrate. In contrast to mycosis fungoides, the epidermis and papillary dermis are completely spared, and on low-power microscopic examination a dense infiltrate will be seen in the deeper part of the reticular dermis, mainly centred around vessels and also both around and destroying the skin appendages. High-power examination will show that the lymphocytes involved are cytologically malignant. The degree of dermal appendage involvement is thought to be of value in making the diagnosis.

Management

If lymphomatoid granulomatosis is suspected on clinical or pathological grounds on examination of cutaneous lesions, complete staging of the patient and examination for other organ involvement, particularly the lungs, is essential. Patients with predominantly pulmonary involvement have been reported to respond well to cyclophosphamide and prednisolone, but those with cutaneous lesions do not appear to respond as well on this regime as those with no cutaneous lesions. Further information is needed on long-term follow-up of patients with cutaneous involvement with lymphomatoid granulomatosis to determine the value of currently advocated treatment regimes.

B-cell cutaneous lymphoma

B-cell infiltration of the skin is less common than T-cell infiltration. This applies to both benign and malignant cutaneous lymphocytic infiltrates. Before the availability of monoclonal antibodies, it was suggested that T-cell and B-cell lymphocytic patterns of infiltrate in the skin could be recognized as discrete entities. The T-cell pattern was the epidermotropic, 'top-heavy' infiltrate involving the epidermis and the papillary dermis, while the B-cell infiltrate pattern involved a relative sparing of the epidermis, a lymphocyte-free Grenz zone in the papillary dermis, and the bulk of the infiltrate seen in the deeper parts of the reticular dermis. With the advent of monoclonal antibodies it has been found that, although the so-called T-cell pattern does appear to contain almost exclusively T-lymphocytes, infiltrates with a so-called B-cell pattern may in fact be composed of T-cells. A good example of this is Jessner's lymphocytic infiltrate, which has been shown to be a T-cell disorder, although the pattern of dermal involvement is what used to be described as a B-cell pattern.

Clinical features

B-cell lymphoma in the skin is rare and may involve B-cells at various stages of differentiation. The usual cutaneous appearance is of large indurated nodules, and these nodules are usually present at a time when lymphadenopathy has already developed (Figures 11.27 and 11.28).[75] It is unusual for cutaneous lesions to be the first presenting feature of a B-cell lymphoma.

Pathology

As described above, a B-cell lymphocytic infiltrate in the skin will be characterized by a relative absence of epidermotropism, and a dense 'bottom-heavy' infiltrate (Figure 11.29). The B-lymphocytes may have a wide range of cytological characteristics depending on the degree of malignancy (Figure 11.30). Once again, cell marker studies are strongly advocated to confirm the type of cell present.

Management

The management of cutaneous B-cell lymphoma involves screening for liver, spleen and bone marrow involvement. Usually these will be present, and patients may respond well to quadruple chemotherapy

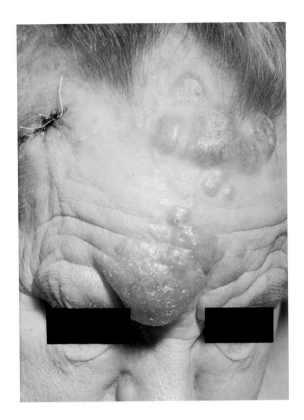

Figure 11.27 Facial nodules of B-cell lymphoma.

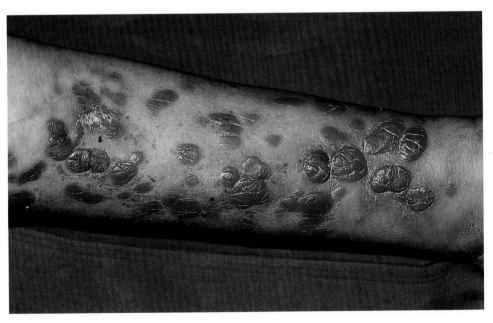

Figure 11.28 Multiple nodules of B-cell lymphoma on the lower leg.

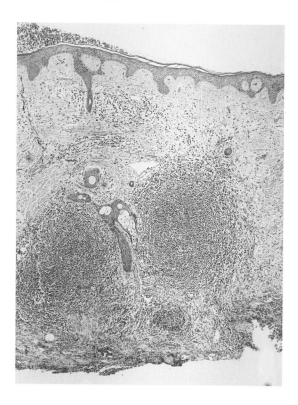

Figure 11.29 Low-power view of the histology of B-cell lymphoma, showing sparing of the epidermis and papillary dermis, but involvement of the deeper reticular dermis.

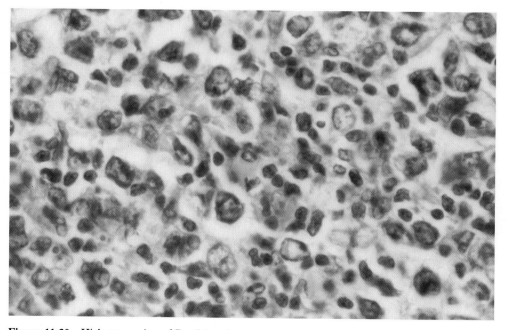

Figure 11.30 High-power view of B-cell lymphoma.

such as CHOP. In general, however, the presence of B-cell infiltrates in the skin is a poor prognostic sign.

Malignant angioendotheliomatosis

A recent development has been the recognition that the condition malignant angioendotheliomatosis, previously of uncertain histogenesis, is a B-cell lymphoma.[76,77]

Hodgkin's disease

Hodgkin's disease may involve the skin with secondary infiltrates (Figure 11.31). In addition, however, it has been suggested that Hodgkin's disease may actually begin in the skin. This is a contentious point and the suggestion of primary cutaneous

Hodgkin's disease as a diagnosis should not be made until an exhaustive search for a primary source in lymph nodes or spleen has been carried out.

A recent paper studying 465 patients with Hodgkin's disease reported the presence of specific secondary cutaneous involvement in 16 (3.4 per cent).[78] This was seen usually as single or multiple dermal or subcutaneous nodules. This paper confirms that poor prognosis is associated with cutaneous involvement.

Clinical features

Clinical features vary. They include papules, nodules, plaques and ulcers. A relatively characteristic site of involvement is the skin around the nipple area, which may be eroded in a striking manner, but not involving the actual nipple tissue. This is well illustrated in Figure 11.31.

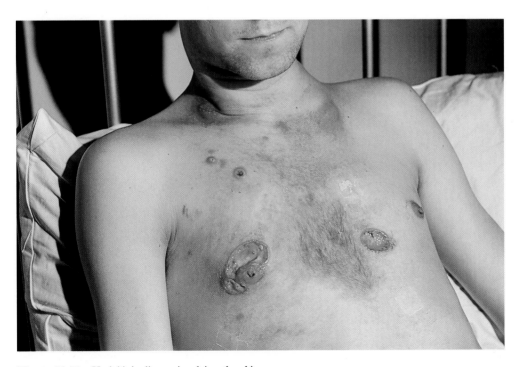

Figure 11.31 Hodgkin's disease involving the skin.

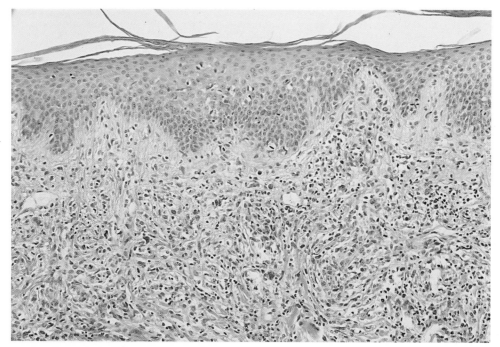

Figure 11.32   Low-power view of the histology of cutaneous Hodgkin's disease.

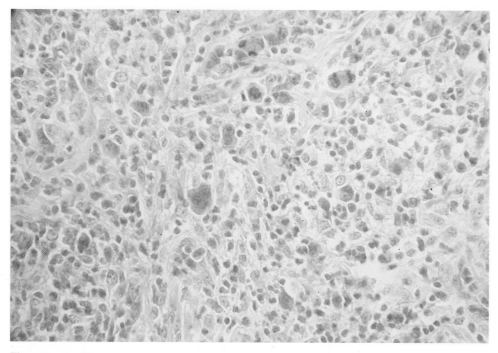

Figure 11.33   High-power view of cutaneous Hodgkin's disease. Two Reed–Sternberg cells are easily seen.

Pathology

The classic Dorothy Reed or Reed–Sternberg cell may be seen in a cutaneous infiltrate that is frequently fairly pleomorphic (Figures 11.32 and 11.33). Recent observations on the presence of cells bearing the Ki 1 (CD 30) marker in both Hodgkin's disease and lymphomatoid papulosis have suggested that these two entities may be aetiologically related.

Management

The management of cutaneous involvement in Hodgkin's disease will depend on the results of staging procedures and the type of Hodgkin's disease present. In general, as with B-cell lymphoma, cutaneous involvement is a poor prognostic sign.

In addition to specific cutaneous involvement, a variable proportion of patients with Hodgkin's disease complain of non-specific cutaneous lesions. These include urticarial lesions and papules and may cause pruritus, which can be severe but may respond to UVB or to PUVA therapy.

Crosti's lymphoma[79,80] and multilobulated T-cell lymphoma of Pinkus[81]

Current evidence would suggest that these two names may describe the same entity.

Clinical features

The clinical presentation is that of an elderly individual, usually male, with large indolent nodules on the trunk.

Pathology

Pathological examination will show a lymphocytic infiltrate sparing the epidermis and papillary dermis, and involving the deeper parts of the dermis in a pattern previously considered to represent a B-cell lymphoma. Despite this, a limited number of marker studies suggest that in some cases the cells are T-lymphocytes. Ultrastructural studies show the presence of a striking multilobulated nucleus.

Management

These lesions respond well to radiotherapy.

Angiolymphoid hyperplasia with eosinophils

A dermal and a subcutaneous variant of this condition were both described in 1969.[82,83]

Clinical features

The clinical presentation is of nodular lesions involving the face and neck, and very often the ear (Figure 11.34). The aetiology is not known, and the lesions are usually asymptomatic.

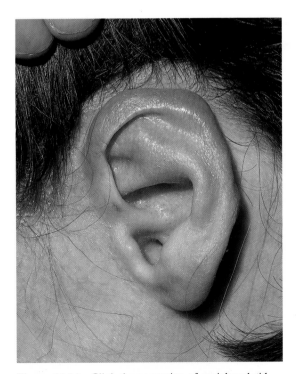

Figure 11.34 Clinical presentation of angiolymphoid hyperplasia.

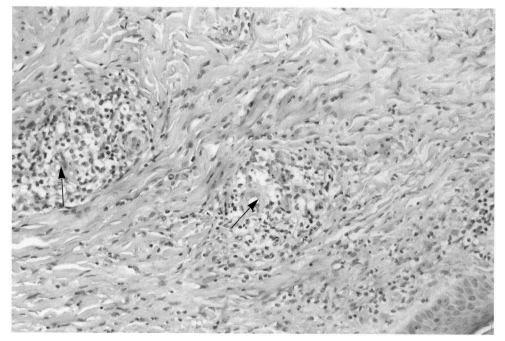

Figure 11.35   Low-power view of the histology of angiolymphoid hyperplasia. Thick-walled vessels are clearly seen (arrows).

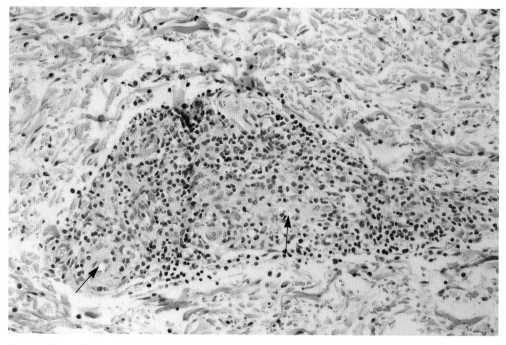

Figure 11.36   Histology of angiolymphoid hyperplasia. Thick-walled vessels are clearly seen (arrows).

Pathology

Biopsy will show a mixture of lymphocytes, often with germinal centre formation, and large numbers of eosinophils, usually at the edge of the lesion. Blood vessels are thickened, with plump endothelial cells. The overall picture is of a benign and reactive process (Figures 11.35 and 11.36).

Management

These lesions are frequently excised to obtain a diagnosis. Multiple local recurrences are seen but further excision or radiotherapy are both satisfactory methods of removal. Spontaneous remission is recorded.

Follicular mucinosis

This condition is included here because it may precede or coexist with cutaneous T-cell lymphoma.

Follicular mucinosis, or alopecia mucinosa, was first described by Pinkus[84] in 1957, and in 1969 Emmerson[85] described 40 patients and divided them into those in whom the follicular mucinosis was associated with lymphoma and those without such an association. Small lesions, and lesions confined to the head and neck, are said not to be associated with lymphoma. Personal experience would suggest that this is not always the case.

Clinical features

The lesions of follicular mucinosis are diffuse boggy plaques, often on the cheeks and neck. They are usually asymptomatic, but thick mucin may be expressed from the lesions. There may be obvious alopecia (Figures 11.37 and 11.38).

Pathology

There is mucinous degeneration of the hair follicles, with a lymphocytic infiltrate (Figures 11.39–11.41).

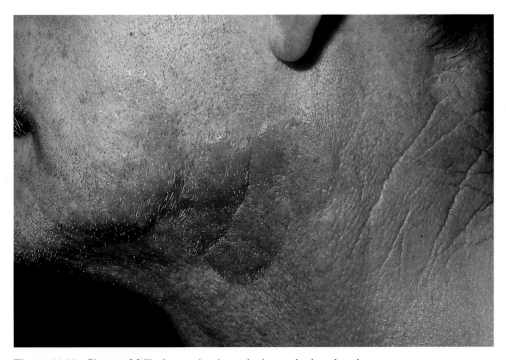

Figure 11.37   Plaque of follicular mucinosis on the lower cheek and neck area.

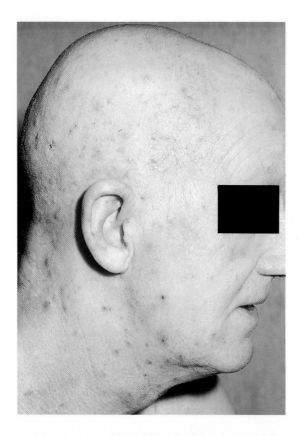

Figure 11.38 Total alopecia has resulted from extensive follicular mucinosis in this patient.

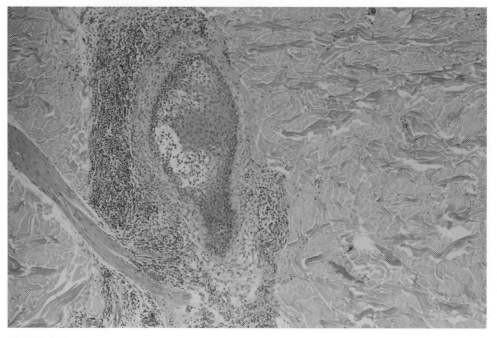

Figure 11.39 Low-power view of hair follicle destruction in follicular mucinosis.

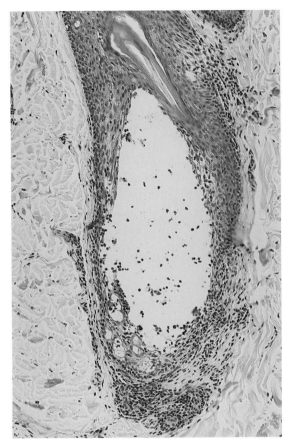

Figure 11.40 High-power view of hair follicle destruction in follicular mucinosis.

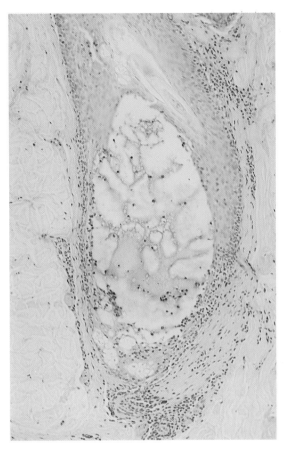

Figure 11.41 Mucin staining of a follicle undergoing destruction in follicular mucinosis.

Management

The aetiology of this process and its association with cutaneous lymphoma are not understood. The lesions respond to radiotherapy.

Histiocytosis X (Langerhans cell histiocytosis)

This term has generally replaced the older trio of Hans Schuller Christian disease, eosinophilic granuloma of bone, and Letterer–Siwe disease.[86,87]

Clinical features

There is little information available on epidemiology and incidence, but a recent publication from a children's hospital in Chicago gave details of 32 cases diagnosed over a 6-year period. Fifty per cent of these children had cutaneous involvement.[88]

The clinical features in children are similar in some cases to those of seborrhoeic dermatitis, but in addition to severe dermatitic lesions in the napkin area, and greasy scaling lesions on scalp and back, these children may have ulcerated or granulomatous lesions, pustules and petechiae (Figures 11.42–11.45).

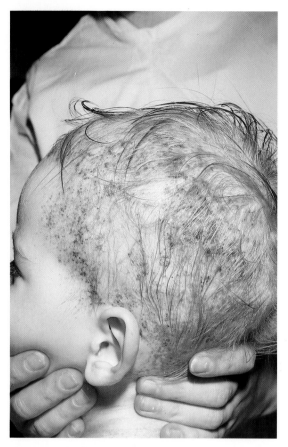

Figure 11.42   Scalp lesions in a child with histiocytosis X.

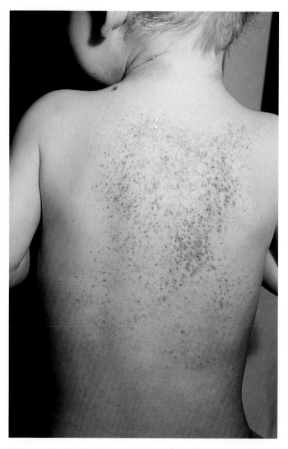

Figure 11.43   Lesions on the back in histiocytosis X.

In the adult, papular crusted lesions, mainly on the trunk, are the usual cutaneous presentation (Figure 11.46).[89,90] In both children and adults, multisystem disease is common.

Pathology

The cutaneous lesions show a proliferation of Langerhans cells. On haematoxylin and eosin staining, a proliferation of large kidney-shaped cells can be seen dropping off from the epidermis into the papillary dermis, with surrounding oedema (Figures 11.47 and 11.48).

The Langerhans cells can be identified at the ultrastructural level by the presence of the specific tennis-racquet-shaped granules, or by immunocytochemistry using monoclonal antibodies of the CD 1 series, or antibody to S 100 protein.

Management

There is doubt as to whether or not histiocytosis X is a malignancy, or a more benign and sometimes self-limiting proliferation.[91] Both radiotherapy and chemotherapy have been reported to be of value, and

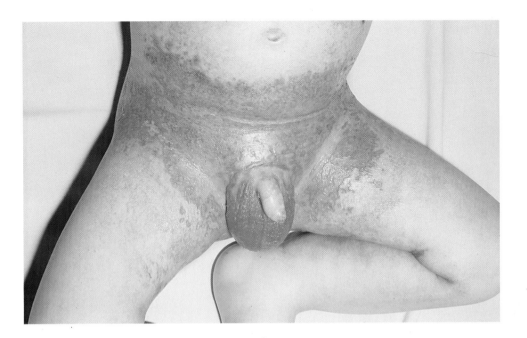

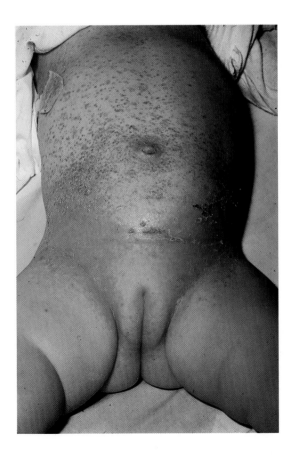

Figures 11.44 and 11.45 Lesions in the napkin area in histiocytosis X.

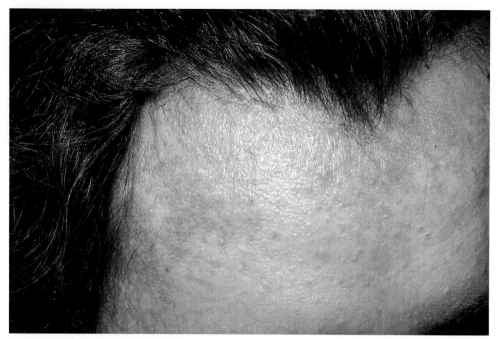

Figure 11.46   Temple area in an adult with histiocytosis X.

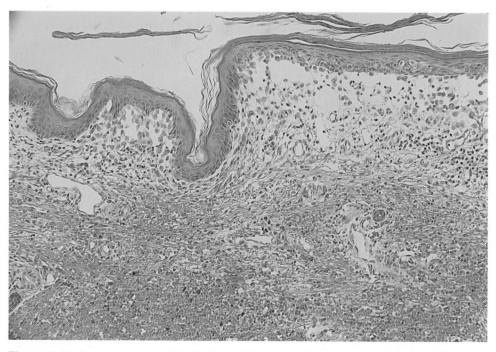

Figure 11.47   Low-power view of the histology of histiocytosis X.

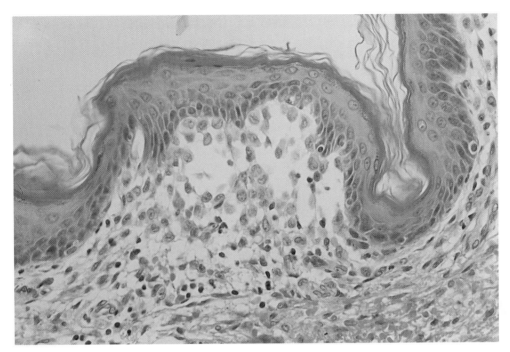

Figure 11.48 High-power view of the histology of histiocytosis X, showing gross oedema of the papular dermis and Langerhans cell proliferation.

more recently immunological therapy with thymic extract has also been reported to induce remission. Patients with lesions confined to the skin may undergo spontaneous remission, but those with multisystem disease have a poorer prognosis. At the present time it would seem prudent to start therapy with less aggressive modalities, and reserve cytotoxic agents for multisystem progressive disease. Long-term follow-up is, however, needed to identify those patients who will relapse.[92]

12
Skin appendage tumours

The following extensive but not comprehensive list of lesions will be discussed in this chapter:

Hair follicle tumours
  Inverted follicular keratosis
  Trichodiscoma
  Tumour of the follicular infundibulum
  Tricholemmoma and tricholemmal carcinoma
  Trichofolliculoma
  Trichoepithelioma
  Pilomatricoma
Sebaceous gland tumours
  Fox–Fordyce anomaly
  Sebaceous gland hyperplasia
  Sebaceous gland adenoma and epithelioma
  Sebaceous gland carcinoma
Apocrine gland tumours
  Supernumerary nipple
  Apocrine hidrocystoma
  Syringocystadenoma papilliferum
  Hidradenoma papilliferum
  Apocrine carcinoma
  Cylindroma
Eccrine sweat gland tumours
  Hidroacanthoma simplex
  Eccrine poroma
  Dermal duct tumour
  Eccrine hidrocystoma
  Eccrine spiradenoma
  Eccrine hidradenoma
  Chondroid syringoma
  Syringoma
Eccrine gland carcinomas
  Mucinous eccrine carcinoma
  Primary cutaneous adenoid cystic carcinoma
  Microcystic adnexal carcinoma

Despite the large number of skin appendage tumours that exist, they are relatively rare and it is therefore difficult for any one individual to gain a significant working experience of these lesions. Their terminology can be confusing to the uninitiated, but this chapter will try to discuss the more common varieties in a logical manner. They are rarely diagnosed clinically, and usually the clinical history is that of a slowly growing cutaneous or subcutaneous nodule, which is removed in order to obtain a pathological diagnosis.

Because of their general lack of distinguishing clinical features, these lesions may be of little initial interest to clinicians, but it is clearly essential that those responsible for communicating with the patient have some knowledge of the biological behaviour and the prognosis of these lesions.

Appendage tumours are of greater interest to the pathologist, possibly because of the difficulty which he or she may have in assigning an appropriate diagnostic label. The majority of skin appendage tumours are locally invasive but do not metastasize. The exceptions to this rule are the sebaceous gland carcinomas, and the primary eccrine gland carcinomas, which are discussed below.

It is not possible to state confidently in every case which particular part of an appendage, or even which cutaneous appendage, a tumour is differentiating from or towards. Histochemistry (Table 12.1) and ultrastructural examination have been used in addition to special stains on conventionally processed material to try to assign as many as possible of these appendage tumours appropriately.[1] Currently there is considerable interest in the use of monoclonal antibodies to keratins of various molecular weights, to epithelial membrane antigen (EMA),

Table 12.1 Enzymes found mainly in eccrine and apocrine structures that can be differentiated by histochemical techniques.

Eccrine-associated enzymes	Apocrine-associated enzymes
Phosphorylase	Beta-glucuronidase
Succinic dehydrogenase	Acid phosphatase
Cytochrome oxidase	Alkaline phosphatase
Indoxyl esterase	Monochrome oxidase
Leucine aminopeptidase	Acetate esterase
	Adenosine triphosphatase

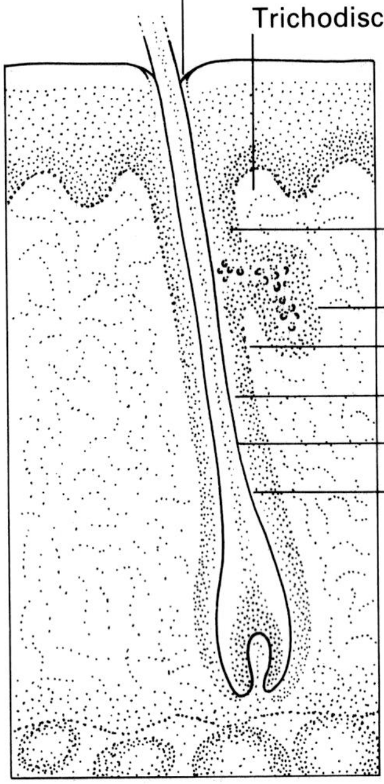

Figure 12.1 Diagrammatic representation of the hair follicle, with sites of origin of the tumours discussed in this chapter.

and to carcinoembryonic antigen (CEA). Both EMA and CEA are positive in the sweat gland lesions but negative in hair follicle tumours, a difference that is of value in distinguishing between the two, and also occasionally in distinguishing malignant skin appendage tumours from metastatic lesions from other body sites.

Hair follicle tumours

The complete range of tumours that can arise from the hair follicle is immense. For a comprehensive pathological review, the reader is referred to the excellent account by Headington.[2] This chapter will concentrate on the most common types of tumour derived from the hair follicle and will tackle them in logical order, beginning with those lesions thought to be derived from the more superficial parts of the hair follicle and moving down to the deeper areas (Figure 12.1). In general, lesions derived from the hair follicle are benign, locally expansive lesions that do not metastasize.

Inverted follicular keratosis[3]

This tumour has been discussed in Chapter 5 in association with the irritated basal cell papilloma (page 69). There is continuing controversy over whether or not the inverted follicular keratosis is a completely separate entity or whether it is a variant of

an irritated basal cell papilloma (seborrhoeic keratosis).[3] Figures 12.2 and 12.3 would suggest that, on occasion, keratin cysts and squamous eddies may be seen in the hair follicle in a pattern which suggests a true inverted follicular keratosis.

Trichodiscoma

This entity was described by Pinkus et al in 1974 and is a small cutaneous tumour of the dermal component of the hair disc.[4] These lesions are usually multiple and appear as skin-coloured papules on the face (Figure 12.4). Rarely, multiple lesions are reported in a familial setting.[5] The pathological appearance is that of a regular dome-shaped non-capsulated fibrovascular lesion in the papillary dermis, with a hair follicle located at the margin of the lesion.

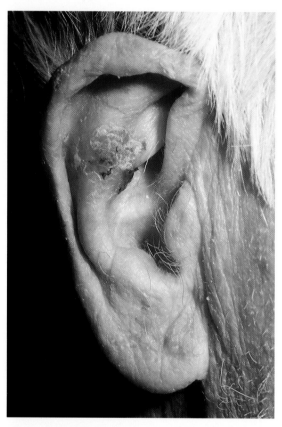

Figure 12.2   Clinical presentation of an inverted follicular keratosis on the ear.

Tumour of the follicular infundibulum

Mehregan and Butler[6] first reported this unusual tumour in 1961 and suggested that it was the hair follicle equivalent of the eccrine poroma in the eccrine sweat duct. The infundibulum of the hair follicle is that component above the entry of the pilosebaceous duct into the hair follicle canal. These lesions clinically present usually on the face as smooth elevated papules.

The pathological features consist of a plate-like mass of epithelial cells connected to the overlying epidermis by a number of pedicles. The cells are usually paler than their overlying epidermal counterparts and are seen to be rich in glycogen on staining with periodic acid–Schiff stain.

Trichilemmoma

These lesions may be solitary or multiple and were first reported as a separate entity by Headington and

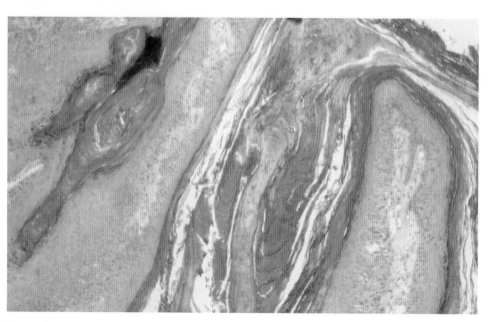

Figure 12.3   Pathological features of an inverted follicular keratosis.

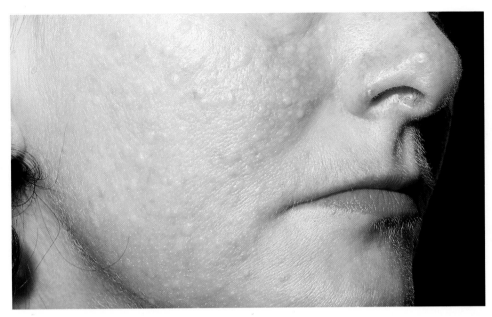

Figure 12.4   Multiple trichodiscomas on the cheek.

French in 1962.[7] They appear as small nodular lesions, usually on the face. Tufts of hair may occasionally be seen to emerge from these lesions.

The pathological features suggest that these lesions are derived from the outer part of the hair sheath. They are found usually in the superficial part of the dermis adjacent to the epidermis as large, well-lobulated masses with a palisading appearance around the lateral margin (Figures 12.5 and 12.6). The cells have large quantities of pale-staining cytoplasm and on periodic acid–Schiff staining will be found to be rich in glycogen. These lesions usually are recognized easily on pathological examination on account of the typical pale cytoplasm, but on occasion a differential diagnosis between them and the pale-staining cells of eccrine derivation may need to be made. Trichilemmomas are CEA- and EMA-negative, whereas eccrine tumours are usually positive to both antibodies.

At present there are approximately 50 malignant trichilemmal carcinomas reported in the world literature.[8] Males appear to be more often affected than females, and the clinical appearance is of slowly expanding plaques or nodules, usually on sun-exposed skin. The usual clinical diagnosis is of a basal cell carcinoma. The microscopic appearance is, however, much more aggressive, with striking cytological atypia, numerous mitoses, and in some cases pagetoid infiltration of the epidermis. Local excision is usually curative and relatively long-term follow-up over several years has not detected recurrences.

Trichofolliculoma

As the name would imply, this tumour appears to be the result of abortive or imperfect attempts at hair follicle formation. It may mark, therefore, a poor interrelationship between the epidermal and dermal components of the hair follicle apparatus.

Clinically these lesions frequently present as papules from which tufts of hair are seen to emerge. They may be multiple, and lesions may be several centimetres at their largest diameter (Figure 12.7).

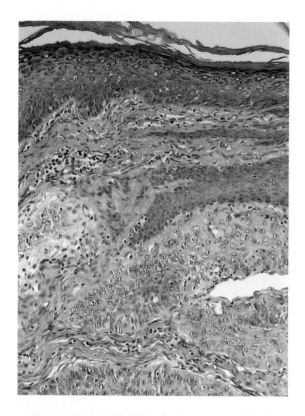

Figures 12.5 and 12.6 Pathological features of trichilemmoma, showing clear cells with a peripheral pseudopalisade.

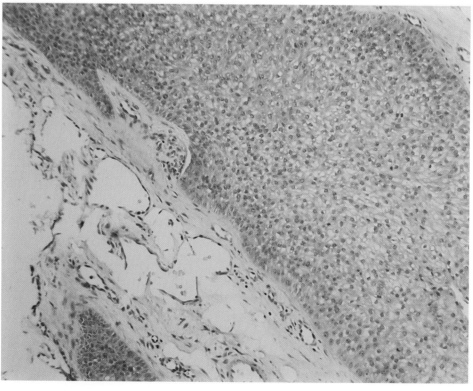

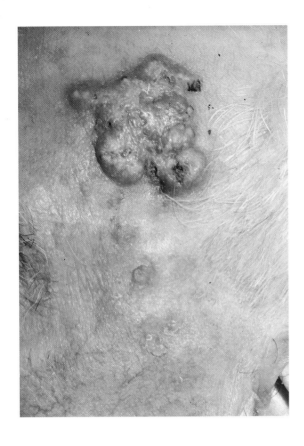

Figure 12.7   Large trichofolliculoma on the temple area.

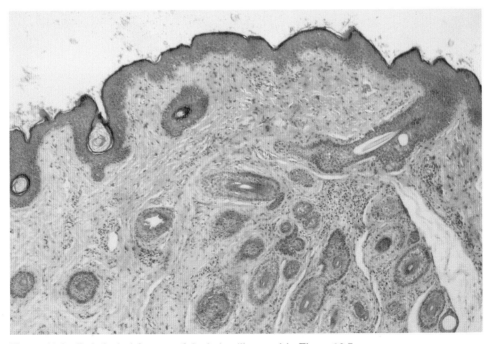

Figure 12.8   Pathological features of the lesion illustrated in Figure 12.7.

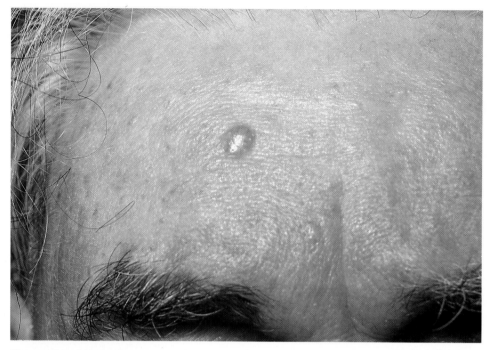

Figure 12.9 Trichoepithelioma on the forehead. Clinically these lesions may be mistaken for basal cell carcinoma.

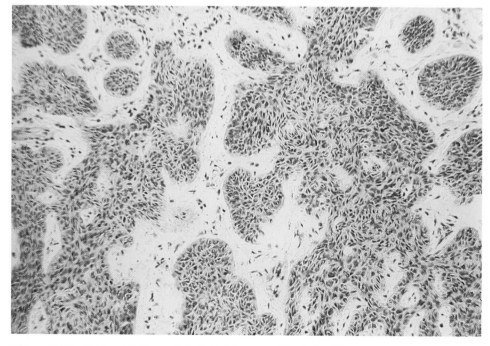

Figure 12.10 Trichoepithelioma. Pathological features of the lesion illustrated in Figure 12.9. Note the nests of basaloid cells without palisading.

On pathological examination, poorly formed hair follicles displaying epithelium-lined tracks filled with imperfectly formed hair can be seen (Figure 12.8). These lesions can usually be distinguished quite easily from other types of appendage tumour.

Trichoepithelioma

This lesion appears to arise from the cells composing the hair shaft deep in the sebaceous gland attachment. Multiple lesions are referred to as epithelioma adenoides cysticum, or Brooke's tumours. The desmoplastic trichoepithelioma, or sclerosing epithelial hamartoma, is thought to be a variant of this lesion (see page 130).

As with other hair follicle tumours, trichoepitheliomas present as single or multiple nodules, usually on the face (Figure 12.9). Pathological examination of the non-desmoplastic variety reveals well-circumscribed nodules of small, darkly stained basaloid cells (Figure 12.10). These cells are set in a fibrous stroma, and the differential diagnosis is usually from a basal cell carcinoma. Palisading, if present, is incomplete in comparison with the true basal cell carcinoma, and the trichoepithelioma contains cysts, which are not seen in true basal cell carcinomas.

Pilomatricoma (calcifying epithelioma of Malherbe)

This is the most common type of hair-follicle-derived tumour to be excised. It was described by Malherbe and Chenantais in the late nineteenth century, and at that time an origination from the sebaceous gland was suggested.[9] It is now known to arise from the hair matrix.

The bulk of these lesions present in children, and 60–80 per cent are said to develop during the first two decades.[10] As with other types of appendage tumour, both single and multiple lesions are seen, and the condition occasionally may be familial.[11] These lesions may reach a considerable size and may be firm, sometimes solid, nodules 2–3 cm in diameter at the time of excision (Figure 12.11). An association with myotonic dystrophy has been reported, and occasionally giant forms are seen.[12,13] The firm texture may be due to calcification.

On pathological examination, a mass of darkly stained basaloid cells will be seen. In parts of the tumour nodule these cells will appear to have undergone an involutional process, giving rise to a shadow or ghost cell configuration (Figure 12.12).

Calcification is frequently seen in and around these areas of ghost cells. Around both the small, darkly stained and the ghost cells, a dense fibrous stroma can be seen. In places, owing to the expansion of the tumour mass, this may form a pseudocapsule. Giant cells are frequently seen in this stroma.

Malignant change in pilomatricomas has been reported but is rare.[14] It can be recognized by the large size of the lesion, and the large number of mitotic figures. Local invasion rather than metastasis has been seen in such lesions.

Sebaceous gland tumours

Both benign and malignant tumours arising from the sebaceous gland apparatus are relatively rare. Minor abnormalities associated with the sebaceous gland are, however, relatively common.

Fox–Fordyce anomaly

The Fox–Fordyce condition, or anomaly, is the presence of ectopic sebaceous glands on mucosal surfaces, most often noticed on the oral mucosa.[15] Because of the lack of hair follicles on this site, these tumours open directly onto the mucosal surface and are recognized clinically as small, yellowish-white papules (Figure 12.13).

Pathologically, these lesions consist of aggregates of sebaceous gland cells.

Organoid or sebaceous naevus

The organoid, or sebaceous, naevus of Jadassohn has already been discussed in Chapter 6. These lesions are relatively common and are usually seen in childhood or adolescence.

The degree of sebaceous gland involvement in the organoid naevus varies, but frequently is considerable.

Sebaceous gland hyperplasia

In older skin, sebaceous gland hyperplasia, sometimes referred to as senile sebaceous hyperplasia, is fairly common, and usually appears on the face and neck

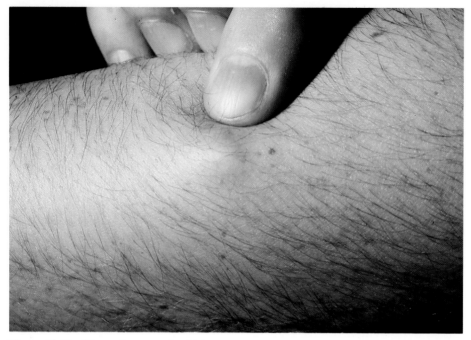

Figure 12.11   Pilomatricoma on the thigh.

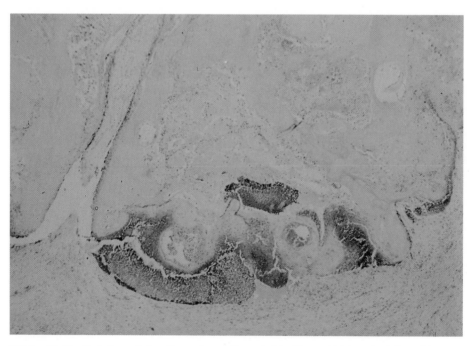

Figure 12.12   Pathology of the pilomatricoma illustrated in Figure 12.11, stained for calcium. Note the dense purple staining at the base, indicating calcification.

area.[16] These lesions may clinically present as translucent glistening papules and clinically there may be confusion with an early basal cell carcinoma (Figure 12.14).

On biopsy these lesions will be seen to consist of large, lobulated aggregates of sebaceous gland cells with foamy cytoplasm (Figure 12.15).

Sebaceous gland adenoma and epithelioma

Sebaceous gland adenomas and epitheliomas are all rare and, if present, the possibility of the Muir–Torre syndrome discussed in Chapter 4 should be considered.[17] All these lesions tend to present as yellow or white elevated papules on the facial skin. The pathology of sebaceous adenoma is similar to that of sebaceous gland hyperplasia, in that aggregates of sebaceous gland cells exhibiting copious foamy cytoplasm are seen. These are usually situated rather deeply and as discrete globules in comparison with the sebaceous gland hyperplasia, which tends to be situated more superficially.

The pathology of sebaceous epithelioma (Figure 12.16) is that of a rather more solid cell mass than the sebaceous adenoma. A proportion of the cells are of the small, dark, basaloid variety, but others are more typically of sebaceous gland origin (Figure 12.17). Cysts are present and, on occasion, there may be problems in differentiating these lesions from tumours of hair follicle origin or, indeed, from basal cell carcinoma. Peripheral palisading, however, is not seen.

Sebaceous gland carcinoma[18,19]

Sebaceous gland carcinoma tends to occur on the eyelids, although the benign tumours of the sebaceous gland apparatus do not appear to be more common on this site.[16,17] The upper lid appears to be involved in the majority of cases and the clinical presentation may be that of a diffuse chronic conjunctivitis or even

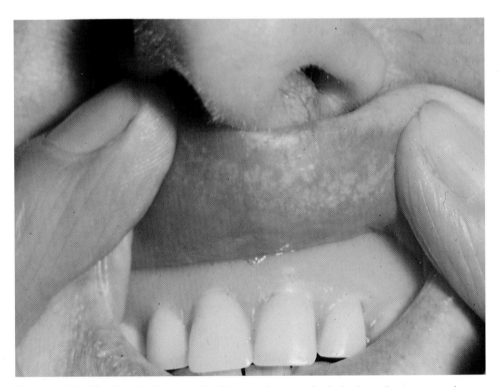

Figure 12.13 The Fox–Fordyce anomaly. Ectopic sebaceous glands in the oral mucous membrane.

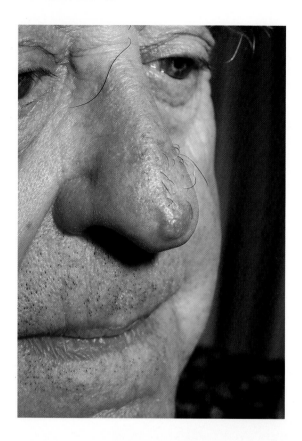

Figure 12.14 Clinical appearance of sebaceous gland hyperplasia on the nose.

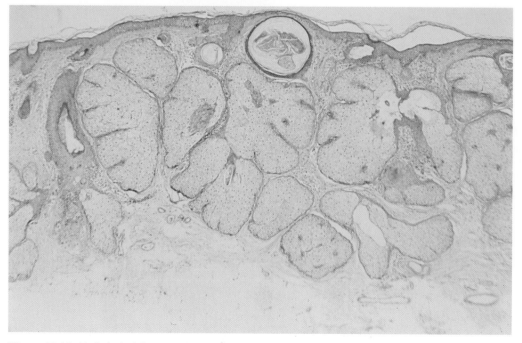

Figure 12.15 Pathological features of senile sebaceous gland hyperplasia.

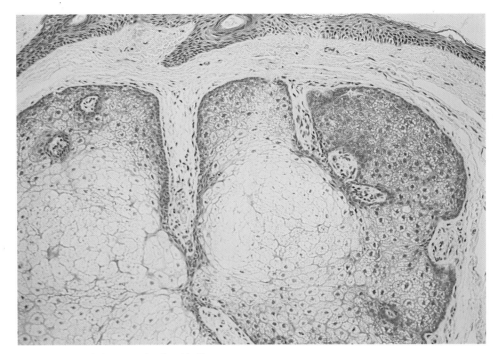

Figure 12.16 Sebaceous gland epithelioma.

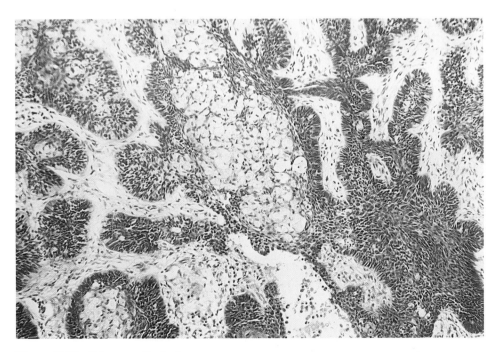

Figure 12.17 Sebaceous gland adenoma.

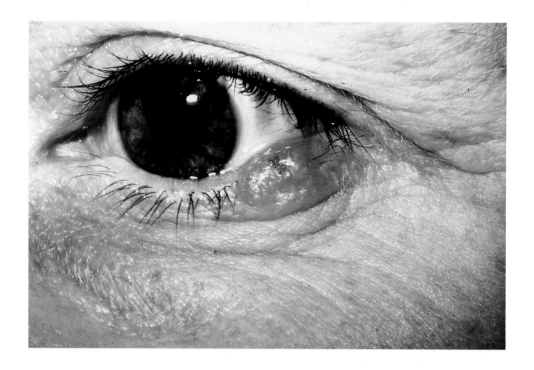

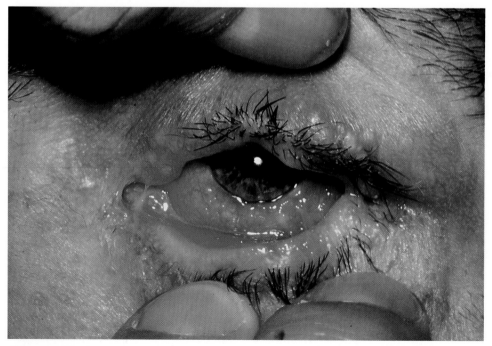

Figures 12.18 and 12.19 Clinical appearance of sebaceous gland carcinoma. (Photographs courtesy of Prof. W Lee.)

a recurrent chalazion (Figures 12.18 and 12.19). Sebaceous gland carcinomas on cutaneous sites other than the eyelid are virtually always seen on the scalp and face (Figure 12.20).

The histology of sebaceous gland carcinoma is that of typical lobules of cells with foamy cytoplasm, having, in addition, large numbers of mitotic figures and atypical mitoses (Figures 12.21 and 12.22). Pagetoid spread of individual malignant cells through the epidermis is frequently seen and is said to be a poor prognostic sign, possibly due to the difficulty in this situation of being certain that excision is complete. If this Pagetoid pattern of spread is present, the pathological differential diagnosis may include true Paget's disease and superficial spreading malignant melanoma. If frozen tissue is available, a fat stain, such as oil red O or Sudan IV, will confirm the sebaceous nature of the cells. Monoclonal antibodies can also be used, and most tumours are positive for both cytokeratins and EMA.

Although sebaceous gland carcinoma is rare, metastatic spread and death are relatively common. A 5-year survival figure of only 50 per cent is reported.[18]

Management

Management of benign sebaceous gland tumours is usually simple local excision to establish a diagnosis. In the case of sebaceous gland carcinoma, controlled excision using the fresh tissue technique to ensure complete removal of tumour at all margins is recommended. Sebaceous gland carcinoma is reported to be radiosensitive, and radiotherapy is therefore an acceptable alternative or adjuvant form of therapy for these rare tumours.

Apocrine gland tumours

Supernumerary nipple[20]

The supernumerary nipple is a relatively common problem and is recognized as a firm nodule of tissue on the nipple line (Figure 12.23).

Bilateral supernumerary nipples are not uncommon, and the symmetry may be helpful in the clinical diagnosis; otherwise these lesions may be confused clinically with a simple intradermal naevus

or a skin tag. In some cases there is a positive family history.

On pathological examination, ectopic breast tissue will be seen, including dilated mammary glands, hair follicles, and large numbers of isolated strips of smooth muscle. These lesions are usually removed for diagnostic purposes.

Apocrine hidrocystoma

The apocrine hidrocystoma is seen most often on the face and presents as a translucent bluish lesion

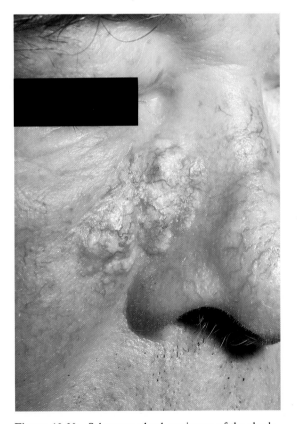

Figure 12.20   Sebaceous gland carcinoma of the cheek.

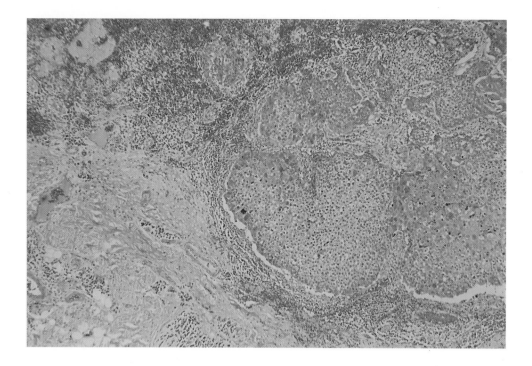

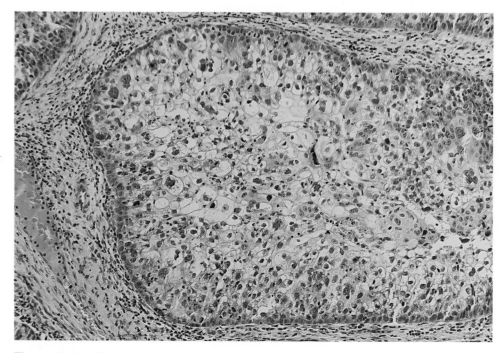

Figures 12.21 and 12.22 Pathological appearance of sebaceous gland carcinoma. Note the foamy cytoplasm and atypical mitotic figures.

(Figures 12.24–12.26).[21] Pigment is frequently present and the lesion may be confused with a pigmented basal cell carcinoma or even a lesion of melanocytic origin.

On pathological examination, spaces filled with cystic fluid will be seen. These cystic lesions are lined with characteristic apocrine epithelium, having tall columnar cells that have small round nuclei at the base. Deep to these cells is a layer of myoepithelial cells. Apparent decapitation secretion is seen in the lumen of the cystic spaces (Figures 12.27 and 12.28).

Syringocystadenoma papilliferum[22]

The syringocystadenoma papilliferum is seen most often on the scalp and face. As previously mentioned (Chapter 6), these lesions may develop on a pre-existing organoid naevus. Usually they present as fairly extensive verrucous lesions (Figures 12.29 and 12.30). About one-half are reported to be present at birth, and a further 25 per cent appear in the first decade. With hormonal stimulus at puberty, they tend to become verrucous and thus easily traumatized.

On pathological examination, the lesions will be seen to comprise papillary structures projecting into a cystic invagination. The papillary structures are lined with a double layer of columnar epithelial cells that show decapitation secretion (Figures 12.31 and 12.32). Beneath this columnar epithelium is a stroma rich in plasma cells. The overall pattern of the syringocystadenoma papilliferum is virtually diagnostic.

Hidradenoma papilliferum[23]

The hidradenoma papilliferum is found almost exclusively in the vulvar area. It is a relatively common tumour and presents as a palpable lesion, usually on the labia majora.

On pathological examination, it will have a superficial similarity to the syringocystadenoma papilliferum, having thin papillary projections lined by cells of the apocrine type with apparent decapitation secretion. On low-power microscopic examination, an almost villous pattern will be seen in this lesion (Figure 12.33), and on higher power an associated stroma will be seen to be present (Figure 12.34).[24] In contrast to the syringocystadenoma papilliferum, a plasma cell infiltrate is not seen in the hidradenoma papilliferum.

Paget's disease

Many cases of Paget's disease appear to be of apocrine gland derivation. They have already been discussed in Chapter 6 (page 96).

Apocrine carcinoma[25]

Apocrine carcinomas are rare, with at present less than 30 well-recorded cases in the world literature.

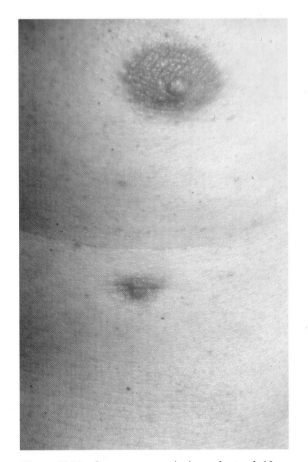

Figure 12.23 Supernumerary nipple on the trunk 10 cm below the 'normal' nipple.

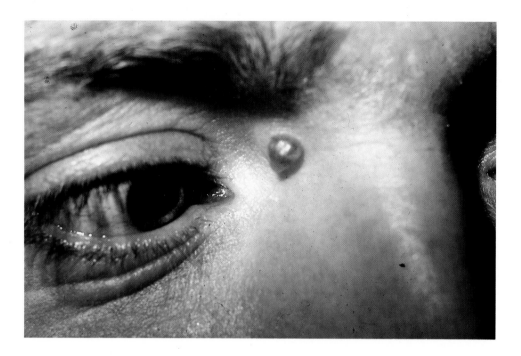

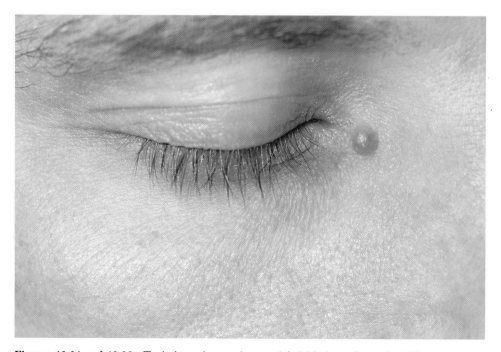

Figures 12.24 and 12.25   Typical translucent pigmented facial lesions of apocrine hidrocystoma.

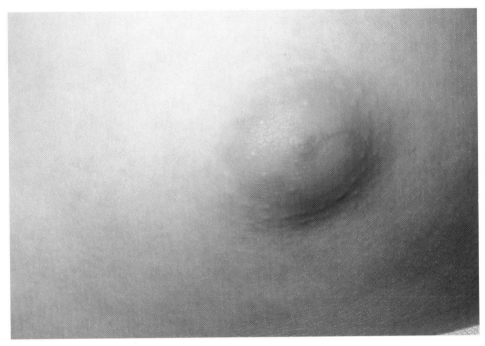

Figure 12.26   Apocrine hidrocystoma on the nipple.

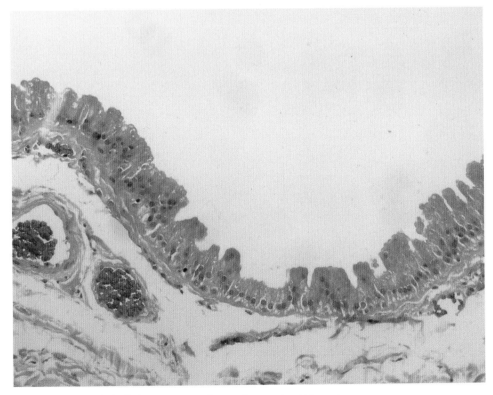

Figure 12.27   Pathological appearance of a cyst in apocrine hidrocystoma.

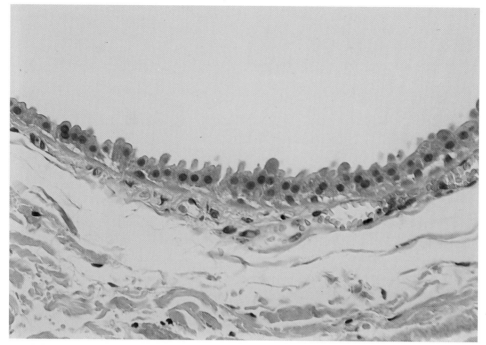

Figure 12.28   High-power view of an apocrine hidrocystoma, showing the apocrine-type cells lining the cyst.

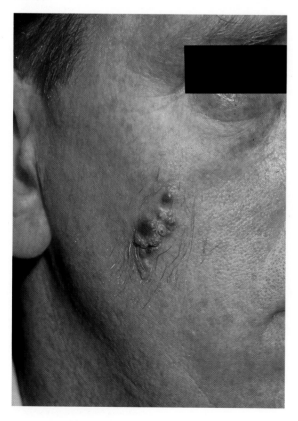

Figure 12.29   Clinical appearance of naevus syringocystadenoma papilliferum.

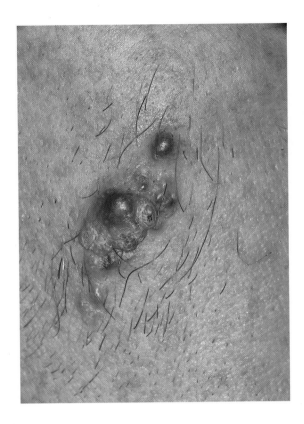

Figure 12.30   Close-up view of the lesion illustrated in Figure 12.29, showing the translucent appearance of the lesion.

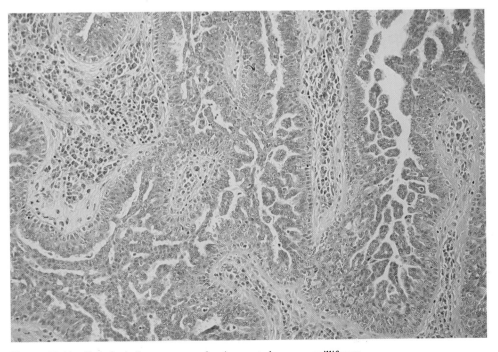

Figure 12.31   Pathological appearance of syringocystadenoma papilliferum.

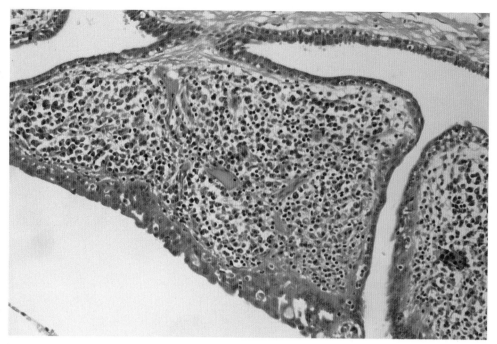

Figure 12.32   High-power view of the pathological features of syringocystadenoma papilliferum, showing apocrine-type lining to the channels and the underlying plasma cell infiltrate.

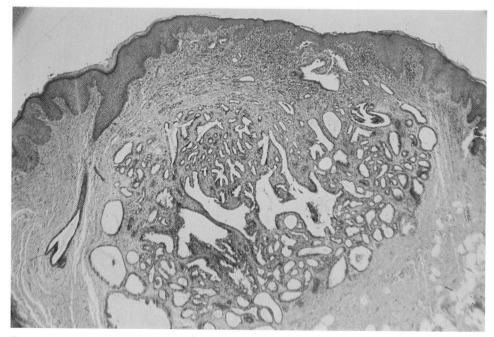

Figure 12.33   Low-power view of hidradenoma papilliferum.

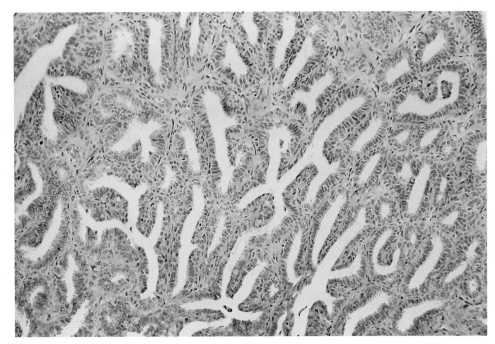

Figure 12.34   High-power view of hidradenoma papilliferum.

The majority arise in the axilla, and are thought to originate from normal apocrine glands, although eccrine sweat glands are often seen adjacent to apocrine carcinomas. There is no distinctive clinical presentation, and the microscopic features suggesting the diagnosis include decapitation secretion, periodic acid–Schiff-positive, diastase-resistant material in the lumen, and immunoreactivity with gross cystic disease fluid protein. Local recurrence and metastatic spread to draining lymph nodes have both been reported.

Cylindroma, or turban tumours[26,27]

The origin of these tumours is debated. In the past, an eccrine origin was postulated, but at present there is considerable evidence to suggest that they are of apocrine origin, which is the reason for their inclusion at this point.

These lesions may be single or multiple (Figures 12.35 and 12.36), and occur mainly on the scalp. They may grow to a considerable size and present as large, dome-shaped nodules. In some families there is a history of autosomal dominant inheritance of these lesions.[28] On pathological examination, the appearance on low-power microscopy is characteristic. Isolated islands of epithelial cells are seen, visibly demarcated by a surrounding band of hyalinized material. Usually this shows up clearly with conventional haematoxylin and eosin staining, but if there is any diagnostic doubt, periodic acid–Schiff staining will indicate the pattern very strikingly (Figure 12.37).

The cells within these demarcated lobules are of two types. At the edge of the lobules, forming an almost palisading pattern, are small, dark cells with deeply stained nuclei and scanty cytoplasm. Within these pseudopalisaded areas are larger cells with paler nuclei. In some areas an impression of apocrine-type decapitation secretion may be seen.

Malignant degeneration of cylindroma has been reported but is extremely rare.[29] Large numbers of mitotic figures and atypical mitoses within a lesion should arouse the suspicion of this possibility. Malignant cylindromas have been reported to metastasize.

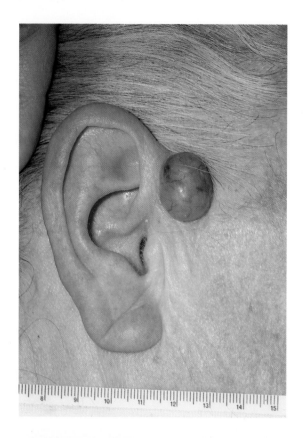

Figure 12.35 Single cylindroma in front of the ear.

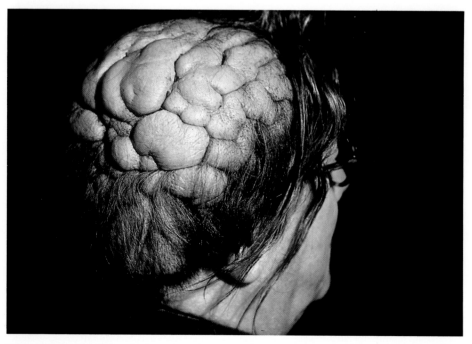

Figure 12.36 Multiple cylindromas on the scalp. The term 'turban tumours' is easily understood.

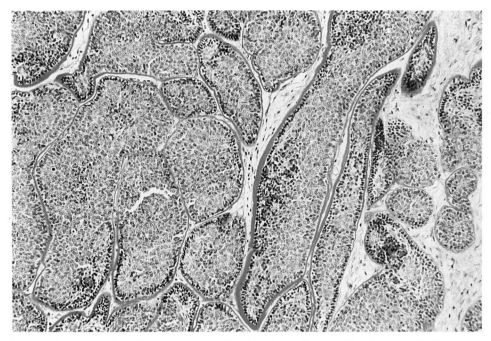

Figure 12.37   Periodic acid–Schiff-stained slide of the lesion illustrated in Figure 12.35. The periodic acid–Schiff-positive band around nests of cells is clearly seen.

Eccrine sweat gland tumours

A large number of lesions may be derived from the eccrine sweat gland apparatus.[30] Figure 12.38 lists these in a logical progression according to their position within the epidermis and dermis.

Hidroacanthoma simplex[31]

This lesion appears to be a benign proliferation within the epidermis of the keratinocytes associated with the intraepidermal portion of the eccrine sweat duct. Its clinical presentation is usually as a facial plaque.

The pathological presentation is that of clearly demarcated nests of intraepidermal cells that are usually smaller, darker and with a clearer cytoplasm than the surrounding normal epidermal keratinocytes (Figures 12.39 and 12.40). This pattern has been described in the past as the Borst–Jadassohn phenomenon. No abnormality is seen in the underlying dermis.

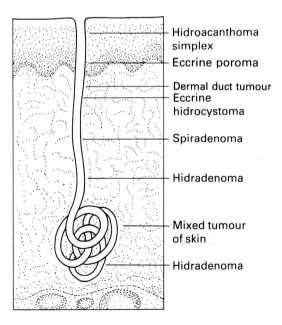

Hidroacanthoma simplex

Eccrine poroma

Dermal duct tumour
Eccrine hidrocystoma

Spiradenoma

Hidradenoma

Mixed tumour of skin

Hidradenoma

Figure 12.38   Diagrammatic representation of the sites of origin of eccrine-sweat-gland-derived tumours.

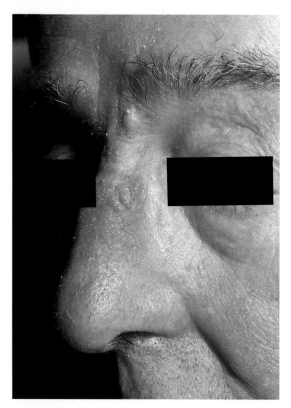

Figure 12.39 Hidroacanthoma simplex on the bridge of the nose.

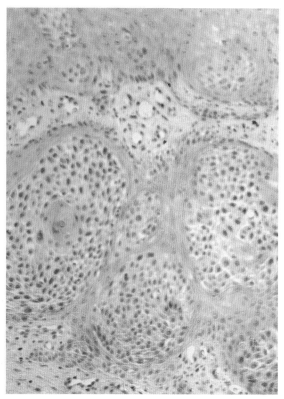

Figure 12.40 Pathology of the lesion illustrated in Figure 12.39. Note the population of smaller, darker cells within the epidermis.

Eccrine poroma

This lesion can be considered as a more advanced form of the hidroacanthoma simplex. Clinically, these lesions are usually recognized as moist, pink, elevated lesions, most frequent on the soles of the feet (Figure 12.41).

The pathological features were described by Pinkus et al in 1956.[32] A mass of small, darkly staining cells is seen in contiguity with the overlying epidermis but extending downward into the dermis. The cells comprising the lesion have a relatively clear cytoplasm, but there is no palisading at the periphery of the lesion (Figures 12.42 and 12.43).

Malignant eccrine poroma is reported, and between 30 and 40 cases are recorded in the world literature.[33,34] The majority of these were found on the lower limb, and metastases to both lymph nodes and viscera are reported. Features suggestive of malignant change in an eccrine poroma include acantholytic areas, multiple atypical mitotic figures, apparent duct formation, and dermal lymphatic spaces filled with malignant cells. The differential diagnosis may include Paget's disease, acantholytic squamous cell carcinoma, and metastatic carcinoma.

The management of eccrine poroma is excision with a narrow margin of normal tissue. If there is any possibility of malignant change, excision with microscopic control of clearance is recommended.

Dermal duct tumour

This tumour was described by Winkelmann and McLeod in 1966.[35] The clinical features are not well described, but the lesions are recognized histologically as isolated groups of cells in the dermis that have the

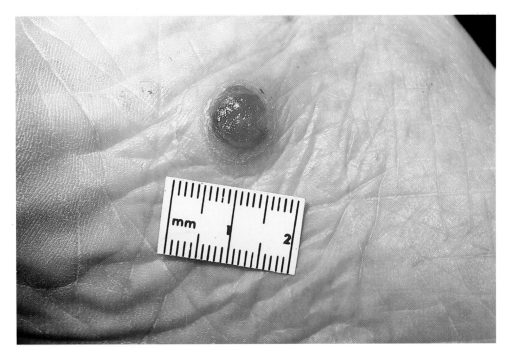

Figure 12.41   Eccrine poroma on the sole of the foot.

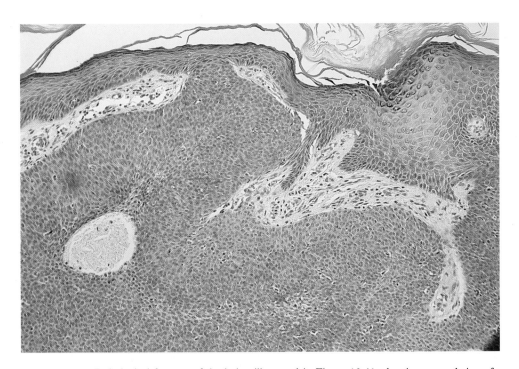

Figure 12.42   Pathological features of the lesion illustrated in Figure 12.41, showing a population of small, dark cells in direct contact with the epidermis.

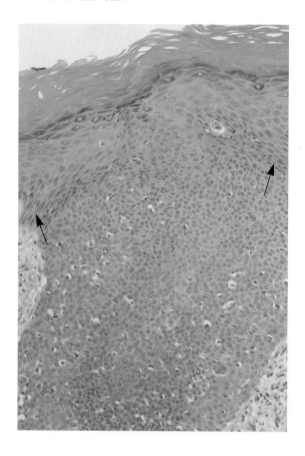

Figure 12.43 High-power view of eccrine poroma, showing the sharp margin between normal keratinocytes and poroma cells (arrows).

cytological characteristics of the cells that compose the eccrine poroma. The dermal duct tumour has, however, no visible connection with the overlying epidermis. The cells are usually distributed in circular aggregates and have clear cytoplasm with small regular nuclei. Staining with periodic acid–Schiff will show large quantities of glycogen to be present and there is a great deal of phosphorylase activity, implying a derivation from the eccrine duct.

These lesions are usually excised to obtain a pathological diagnosis.

Eccrine hidrocystoma[36]

These lesions occur most frequently on the face and may be either single or multiple. Clinically, they are very similar to the apocrine hidrocystomas and consist of small, translucent nodules under 5 mm in diameter. As with the apocrine hidrocystomas, some bluish or black discoloration is frequently seen (Figure 12.44).[37]

Pathological examination shows a single cystic cavity, usually located in the papillary dermis. The cyst is lined with two layers of small cuboidal epithelial cells and there is no evidence of apocrine-type secretion (Figure 12.45). The individual cells are more cuboidal than columnar, and, in contrast to the apocrine-derived lesions, decapitation secretion is not seen.

Eccrine spiradenoma[38]

These lesions frequently present in early adult life as isolated painful nodules on any body site (Figure 12.46).

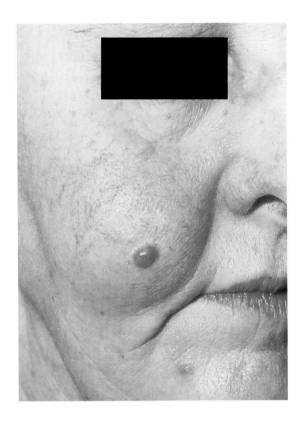

Figure 12.44 Eccrine hidrocystoma on the cheek.

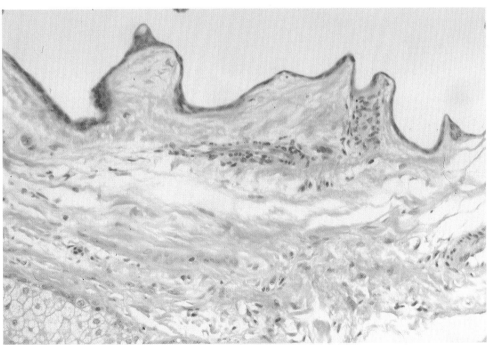

Figure 12.45 Pathological appearance of eccrine hidrocystoma. Note the absence of the apocrine-type lining seen in Figure 12.28.

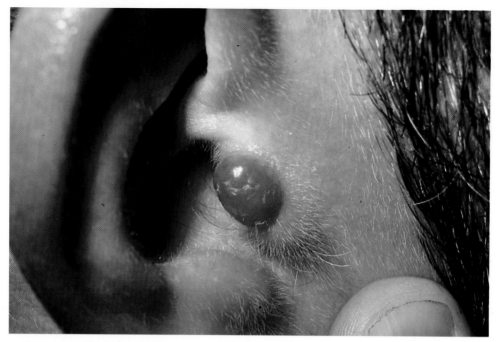

Figure 12.46 An eccrine spiradenoma. This patient complained bitterly of spontaneous pain.

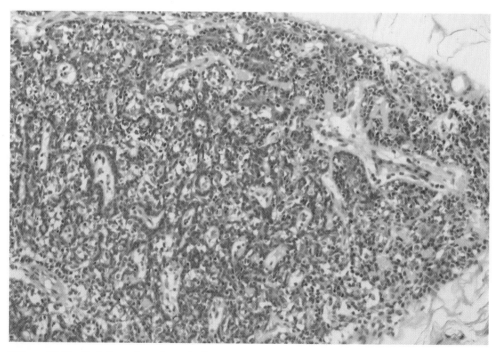

Figure 12.47 Pathology of eccrine spiradenoma, showing pseudocapsule formation.

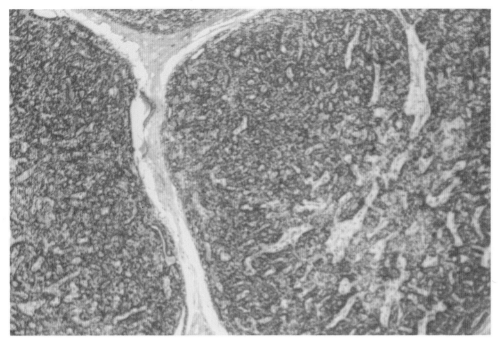

Figure 12.48   High-power view of eccrine spiradenoma, showing cords of cells and oedematous stroma.

On pathological examination, lobules of cells can be seen lying in the dermis with no overlying epidermal connection. There may be an impression of capsule formation (Figure 12.47) due to pressure on the surrounding structures, and the components of the cellular lobule are cords of intertwining epithelial cells enclosing an oedematous stroma (Figure 12.48). Two kinds of epithelial cell can be seen clearly. The first is a population of cells with small, dark nuclei lying at the periphery of the cords, and the second are larger cells with larger, paler nuclei lying within the cords or around small apparent lumina. Staining with periodic acid–Schiff will show large quantities of granular eosinophilic material within these lumina. Histochemical studies in the past have shown evidence of large quantities of phosphorylase activity, which confirms that this tumour is of eccrine origin.

Eccrine spiradenomas are usually treated by excision both to obtain a diagnosis and because of symptoms. Malignant eccrine spiradenoma has been recorded but is rare.[39]

Eccrine hidradenoma[40]

This eccrine-derived lesion suffers from a variety of alternative eponyms. It is recognized clinically as a usually isolated red or bluish nodule on any body site (Figure 12.49). On pathological examination, an aggregate of well-circumscribed tumour cells can be seen within the dermis with no overlying epidermal connection (Figure 12.50). Within the tumour mass there are often cystic or duct-like spaces. Two main cell types compose the tumour mass. The first is a small cuboidal cell with a small, round nucleus and basophilic cytoplasm. The second cell is usually slightly rounder with a distinct, clear cytoplasm and a small, dark nucleus. The proportions of these cells seen in different lesions are very variable. The clear cells show periodic acid–Schiff-positive diastase-resistant staining. The clear cell component of these hidradenomas may be similar cytologically to the cells composing the tricholemmoma, or even to a metastatic deposit from a clear cell carcinoma of the

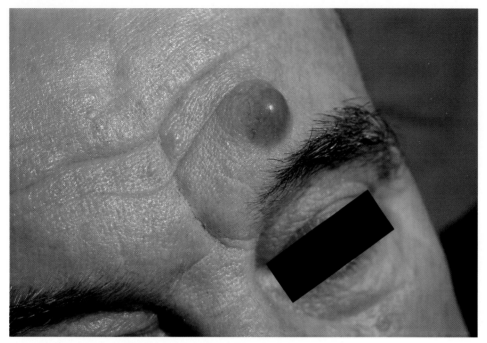

Figure 12.49 Eccrine hidradenoma – clinical appearance.

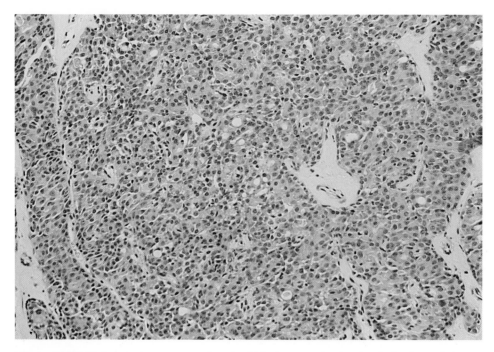

Figure 12.50 Pathological appearance of eccrine hidradenoma, showing the dual cell population.

kidney. The presence of cystic spaces and tubular lumina is characteristic of the hidradenoma rather than the tricholemmoma. These tubular lumina may be lined with small cuboidal cells similar to those seen in eccrine secretory lesions, but, on occasion, an additional component of taller, columnar cells displaying apparent apocrine secretory features may be seen in small areas. Thus, these lesions may have either a predominantly tubular appearance or a predominantly nodular and clear cell appearance. Immunopathology may be helpful, as the cells stain positively with CEA.

Local excision is the usual method of choice, both to obtain a diagnosis and as a therapeutic measure.

Chondroid syringoma

The alternative name for this lesion is mixed tumour of the skin. It usually presents as a subcutaneous nodule, which may reach a considerable size, and is seen most frequently on the head and neck areas.[41]

On pathological examination, a mixed, irregular aggregate of cells can be seen with ill-defined peripheral borders. The individual components of chondroid syringomas vary, with some lesions containing large numbers of tubular structures (Figure 12.51) and others being rather more solid (Figure 12.52) and very similar to the hidradenoma. The cells and tubular structures are situated in an irregular and dense fibrous stroma. The tubular structures have a double lining of cuboidal epithelial cells and a more peripheral layer of flattened cells. The lumen of the tubular structures frequently contains periodic acid–Schiff-positive diastase-resistant material. As with the hidradenomas, there may be small areas within the chondroid syringomas more suggestive of apocrine than eccrine differentiation. As the name implies, in places the stroma has a striking resemblance to true cartilage.

Malignant change in chondroid syringomas has been recorded.[42]

Syringoma

As with cylindromas, the exact histogenesis of these lesions is debated, but the majority of reports suggest that they are of eccrine origin.[43]

The most common clinical presentation is of multiple small papules below the eyes (Figure 12.53). Other sites, such as the neck, may also be involved (Figure 12.54). The lesions are asymptomatic, and

the majority of patients presenting for treatment are young females. A linear variant has been reported,[44] as has an association with Down's syndrome.[45]

The pathology is that of a dense dermal stroma in which numerous small comma-shaped ducts are embedded (Figure 12.55). The ducts have a double lining of cells, and frequently contain periodic acid–Schiff-positive material (Figure 12.56).

Eccrine gland carcinomas

Mucinous eccrine carcinoma

This may be misdiagnosed as a secondary deposit.[46] It is seen most frequently on the head and neck, and presents as a raised nodule.

The striking observation on pathological examination is the presence of large quantities of sialomucin in a honeycombed mass of malignant cells. Local recurrence is common, but metastases are relatively rare.

Primary cutaneous adenoid cystic carcinoma

This tumour is extremely rare, with fewer than 20 cases recorded in the world literature. Most patients described to date are middle-aged females who have slowly growing painful nodules, with, in some cases, associated alopecia.

The pathological features of the tumour are very similar to those of the adenoid cystic carcinoma found in the salivary gland. A population of small basaloid cells forms striking tubular structures. There is no connection with the overlying dermis, and both mucin and hyaline are present around the cell masses.[47,48] Some features of this tumour are very similar to those seen in the cylindroma.

Microcystic adnexal carcinoma

The lesion is a particularly aggressive one, with a tendency to relentless local recurrence. The majority of cases recorded to date are on the upper lip area, and may be clinically rather inconspicuous lesions in comparison with their aggressive biological behaviour.[49–51]

The pathological features are the presence of small, adnexal-type keratinocytes in the dermis, with

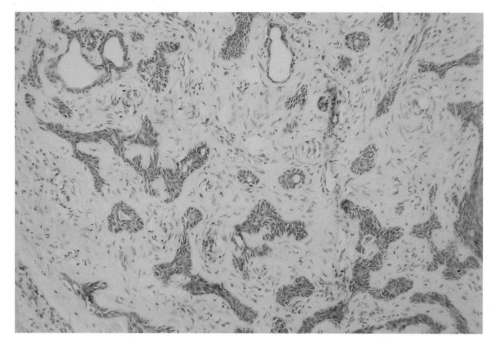

Figure 12.51 Chondroid syringoma – tubular variant.

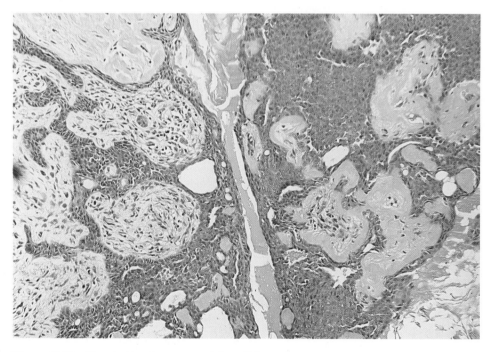

Figure 12.52 Chondroid syringoma – nodular cellular variant.

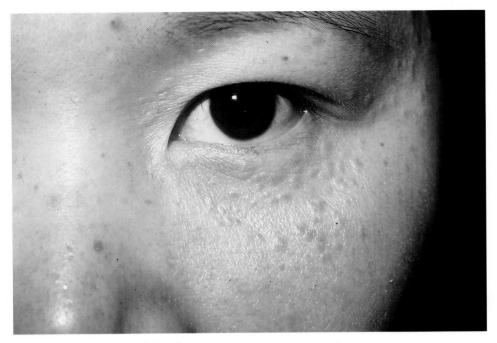

Figure 12.53 Syringomas below the eyes.

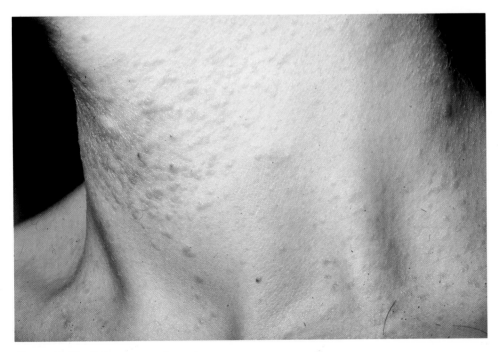

Figure 12.54 Syringomas on the neck.

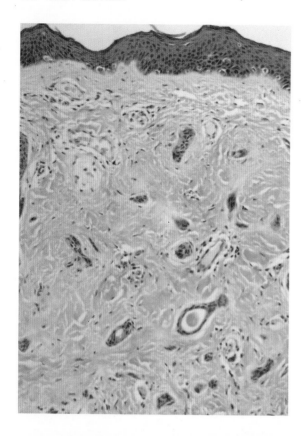

Figure 12.55 Low-power view of the pathology of a syringoma, showing comma-shaped structures.

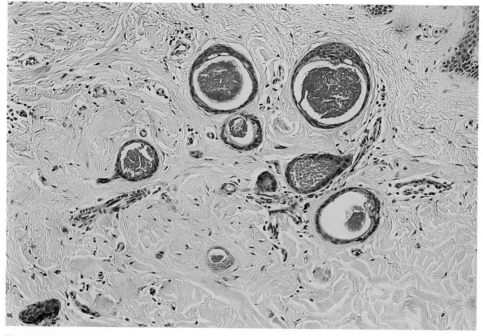

Figure 12.56 High-power view of a periodic acid–Schiff-stained section of a syringoma, showing striking positivity.

duct-like structures lined by two layers of cuboidal cells and large numbers of horn cysts. The lesions are rich in glycogen. The lesions tend to invade fat, and perineural spread is seen frequently.

Conclusion

The appendage tumour group is of great interest to the pathological enthusiast, but happily the population affected is small. As more specific monoclonal antibodies become available that react with only small areas of individual ducts and/or secretory components, it may be possible to assign each of these tumours to its cell of origin more rapidly and with greater precision than is currently possible. It should be borne in mind, however, that the phenotypic expression of a tumour does not always mirror that of its benign counterpart, and this approach should therefore be adopted with some caution.

13

Tumours of the dermis

The list below is a representative selection of the very large spectrum of tumours which may arise in the dermis:

Neural tumours
  Neurilemmoma and Schwannoma
  Palisaded and encapsulated neuroma
  Neurofibromas, multiple neurofibromatosis
  Malignant neurofibroma and Schwannoma
  Primary neuroendocrine carcinoma of the skin (Merkel cell tumour)
Fibrohistiocytic tumours
  Keloids and hypertrophic scars
  Dermatofibroma
  Angiofibroma
  Dermatofibrosarcoma protruberans
  Atypical fibroxanthoma
  Malignant fibrous histiocytoma
Vascular tumours
  Pyogenic granuloma
  Angiokeratoma
  Glomus tumour
  Lymphangioma
  Angiosarcoma
  Kaposi's sarcoma
Leiomyosarcoma
Liposarcoma
Malignant melanoma of soft parts
Differential diagnosis of spindle cell tumours
Cutaneous metastatic deposits

A wide range of tumours can arise in the dermis, derived from fibroblasts and neural, vascular, muscle and fat cells. In addition, secondary tumours may metastasize to the dermis from non-cutaneous sites, causing diagnostic difficulties.

The clinical presentation of all these lesions is, in general, a non-specific lump, and accurate diagnosis is only possible after excision and pathological examination. For a detailed account of the histological features of a wide range of these lesions, the reader is referred to the excellent text by Enzinger and Weiss.[1] This chapter will concentrate on a selected group of the most common lesions.

Neural tumours[2]

Benign neurilemmoma and Schwannoma

These lesions develop as slowly growing, usually isolated, nodules which are attached to the long axis of a peripheral nerve. A number of affected patients have associated von Recklinghausen's disease.[3] On pathological examination, a densely cellular mass will be seen. At low power, the appearance may be almost sarcomatous. At higher power the diagnostic mixture of Antoni A and Antoni B areas will be seen (Figure 13.1). The former are areas of spindle cells that are closely packed and appear to form a syncytium, with elongated nuclei, and poorly differentiated cytoplasmic margins. Verocay bodies are seen in these areas (Figure 13.2). Antoni type B areas are less cellular, and have a rather oedematous-looking myxoid stroma with large vascular channels. These areas are similar to the cellular pattern seen in neurofibroma, but, in contrast to neurofibromas, mast cells are not seen.

A plexiform schwannoma has been recorded,[4] and should be distinguished from plexiform neurofibroma,

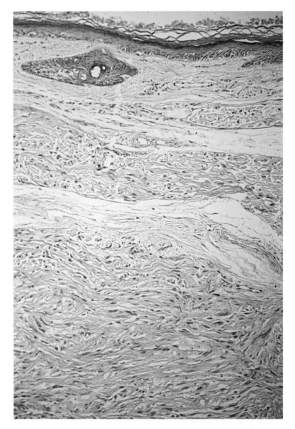

which is found exclusively in von Recklinghausen's disease and has the potential for malignant change; this has not yet been reported in plexiform schwannoma. A cellular schwannoma is also recorded, and as this may show considerable cellular atypia, care should be taken not to confuse the lesion with a sarcoma.[5]

Palisaded and encapsulated neuroma[6,7]

Palisaded and encapsulated neuromas are usually asymptomatic flesh-coloured nodules on the face of middle-aged individuals of either sex. They are not associated with von Recklinghausen's disease and are encapsulated, well-differentiated clusters of spindle cells situated in the dermis. Local excision is curative (Figures 13.3 and 13.4).

Figure 13.1 Low-power view of a neurilemmoma, showing the spindle cell population.

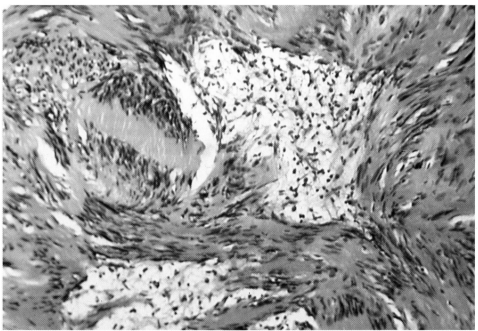

Figure 13.2 High-power view of a neurilemmoma, showing Verocay bodies.

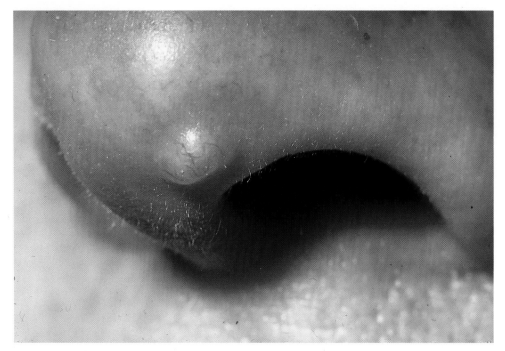

Figure 13.3   Clinical appearance of a palisaded encapsulated neuroma on the nose.

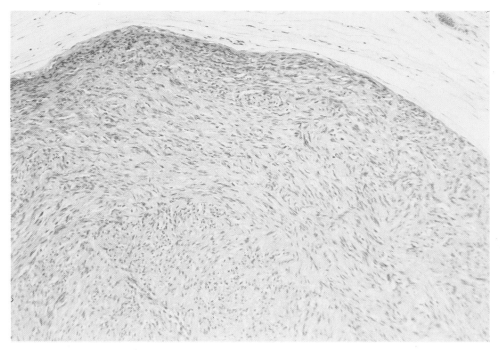

Figure 13.4   Pathological features of the palisaded encapsulated neruoma illustrated in Figure 13.3.

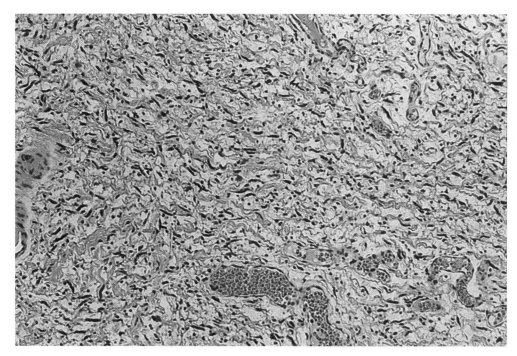

Figure 13.5   Neurofibroma showing the striking spindle cell pattern with no Verocay bodies.

Neurofibroma[8]

Neurofibromas may be solitary or multiple lesions. Multiple lesions are found in von Recklinghausen's disease. Solitary lesions are relatively common, and present as slowly growing asymptomatic lesions, usually in young adults.

The characteristic pathological picture is of a network of collagen fibrils and mucinous stroma with Schwann cells set in this network (Figure 13.5). A cellular variant is seen, in which the proportion of Schwann cells is high, and rarer variants include the myxoid and diffuse types. Numerous mast cells are seen, but, in contrast to the neurilemmomas, Verocay bodies are not present.

Malignant change is very rarely reported in solitary lesions.

von Recklinghausen's disease (multiple neurofibromatosis)

This condition is inherited by autosomal dominant transmission, with a high degree of penetrance. Spontaneous mutations appear to be extremely common, and recently the genes for NF 1 and NF 2 have been mapped to chromosomes 17 and 22 respectively.[9] The clinical presentation may be of a peripheral or a central type of involvement.

The peripheral type is usually recognized in early childhood because of the presence of 'café au lait' spots. Solitary café au lait spots should alert the physician to search for other evidence of von Recklinghausen's disease, and the presence of six or more lesions measuring 1.5 cm or more in diameter is virtually diagnostic (Figure 13.6).

The neurofibromas may not appear until adolescence, and may involve any body site, and be both numerous and disfiguring (Figure 13.7). Very large, pendulous fibroma molluscum may develop. New lesions appear, and existing lesions tend to expand, during periods of hormonal stimulation such as pregnancy and puberty. Bony defects of various types are extremely common.

The central type of von Recklinghausen's disease presents with intracranial or intraspinal neural tumours, and few of the peripheral features described above.

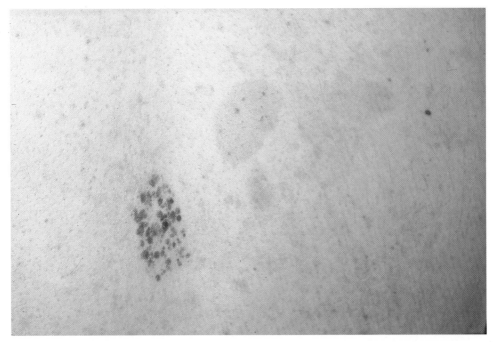

Figure 13.6 Café au lait spots. These were the only lesions present in an 8-year-old child who developed gross neurofibromatosis in the second decade.

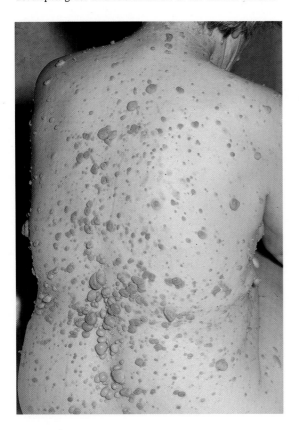

The pathological features of neurofibromas in von Recklinghausen's disease are identical to those of the solitary neurofibroma, although the lesions may be much larger (see Figure 13.5).

The incidence of malignant degeneration in von Recklinghausen's associated neurofibromas varies in reported series from 2 to 13 per cent. The usual presenting feature is of rapid and painful expansion of a pre-existing benign neurofibroma.[10]

Malignant neurofibroma and Schwannoma[11]

These tumours are seen in patients with and without von Recklinghausen's disease. The former group tend to present at a younger age. The classic presentation is that of a rapidly expanding painful nodule.

Figure 13.7 Multiple pendulous fibroma molluscum of von Recklinghausen's disease.

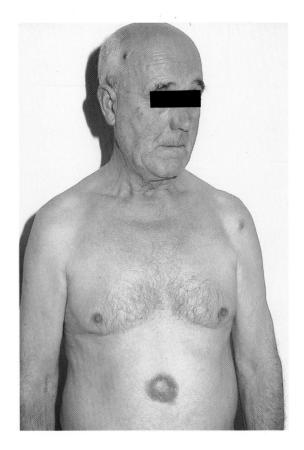

On pathological examination, dark, closely packed fascicles of tumour cells can be seen alternating with less cellular myxoid areas. Individual cell nuclei have a wavy and buckled outline, and this feature may be of value in differentiation from a fibrosarcoma. Hyaline bands, nodules and both perineural and intraneural metastatic spread are all useful diagnostic features.

Primary neuroendocrine carcinoma of the skin (Merkel cell tumour or trabecular cell carcinoma)

The exact ontogeny of this lesion is not yet established. As it shows features of differentiation towards a Merkel cell, and as Merkel cells are thought to be a type of mechanoreceptor converting mechanical to humoral stimuli, the lesion would at present appear to merit inclusion in this section on neural tumours.[12]

Figure 13.8 Primary neuroendocine carcinoma on the trunk of an elderly male.

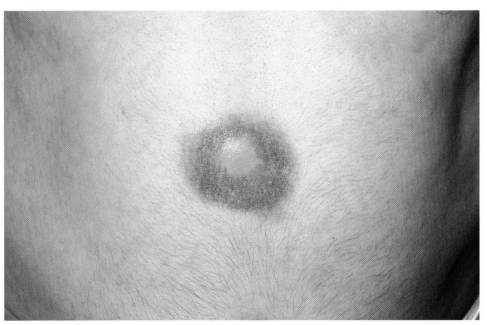

Figure 13.9 Close-up view of the lesion illustrated in Figure 13.8.

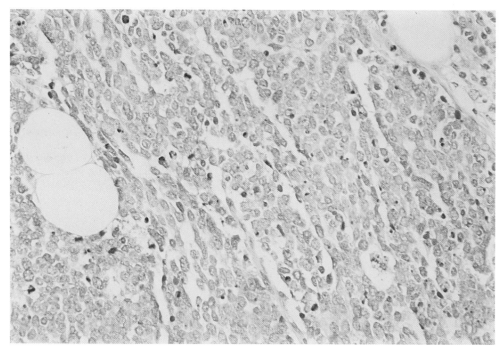

Figure 13.10 Primary neuroendocrine carcinoma. The section is stained with haematoxylin and eosin, showing a trabecular appearance and numerous mitotic figures.

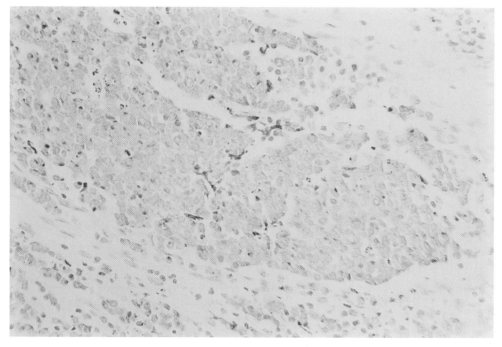

Figure 13.11 Primary neuroendocrine tumour stained with Campath 5.2 anticytokeratin monoclonal antibody. The positive staining is seen with the brown dots in numerous cells.

The Merkel cell was first identified in 1875 on the mole's snout.[13] It is seen in the basal layer of the epidermis, and forms the third member of the triad of branched epidermal cells, the other two being the melanocyte and the Langerhans cell. Until recently, a Merkel cell could only be seen using electron microscopy to reveal the numerous electron-dense Merkel granules in the cytoplasm. In the past two years the monoclonal antibody Campath 5.2 has proved to be a useful marker of Merkel cells, as a very characteristic dot pattern of staining appears to be relatively, but not totally, specific for the Merkel cell.

Large numbers of Merkel cells are seen in animals in association with hairs, and in humans they are frequently seen in association with cutaneous nerves.[14] Histochemical techniques have indicated that they are a member of the APUD (amine precursor uptake and decarboxylation) cell system.

In 1972 Toker described a dermal tumour which he called trabecular cell carcinoma of the skin.[15] At that time he suggested an origin from the eccrine sweat gland, but six years later he published a second paper describing the electron-dense granules seen in the cytoplasm of these tumours.[16] Since this second paper, a Merkel cell origin for these tumours has been postulated but not proven.

The usual clinical presentation of primary neuro-endocrine carcinoma of the skin is an expanding red nodule in an elderly patient (Figures 13.8 and 13.9).[15] A number of these lesions have been reported to coexist with squamous cell carcinoma.[12] Ulceration is said to be rare.

On pathological examination a cellular mass will be seen in the mid to deep dermis (Figure 13.10). The cells are embedded in a vascular stroma, and may give an appearance of anastomosing trabeculae, with no apparent duct formation. The cytoplasm is scanty, pale and granular, and the nuclei are large with multiple small prominent nucleoli. Normal mitotic figures are numerous, and apoptosis is a common feature. Silver stains may be positive, but are not always so on routinely fixed material.

The pathological differential diagnosis using light microscopy will include lymphoma, squamous cell carcinoma, malignant melanoma, and secondary tumour, particularly oat cell carcinoma of the bronchus. Ultrastructural examination will reveal the characteristic electron-dense granules.

If electron microscopy is not available, or if all tissue has been processed, the use of immunopathology may be helpful. Neurone-specific enolase positivity is reported in the majority of lesions,[17] and staining with anticytokeratin antibodies, notably Campath 5.2,

will show a characteristic dot-like positivity (Figure 13.11).[18]

Management

Both local recurrence and distant metastases are recorded, the former in up to 75 per cent of published cases and the latter in 25 per cent. For this reason, wide local excision and a search for metastatic spread is recommended.

Fibrohistiocytic tumours

Keloids and hypertrophic scars

Keloids and hypertrophic scars are seen clinically as large, erythematous and elevated, cosmetically unacceptable scars that are frequently tender (Figure 13.12).[19] The clinical difference between these two lesions is somewhat debatable, although it has been suggested that keloids are painful and do not vanish spontaneously. Many scars go through a period of apparent hypertrophy during the first 6–12 months of their development and then resolve spontaneously.[20]

On pathological examination, foci of dense hyalinized collagen bundles running in various directions through the dermis will be seen. Giant cells may be seen in association with these collagen fibrils (Figure 13.13).

Dermatofibroma (sclerosing angioma, subepidermal nodular fibrosis)

There is still some debate as to whether this lesion is a traumatic reaction to stimuli such as an insect bite or whether it is a true neoplasm. It has recently been postulated that the dermatofibroma may be a tumour of the so-called dermal dendrocyte.[21]

The majority of these lesions are seen on the limbs, particularly the legs, of younger individuals and present as firm, sometimes slightly pruritic nodules.[22] They may have a slightly yellow tinge, and some are deeply pigmented, particularly at the periphery, giving rise on occasion to clinical concern about malignant melanoma (Figures 13.14 and 13.15). A small number of dermatofibromas have been reported in association with basal cell carcinomas.[23]

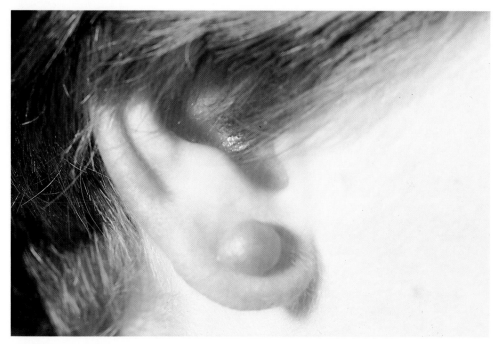

Figure 13.12 Keloidal reaction to ear piercing. This phenomenon is seen more commonly in dark-skinned races.

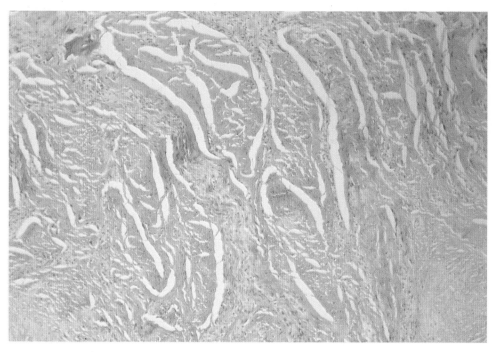

Figure 13.13 Pathology of a keloid, showing coarse, dense collagen bundles.

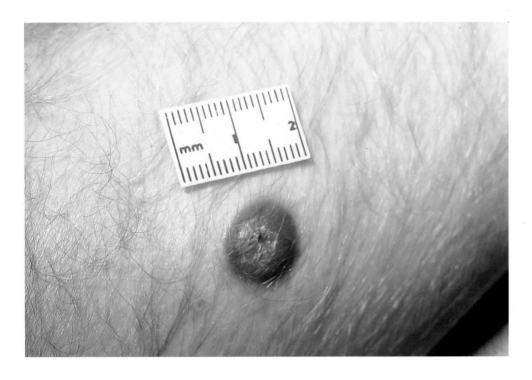

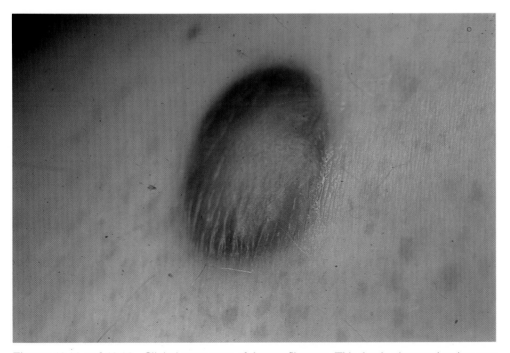

Figures 13.14 and 13.15   Clinical appearance of dermatofibromas. This deeply pigmented variant may be clinically confused with a melanocytic lesion, possibly melanoma.

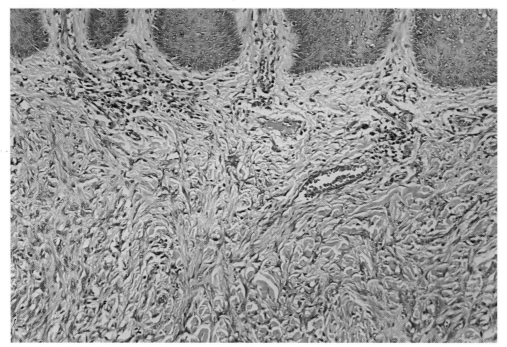

Figure 13.16 Cellular characteristics of dermatofibroma.

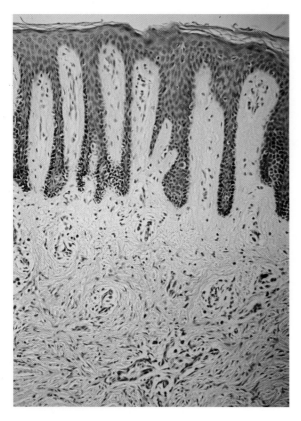

On pathological examination, the characteristic pattern is that of dermally situated cellular aggregate (Figure 13.16) underneath an area of epidermal hyperplasia (Figure 13.17).[24] This epidermal hyperplasia may be very striking indeed and at times be frankly pseudoepitheliomatous.

The dermal component of a lesion biopsied early in its development shows a large number of histiocytic cells and also Touton-type giant cells. A surprising amount of lipid may be present and this will be apparent only if frozen sections are stained for fat. Varying quantities of haemosiderin-containing macrophages may be seen, and the presence of iron explains the clinical pigmentation (Figure 13.18).

In an older lesion there will be a higher proportion of fibroblasts and collagen, and the lesion may be more vascular than the younger lesion, and contain even larger quantities of haemosiderin. The histiocytic cells and collagen fibres are seen as an intertwined mesh which does not have the characteristic cartwheel or

Figure 13.17 Pseudoepitheliomatous hyperplasia overlying dermatofibroma.

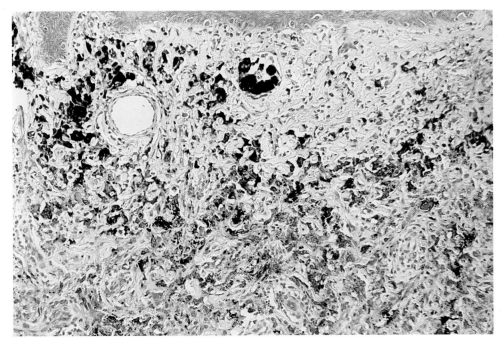

Figure 13.18   Iron stain in dermatofibroma. The blue reaction indicates strong positivity.

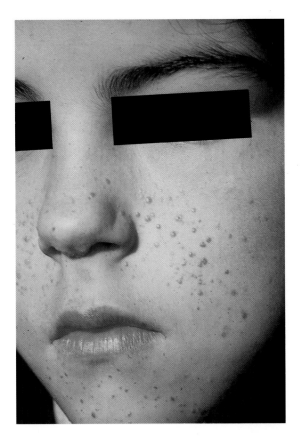

Figure 13.19   Multiple angiofibromas in the centre panel of the face of a child with tuberous sclerosis.

storiform pattern of the dermatofibrosarcoma protruberans discussed below. Mitotic figures are rare, but the pattern of infiltration of the lateral margin of the dermatofibroma into the surrounding normal collagen may give rise to concern about malignancy.

Angiofibroma, or perivascular fibroma[25]

Angiofibromas are most often identified in association with tuberous sclerosis. In the past, a number of pathologically inappropriate terms have been used to describe these lesions.

The clinical presentation is of multiple firm, red, papular lesions, usually on the face and generally concentrated around the nasolabial folds (Figure 13.19). These lesions are frequently not present at birth but develop and become multiple at puberty. Patients with such lesions may be referred inappropriately as cases of

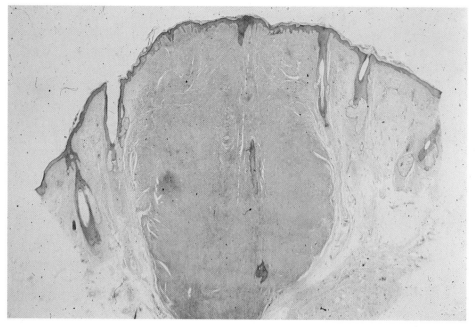

Figure 13.20   Perivascular fibroma or angiofibroma – pathological appearance.

atypical acne vulgaris because of their age at the time of the expansion of the lesions.

On pathological examination, fibrous lesions will be seen concentrated around small blood vessels in the papillary dermis (Figure 13.20).

Usually, the large number of the lesions makes excision of all lesions impractical. Some success has been observed with cryotherapy, and possibly laser therapy may be of value in the future.

Dermatofibrosarcoma protruberans[26]

The clinical presentation of this lesion is as a slowly expanding lump on any body site, most commonly the thigh (Figure 13.21).

On pathological examination, a spindle cell dermal mass will be seen underlying an area of epidermal thinning.[27] This is in contrast to the pseudoepitheliomatous hyperplasia seen in the dermatofibroma. Ulceration is, however, rare, and there is usually a Grenz zone of normal dermis between the epidermis and the actual lesion. The spindle cells are arranged in a storiform, rushmat or cartwheel pattern, with intertwining fascicles of spindle cells being a striking feature of this lesion (Figure 13.22). This storiform pattern is not, however, diagnostic of or specific to dermatofibrosarcoma protruberans and may be seen in a number of other soft tissue tumours. Mitotic figures are rare, and the lateral margin of the lesion may be difficult to identify because of the way in which the cells composing the lesion merge with surrounding normal dermal tissue.

A rare variant of the dermatofibrosarcoma protruberans is the pigmented variant, or so-called Bednar tumour.[28] This could be confused with a spindle cell melanoma metastasis. With the use of immunopathology, these two conditions can be differentiated, as the melanoma will stain positively with S 100 antibody whereas the dermatofibrosarcoma protruberans will not stain with this antibody.

The high frequency of local recurrence – up to 50 per cent in some series – means that wide local excision should be carried out, with 3 cm of normal tissue around the apparent margins of the lesion. Erosion must also be adequate in depth, and many authorities suggest that this should be to the muscular aponeuroses.

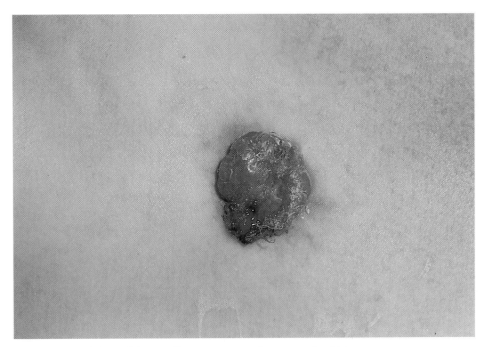

Figure 13.21 Ulcerated dermatofibrosarcoma protuberans on the thigh.

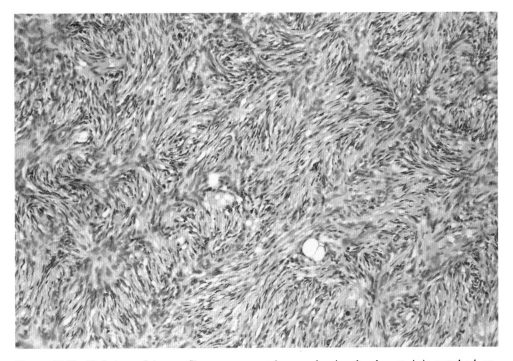

Figure 13.22 Pathology of dermatofibrosarcoma protuberans, showing the characteristic cartwheel, or storiform, pattern of cells.

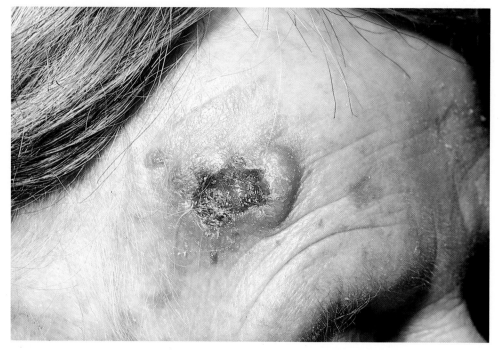

Figure 13.23   Ulcerated atypical fibroxanthoma on the forehead of an elderly female.

Atypical fibroxanthoma (AFX)[29]

This tumour is most often seen on sun-exposed skin in elderly individuals. The ears, cheeks and nose are all common sites, and the tumour is also reported in sites of previous X-ray therapy. Ulceration is frequently seen (Figure 13.23).

On pathological examination, the epidermis will be seen to be thin, or even ulcerated, and under this area a striking and alarming population of atypical fibrohistiocytic cells will be seen (Figure 13.24). Nuclei tend to be very large, and grossly abnormal mitotic figures are numerous (Figure 13.25).[30] Depending on whether flow cytometry or image analysis is used, these cells may appear to be diploid[31] or aneuploid,[32] but the pathological appearance is usually rather more alarming than the biological behaviour, as local recurrence is usually curative (although metastatic spread has been reported in a small number of these lesions).

It is currently considered that the atypical fibroxanthoma should be treated as a low-grade malignancy, and that it is related to malignant fibrous hystiocytoma. In comparison with malignant fibrous histiocytoma, atypical fibroxanthoma is more superficially situated in the dermis, and usually comprises a smaller cellular mass. In contrast to both malignant fibrous histiocytoma and dermatofibrosarcoma protruberans, atypical fibroxanthoma does not usually show the storiform pattern of the involved spindle cells.

Malignant fibrous histiocytoma (MFH)

At the time of writing, malignant fibrous histiocytoma is a fashionable diagnosis and is said to be the most common dermal tumour of late adult life.[33–35] There is perhaps a tendency at the present time to overdiagnose this lesion.

The majority of malignant fibrous histiocytomas to date are reported on the thighs and buttocks, but are seen on any body site, usually in individuals aged 50 years or older (Figure 13.26).

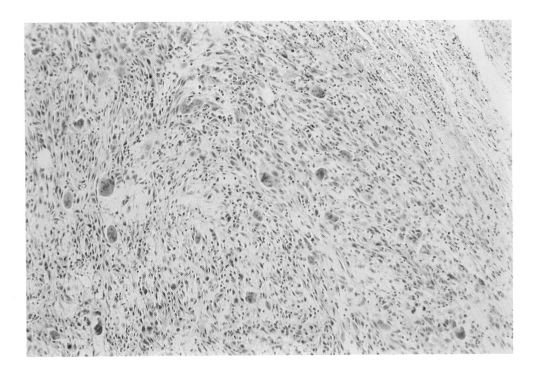

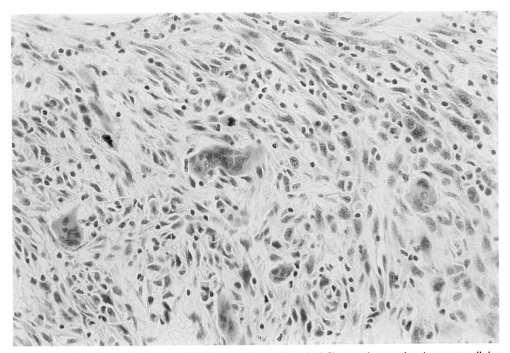

Figures 13.24 and 13.25   Low- and high-power views of atypical fibroxanthoma, showing gross cellular atypia and abnormal mitoses.

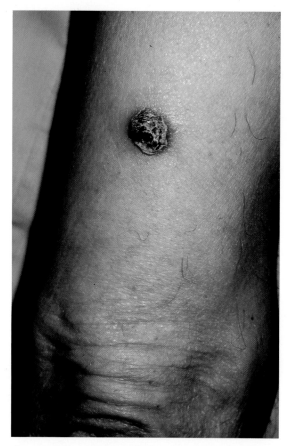

Figure 13.26 Malignant fibrous histiocytoma on the upper arm of an elderly male. This lesion recurred locally twice after wide local excision.

On pathological examination, a poorly demarcated, deeply situated dermal mass will be seen. Subcutaneous fat and muscle are frequently involved (Figure 13.27). The lesion is a cellular pleomorphic tumour (Figure 13.28). Myxoid, inflammatory, angiomatoid and giant cell variants have all been reported. A storiform or rushmat-like pattern is frequently seen, but in contrast to the dermatofibrosarcoma protruberans, the cells comprising these masses have pleomorphic nuclei with frequent abnormal mitotic figures.

The prognosis of malignant fibrous histiocytoma is said to be related to both the volume and the depth of the tumour, and 44 per cent local recurrence with 42 per cent metastatic spread is reported. Thus, this is a fully developed malignant tumour with the capacity to metastasize and kill the patient. As with other fibrohistiocytic tumours, the lateral margins of this lesion are poorly demarcated, a factor which may explain the high local recurrence rate.

Wide local excision and careful follow-up is essential in this aggressive group of tumours.

An important variant of malignant fibrous histiocytoma is the angiomatoid variant.[36] This is a distinct fibrohistiocytic tumour seen in children and young adults, with the median age at presentation of 13 years. This lesion simulates a vascular neoplasm and can be locally aggressive. Wide excision and careful follow-up is again required.

Vascular tumours

Pyogenic granuloma

This common tumour usually arises on the fingers after minor trauma, the classic injury being the trauma to gardeners' fingers after pruning roses. These lesions present clinically as rapidly expanding, painful, moist, vascular lesions (Figure 13.29). The rate of growth can lead to concern about frank malignancy, and because of their site the lesions can give rise to considerable discomfort and temporary disability.

On pathological examination, a network of vascular capillary channels will be seen, set in an extremely oedematous stroma (Figure 13.30). Mitotic figures are rare and usually there is virtually no inflammatory reaction. Careful examination of the depth of the lesion may identify a thick-walled feeder vessel from which the tumour has presumably arisen.

These lesions are usually excised locally, both to confirm the diagnosis and for comfort. Recurrence of the lesion after local excision is not infrequent, and multiple small satellite lesions may develop, giving rise to alarm about a rapidly metastasizing malignant lesion (Figure 13.31). These lesions, however, do not spread beyond the site of local recurrence and are benign.[37]

Angiokeratoma[38]

Several types of angiokeratoma are recognized.[39] These include isolated lesions (Figure 13.32), the localized angiokeratoma of Mibelli found on the fingers (Figure 13.33), the angiokeratoma of Fordyce found on the scrotum (Figure 13.34), and the rarer systemic disease, the angiokeratoma of Fabry.

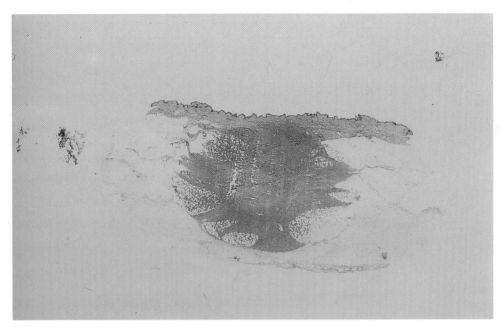

Figure 13.27 Low-power view of malignant fibrous histiocytoma, showing the extension of the lesion through the dermis to subcutaneous fat.

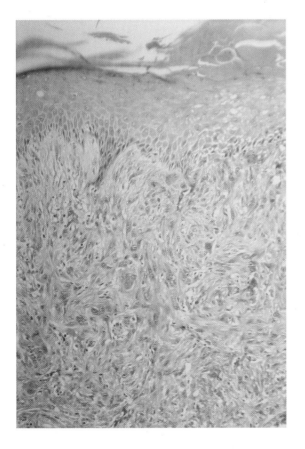

Figure 13.28 High-power view of the malignant fibrous histiocytoma illustrated in Figure 13.27, showing gross cellular atypia in cells in the papillary dermis. Note the similarity to Figures 13.24 and 13.25.

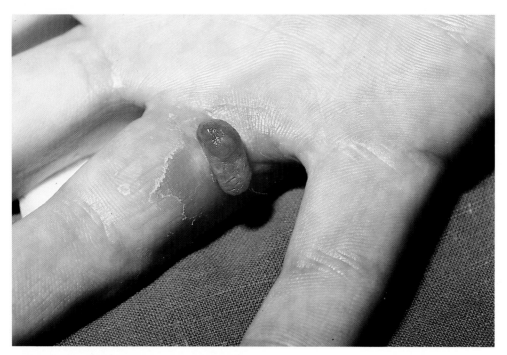

Figure 13.29 Classic solitary moist pyogenic granuloma on the finger.

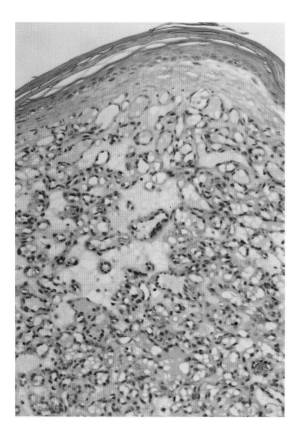

Figure 13.30 Pathology of pyogenic granuloma, showing wide, thin-walled vascular channels.

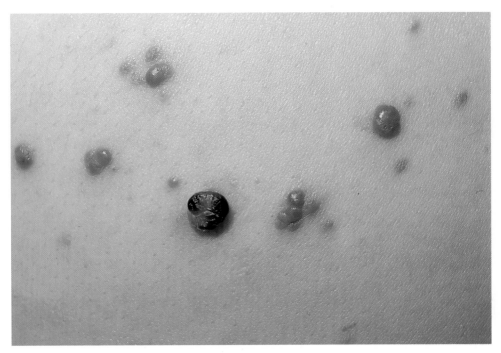

Figure 13.31 Clinical appearance of a recurrence of multiple pyogenic granulomas after diathermy to a solitary lesion. All regressed spontaneously.

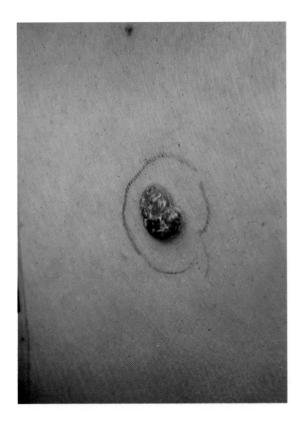

Figure 13.32 A solitary angiokeratoma.

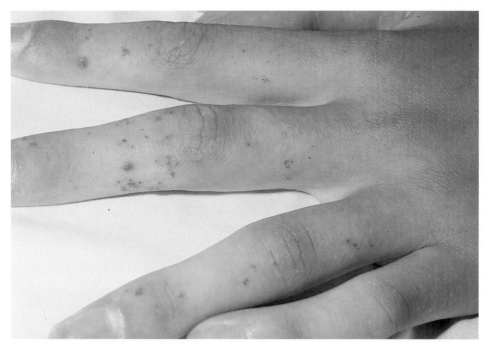

Figure 13.33 Angiokeratoma of Mibelli on the fingers.

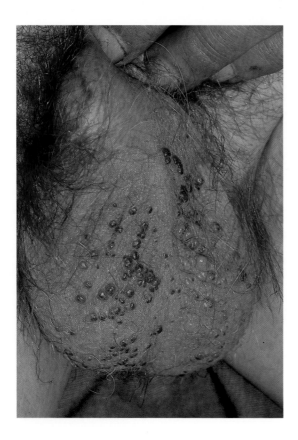

Figure 13.34 Angiokeratoma of Fordyce on the scrotum.

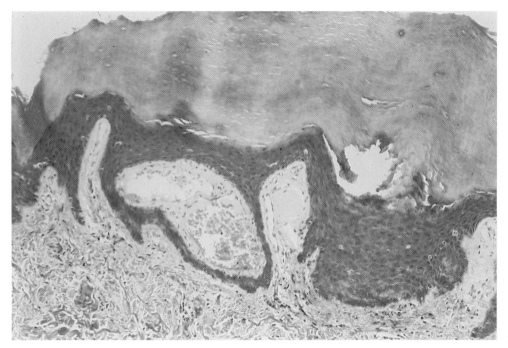

Figure 13.35   Pathology of the angiokeratoma illustrated in Figure 13.32, showing wide vascular channels under hyperkeratosis.

On pathological examination, large, thin-walled vascular channels will be seen underneath an area of gross hyperkeratosis (Figure 13.35).

Glomus tumour

Glomus tumours were first described by Masson in 1924 and may be isolated or multiple.[40] The latter are rare and may be familial.[41,42] Both types are painful. The isolated lesions are most frequently reported in the subungual area (Figure 13.36), and the multiple lesions may be seen on any body site, with lesions on the thigh being reported relatively frequently (Figure 13.37).[43] The subungual lesions present as firm, tender, vascular nodules, and the multiple glomus tumours present as bluish-black, multiple nodules, a factor which may give rise to concern about melanoma.

On pathological examination, the tumour mass will be seen to be composed of multiple, small, regular, cuboidal cells. These are the so-called glomus cells and are thought to be part of the Suquet–Hoyer canals, which are associated with arterial venous anastomoses. Solitary lesions have a capsule, and contain a mesh of endothelium-lined vessels around which large numbers of glomus cells are situated. Multiple lesions have larger vascular spaces (Figure 13.38), do not usually have a capsule, and contain relatively fewer glomus cells, with perhaps only three or four cell layers around the vascular spaces.

These lesions are frequently removed because of spontaneous pain, and also to obtain a diagnosis.

Lymphangioma circumscriptum

Lymphangiomas are seen most often in children and young adults. They usually present clinically as linear polypoid lesions comprising large numbers of thin-walled vesicles on the skin (Figure 13.39). These vesicles are ruptured easily by friction from clothing, but new lesions develop fairly rapidly.

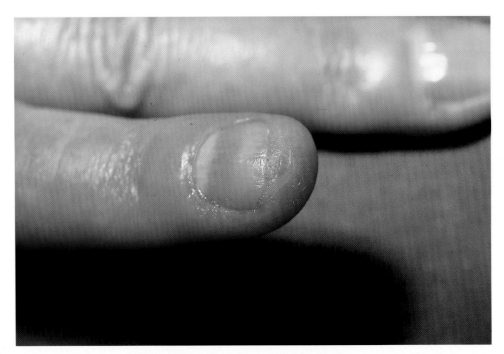

Figure 13.36   Solitary painful glomus tumour proximal to the nail-bed.

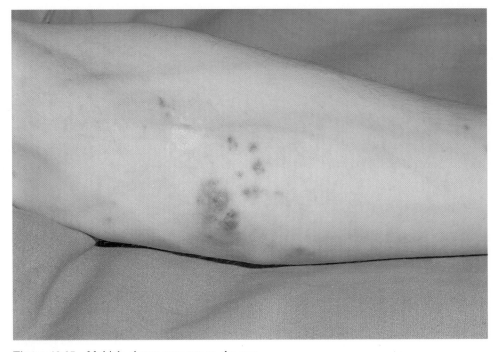

Figure 13.37   Multiple glomus tumours on the arm.

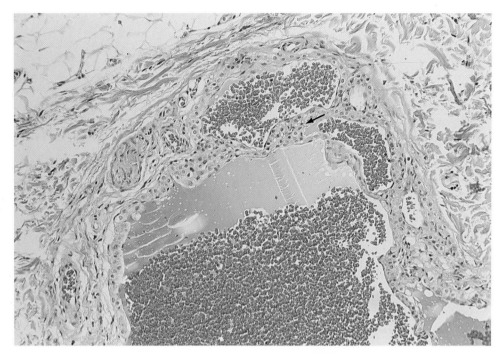

Figure 13.38 Pathology of the glomus tumours illustrated in Figure 13.37, showing wide vascular channels with glomus cells (arrow).

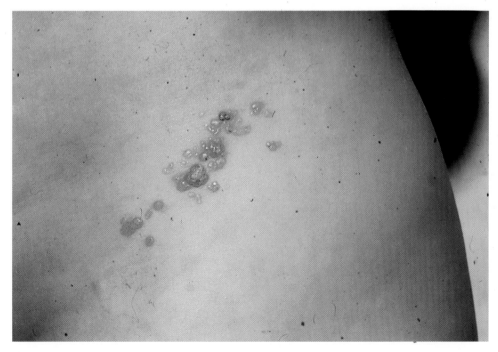

Figure 13.39 A linear lymphangioma in the groin area.

On pathological examination, large numbers of extremely thin-walled lymphatic channels will be seen in the superficial dermis, with only one layer of lining endothelial cells.

In contrast to lesions arising from the vascular channels, no associated myoepithelial cells will be seen around the lymphangiomatous vessels.

Whimster carried out a valuable detailed pathological study of lymphangioma and showed that, in addition to the superficial lesions that give rise to the clinical problem, there are deeply situated cisternae in the deep dermis that supply the superficial vessels.[44] This study provided a logical explanation for the observation that lymphangiomas tended to recur after local excision.

Clearly, wide and deep local excision is necessary to remove the feeder vessels and cure the lesion completely.

Angiosarcoma

Cutaneous angiosarcoma is a relatively rare condition.[45] The clinical presentation may be misleading. The majority of reported cases have lesions on the forehead and scalp and may present as an extensive bruise-like lesion, or even as a persistent cellulitis-like swelling around the eyes. Most reported cases are in elderly males, and a history of excessive sun exposure is common (Figure 13.40).

On pathological examination, large, thin-walled vascular channels will be seen dissecting through the collagen in a very irregular fashion.[46] The endothelial cells lining these irregular vessels show frequent mitoses, and gross haemorrhage is present (Figure 13.41). Occasional tufts of endothelial cells will be seen projecting into the vascular channels. The use of

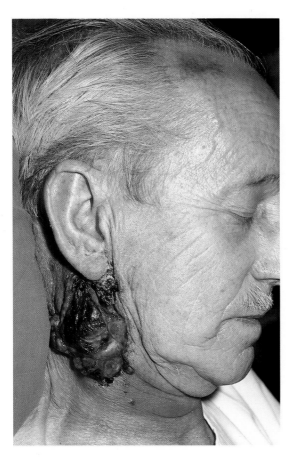

Figure 13.40 Angiosarcoma on the neck of an elderly male.

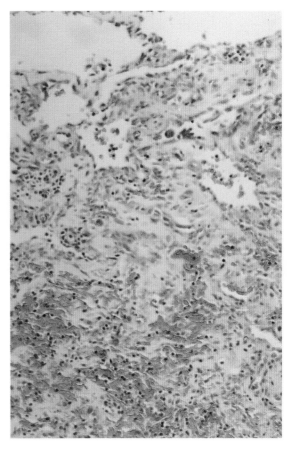

Figure 13.41 Gross haemorrhage in the dermis of an angiosarcoma.

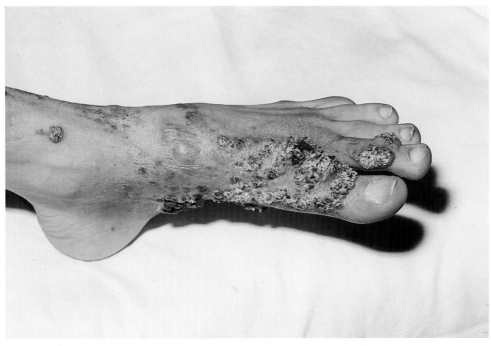

Figure 13.42   Clinical appearance of Kaposi's sarcoma in an elderly male of central European background.

monoclonal antibodies to factor-VIII-related antigen will show these cells to be of vascular origin. Similar confirmation can be obtained using the lectin *Ulex europaeus*, which also stains vascular tissue. In general, factor-VIII-related antigen is relatively specific but not sensitive for vascular tissue, whereas *Ulex* is sensitive but not specific.[47]

The most probable differential diagnosis will be from Kaposi's sarcoma. The larger vascular spaces in the angiosarcoma and the presence of endothelial cells in mitoses, together with a relative lack of the spindle cells seen in Kaposi's sarcoma should all be helpful pointers.

These tumours metastasize frequently, and a very poor 2-year survival rate is quoted.[48] Once the diagnosis is made, a search for involvement of lymph nodes and other organs is necessary. Radiotherapy may provide worthwhile temporary remission, but tumour recurrence is the usual rule.

Kaposi's sarcoma

Kaposi's sarcoma (KS) may develop in four clinical situations. These consist of:

1. a rather indolent form, usually seen on the lower legs of elderly males (Figure 13.42);
2. the type seen in immunosuppressed patients after cytotoxic therapy (Figures 13.43 and 13.44);
3. an endemic form seen in Africa; and
4. the type found in the acquired immunodeficiency syndrome (AIDS).

With the current public awareness of this last situation, patients are presenting with very small vascular lesions, and it is necessary to be able to differentiate between the early patch or lymphangioma-like form of KS and benign vascular lesions. This can be difficult, and at times impossible.

The usual clinical presentation is of multifocal vascular lesions with raised, reddish nodules on any site, but most frequently the lower legs.[49] Patients with the AIDS-related form may, in addition, have lesions on the hard palate. In the non-AIDS-related forms the lesions usually grow very slowly, but in the AIDS-related form there may be explosive growth and rapid development of unsightly and painful lesions with metastatic spread.[50,51] Recent evidence suggests that in addition to HIV infection, the presence of a novel

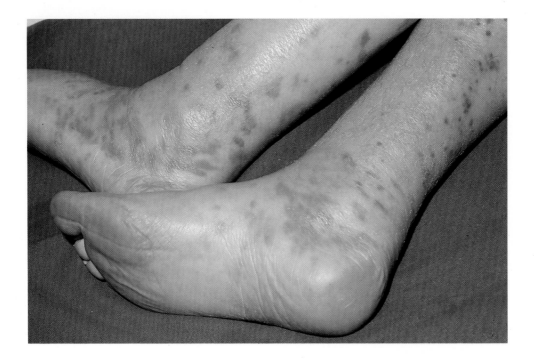

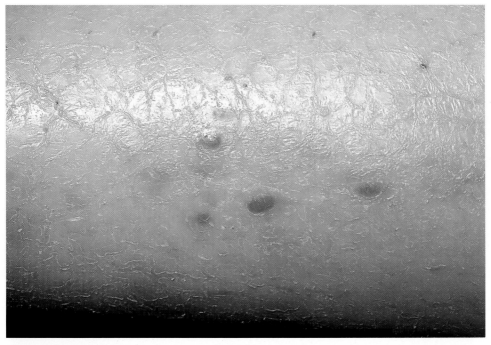

Figures 13.43 and 13.44 Kaposi's sarcoma arising on the legs of an elderly female after cytotoxic chemotherapy.

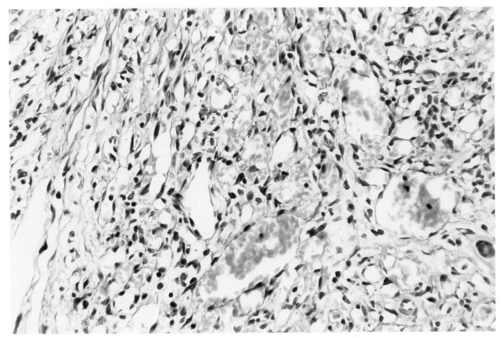

Figure 13.45   Pathology of Kaposi's sarcoma, showing thin-walled, 'back-to-back' capillaries.

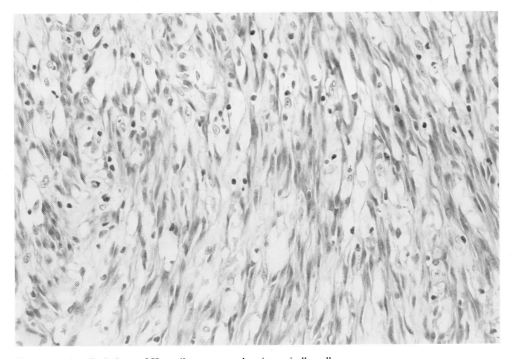

Figure 13.46   Pathology of Kaposi's sarcoma, showing spindle cells.

herpes virus may be needed in HIV-positive men for clinical manifestations of KS to develop.[52] On pathological examination, numerous very thin-walled 'back-to-back' capillaries will be seen in the dermis with an associated proliferation of spindle cells (Figures 13.45 and 13.46).[53] Erythrophagocytosis is a characteristic feature, and eosinophilic globules or hyaline bodies are seen in these spindle cells. These give a striking appearance if the phloxine tartrazine stain is used, and are thought to be disintegrating erythrocytes. A mild lymphocytic infiltrate may be seen in early lesions.

The differential diagnosis will include stasis dermatitis, dermatofibroma, scar tissue, and haemangiomas.[54] In stasis, the vessels are thick-walled, whereas in KS they are thin-walled. Also, in stasis one does not see vessels back to back but separated by proliferating fibrous tissue similar to scar tissue. This is not seen in KS. The combination of spindle cells and erythrophagocytosis is virtually diagnostic of KS.

Immunopathological studies have shown that the malignant cells in KS are positive for factor VIII antigen, and are positive when stained with antibody to *Ulex europaeus* lectin, both confirmatory signs of a vascular origin.[54]

In non-AIDS-related KS, the progress of the disease may be so slow that treatment may be more distressing for the patient than the condition, and in AIDS-related KS, the patient's other problems may be of more pressing importance. The lesions do respond well to radiotherapy, which is currently the treatment of choice, if treatment is considered necessary. It has been observed that patients with AIDS who develop KS have a longer survival than those who do not. The reason for this is not at present known.

Patients with all types of KS have a greater than expected incidence of second malignancies, and investigations should be carried out as appropriate, depending on the patient's age and general clinical condition.[55]

Leiomyosarcoma

Smooth muscle tumours are relatively rare in the dermis and, once again, tend to present as rapidly enlarging nodules.

On pathological examination, the striking features are the presence of a spindle cell neoplasm with interlacing bundles.[56] The subcutaneous tissues and fat may be involved. The cytology is that of spindle cells

with elongated, blunt-ended nuclei having clearly visible chromatin. Unlike those in tumours of nerve origin, the nuclei are uniform and smooth rather than having a wavy outline. If polarized light is used, birefringent fibrils can be demonstrated in the surrounding cytoplasm. Mitotic figures are extremely rare in benign smooth muscle lesions, and it is said that if as few as one mitotic figure is found in every five high-power fields the tumour is likely to be malignant. These mitoses, however, may be non-randomly distributed throughout the tumour and a careful search for mitoses is essential.

Until the advent of immunopathology it was considered that for such a spindle cell tumour ultrastructural examination was necessary to determine its histogenetic type. Now, however, the use of antibodies raised against desmin can be used as a positive marker of muscle-derived lesions.

These lesions require excision. There appear to be relatively few reports of leiomyosarcomas metastasizing and the prognosis, therefore, is relatively good.

Liposarcoma

Liposarcomas are relatively common soft tissue tumours in adults, more frequently arising in interfascial muscle planes than in the subcutaneous fat.

The thigh is a well-known site, and, once again, the tumours present as rapidly expanding, painless nodules. They may become extremely large before help is sought.

On pathological examination of an excised specimen, the presence of balloon-like cells displaying the typical foamy cytoplasm of fat cells will be seen.[57] Only a small proportion of these tumours are well differentiated, so there may be differential diagnostic confusion with a benign lipoma. High-power microscopic examination will, however, reveal cytologically atypical cells with atypical mitotic figures. The majority of liposarcomas have a somewhat myxoid appearance, with atypical lipoblasts embedded in a richly vascular myxoid stroma. A few liposarcomas are extremely pleomorphic, with grossly dilated cells, foamy cytoplasm, and atypical nuclei. The malignancy of these lesions and their lipomatous origin are immediately apparent.

These tumours should be excised locally with a wide margin of apparently normal tissue. The pleomorphic variety has a poor 5-year survival rate, but the prognosis for survival with the other types is reasonably good.

Melanoma of soft parts (clear cell sarcoma of tendons and aponeuroses)

In 1968 Enzinger published details of 21 cases of clear cell tumours intimately associated with the tendons and aponeuroses, and suggested that they were sarcomatous.[58] Work since this time, and in particular the observation of the presence of melanosomes in 50 per cent of these lesions, has suggested that the term melanoma of soft parts may be more appropriate.[59,60] Over 75 per cent of reported cases arise on the lower limbs, usually around the ankles. There are no changes in the epidermis, and the patient will complain of an expanding painful nodule. It is most often seen in young adults.

The pathological features are those of a tumour mass comprising fascicles of pale-staining, uniform, fusiform cells embedded in a dense stroma (Figure 13.47). Mitotic figures are rare, and silver stains will reveal the presence of melanin in approximately 50 per cent. The cell mass may be attached to tendons and aponeuroses. Electron microscopy will show the presence of melanosomes in some of these lesions.

Despite the relatively bland cytology of these lesions, they tend both to recur locally and to metastasize. Wide local excision, possibly amputation, is therefore required, with investigations as appropriate for metastatic spread.

Differential diagnosis of spindle cell tumours in the dermis

A fairly common problem confronting the pathologist or dermatopathologist is the presence of a malignant spindle cell tumour mass in the dermis. In the past, the identification of the type of cell from which these spindle cells were derived, or towards which they are differentiating, has been difficult and has required ultrastructural study, which has not always been definitive. With the advent of immunopathology and

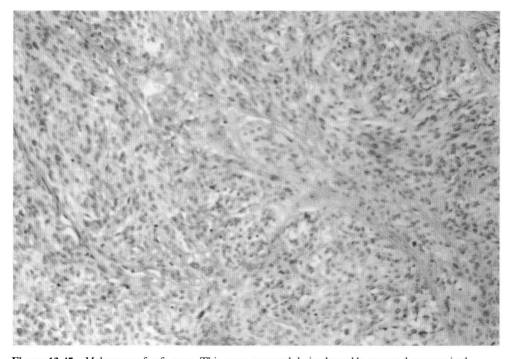

Figure 13.47   Melanoma of soft parts. This arose as a nodule in the ankle area and metastasized.

Table 13.1 Immunopathological identification of undifferentiated dermal spindle cell tumours.

Monoclonal antibody	Cytokeratin	Leucocyte common antigen	S 100	Desmin	Factor VIII
Tumour type if positive	Squamous cell carcinoma	Lymphoma	Melanoma or neural	Muscle	Vascular
		Further tests required with T (UCHT 1) B Histiocytic markers	NKI C 3 positivity also confirmatory — Stain with GFAP		

NB (1) Not all malignant cells derived from these phenotypes will stain strongly or even stain at all. These tests, therefore, are a guide only. A negative result does not exclude the possibility of malignancy.

(2) Other antibodies found, in the author's experience, to be less useful are vimentin, which stains cells of mesenchymal derivation, and alpha1-trypsin, alpha1-antitrypsin and lysozyme, all of which stain cells of histiocytic origin.

monoclonal antibody techniques it has become a great deal easier to identify the spindle cell type accurately. An important point here is that a large number of the antibodies concerned are reactive on conventionally fixed, paraffin-embedded material. This has been a considerable advance in our ability to identify the origin of spindle cell tumours. Table 13.1 gives a reasonable immunopathological working plan for the identification of spindle cell masses in the dermis.

Cutaneous metastatic deposits

Metastatic deposits to the dermis from other body sites are relatively rare. The incidence of cutaneous metastases from solid tumours has been estimated at between 1.0 and 4.5 per cent.[61]

It is very rare for cutaneous metastases to be the first sign of a primary cutaneous tumour, but rather more common for cutaneous metastases to herald recurrence from the previously identified primary tumour in both the dermis and, frequently, sites other than the skin. Metastatic deposits may arise as a result of direct spread from underlying structures, by lymphatic or vascular embolization, or rarely by implantation of tumour cells at surgery (Figures 13.48-13.51).

Virtually any solid tumour may metastasize to the skin. A large published series reports that, in men, lung, large intestine, melanomatous and oral squamous cell carcinomas are the most frequent sources of cutaneous metastases, and that in women the pattern is similar but with the addition of breast and ovarian carcinomas (Figures 13.52–13.55).[62,63]

Metastasis to the scalp may give rise to areas of alopecia with firm underlying papules and nodules. This is reported for a number of tumour types, including breast and kidney. Squamous cell carcinoma from sites such as the bronchus may be difficult at times to differentiate from a primary squamous cell carcinoma of the skin or a metastatic deposit from an adjacent primary cutaneous squamous cell source.

The clinical presentation of tumours metastatic to skin is usually that of multifocal, firm nodules on virtually any body site.

The pathological features will obviously vary according to the site of the primary tumour, as is illustrated in Figures 13.48–13.55. A good clinical history will greatly facilitate diagnosis.

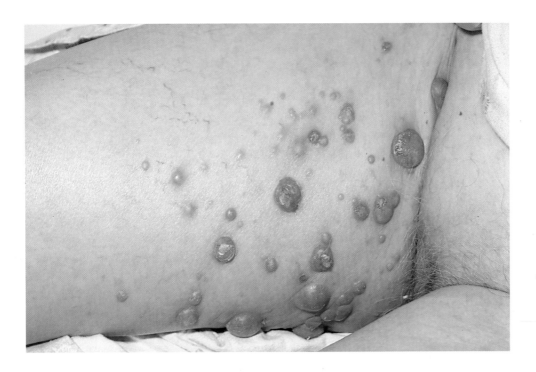

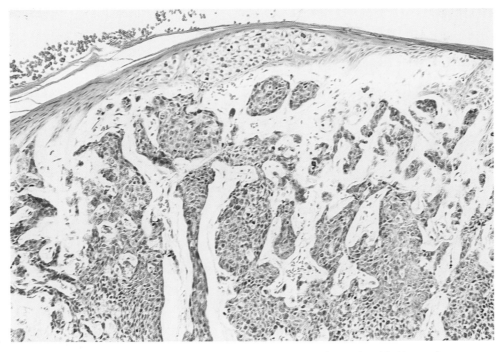

Figures 13.48 and 13.49 Clinical and pathological appearances of secondary bladder carcinoma.

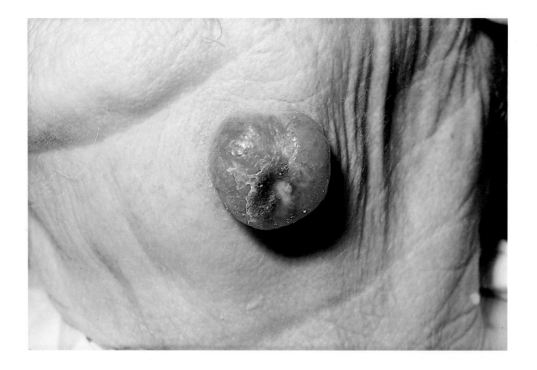

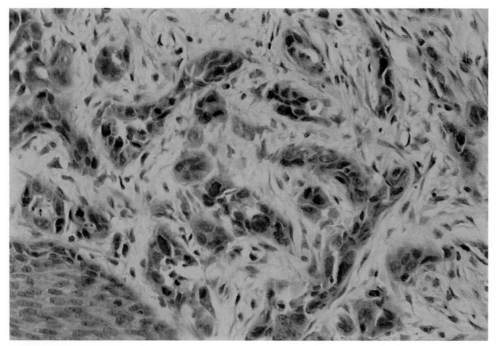

Figures 13.50 and 13.51 Clinical and pathological appearances of a secondary tumour from oesophageal malignancy.

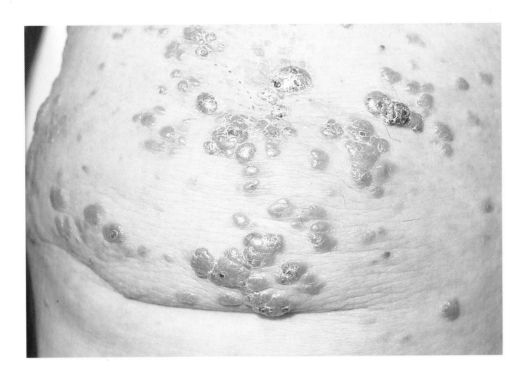

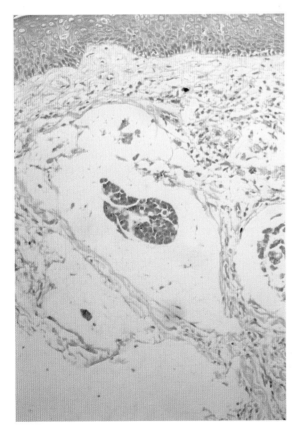

Figures 13.52 and 13.53 Clinical and pathological features of secondary ovarian carcinoma.

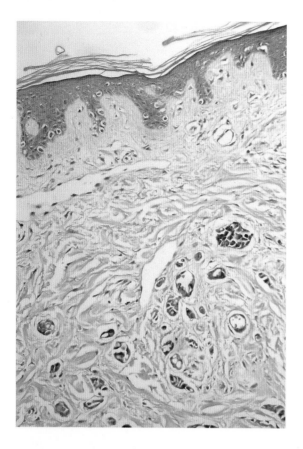

Figures 13.54 and 13.55   Pathological appearance of a carcinoma of the breast which had metastasized to the scalp.

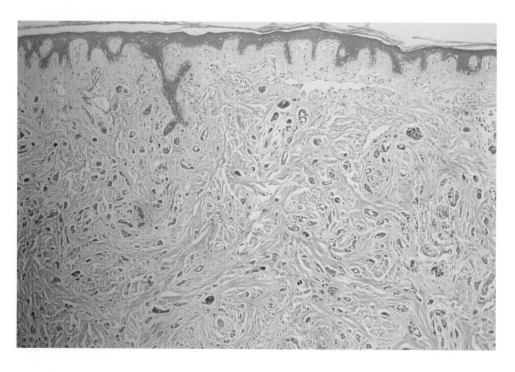

14

Paraneoplastic and putative paraneoplastic cutaneous manifestations of non-cutaneous malignancy

Conditions regarded as cutaneous manifestations of internal malignancy can be divided into what would appear to be a logical grouping of subsets shown below:

Autoimmune paraneoplastic disorders
   Dermatomyositis
   Bullous disorders, paraneoplastic pemphigus
Migratory erythemas
   Necrolytic migratory erythema
   Erythema annulare centrifugum
   Erythema gyratum repens
Disorders possibly mediated by growth factors
   Acanthosis nigricans
   The sign of Leser–Trélat
   Multiple acrochordons or skin tags
   Paraneoplastic acrokeratosis
   Acquired ichthyosis
   Hypertrichosis lanuginosa acquisita
Pruritus

The genodermatoses associated with malignancy discussed in Chapter 4, and the cutaneous diseases associated with ingestion of or exposure to a known carcinogen, such as arsenic, may also be included in this group. Bowen's disease and its possible association with internal malignancy is an example of this latter type.

The interesting group of conditions to be discussed in this chapter are the so-called paraneoplastic group of dermatological disorders that may be the first manifestation of non-cutaneous malignancy. In all the situations discussed below there is at present no established scientific explanation for the coexistence of cutaneous lesions and neoplastic disorder, although there are speculations concerning the output of growth factors and similar substances from the tumour cells.

To label a dermatological disorder paraneoplastic, the appearance of the dermatosis should coincide approximately in time with the malignancy, and should improve spontaneously, at least temporarily, if the tumour is successfully excised.

The great majority of paraneoplastic disorders are relatively rare, and the frequency with which a malignancy is reported to coexist is variable. This is an important point in management when determining the degree of enthusiasm to be adopted in searching for a possible occult malignancy if the dermatosis in question presents in an apparently healthy patient.

At the time of writing, a number of well-conducted case–control studies are appearing in the literature and reporting that the raised incidence of malignancy seen in association with certain of the dermatological disorders discussed below is not statistically significant when compared with that of an appropriate control group. While this may cast doubt on a common or associated aetiological mechanism, it does not, in the author's opinion, remove the need to consider appropriate investigations for an associated malignancy.

Autoimmune paraneoplastic disorders

Dermatomyositis[1]

Dermatomyositis is the predominant paraneoplastic disorder in this group. It is seen in both a childhood

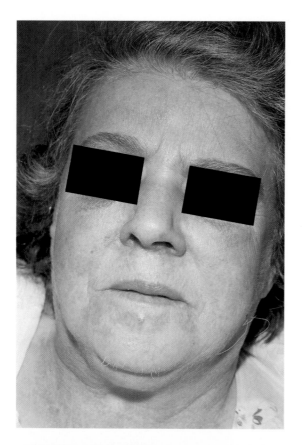

and an adult form, and the controversy with regard to an association with cutaneous malignancy exists only in association with adult-onset dermatomyositis. Childhood dermatomyositis is associated with long-term disability in terms of intramuscular calcification, but no increased incidence of malignancy has been reported.

Clinical features of adult-onset dermatomyositis

Females are affected with dermatomyositis more frequently than are males, and may present with a predominantly dermatological or a predominantly muscular problem. The purely muscular form of the disorder is termed polymyositis, and some reports suggest that the association with malignancy is confined to patients with associated dermatological disorders. Unfortunately, not all series state clearly the exact division of their patients into the two categories.

The dermatological features include a non-specific and diffuse erythema of the face and neck, with a

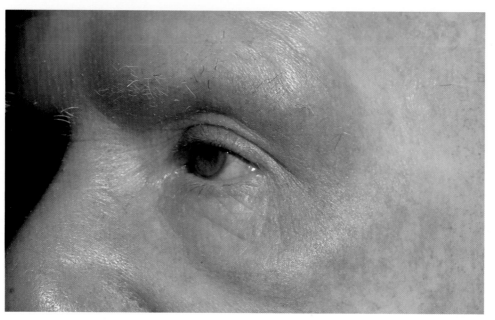

Figures 14.1 and 14.2 Periorbital swelling and erythema in two patients, both with malignancy-associated dermatomyositis.

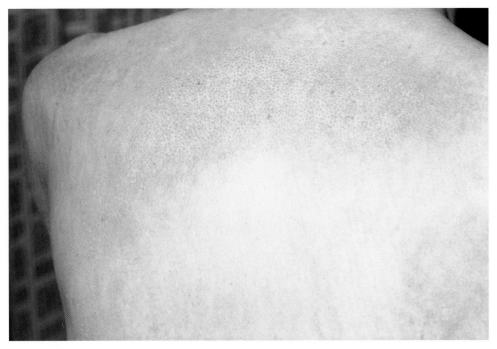

Figure 14.3   Erythema over the shawl area of the upper back in a patient with malignancy-associated dermatomyositis.

rather more specific concentration of this erythema on the eyelid area, which may be associated with oedema (Figures 14.1 and 14.2). The term heliotrope discoloration is sometimes used to describe these eyelids, but the exact definition of heliotrope coloration is hard to come by. A rather more specific feature is the erythema seen on the upper back (Figure 14.3) and the backs of the hands, which, in the latter site, is very often concentrated in a linear streak extending down each finger (Figure 14.4). Both the facial and limb lesions tend to be photosensitive, with exacerbation of the rash on exposure to UV radiation.

The muscular involvement in dermatomyositis is usually greatest in the muscles of the proximal parts of the limb girdles involving the thighs and upper arms. Classic symptoms are those of weakness when climbing stairs or running, or when carrying out tasks involving holding the hands above the head. The diagnosis of dermatomyositis can be confirmed by the presence of raised muscle enzymes in the serum, by abnormalities in electric conduction potential of muscles on electromyography, and on pathological features identified on muscle biopsy.

The cutaneous lesions of dermatomyositis do not have a specific pathological presentation. A biopsy of lesions from the face or hand will show some destruction of the basal layer of the epidermis, with free red cells in the dermis – a pattern described as poikiloderma, which may be seen in other dermatological conditions.

Evidence for an association of dermatomyositis with internal malignancy

The possibility that dermatomyositis or polymyositis might be associated with non-cutaneous and non-muscle malignancy has been discussed for the past 70 years. As with all the conditions discussed in this chapter, the early literature is confined to case reports of an association of the disease in question and the malignancy. Until recently, no case–control studies had been carried out, and therefore assessment of the true statistical significance of these associations is relatively new.

A personal review of a large proportion of published case reports suggests that an association

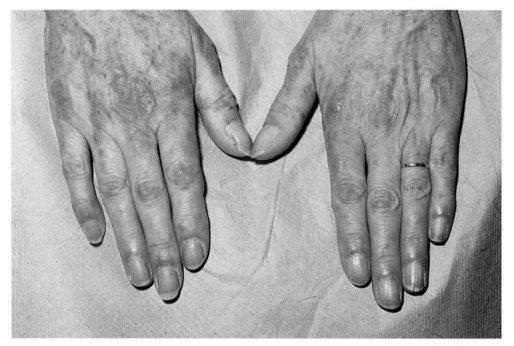

Figure 14.4   Erythema on the backs of the hands in a dermatomyositis patient. Note the linear streaking on the fingers.

with malignancy is more commonly seen in men than in women. The frequency with which the association is reported ranges from 7 per cent (18 cases out of 270, and this result was considered coincidental)[2] to 34 per cent.[3] The association should be suspected if the dermatomyositis is unusually slow in responding to appropriate therapy. One series reports an association with malignancy only with dermatomyositis patients, and not with polymyositis.[4]

The sites of the reported non-cutaneous malignancies mirror the common sites of malignancies in general. This fact could be considered grounds for scepticism about a true causal relationship between the two disorders. In men, malignancy of the gastro-intestinal tract is most often reported, whereas in women the most common site is the breast.

More recent reports of dermatomyositis and malignancy suggest that the coexistence of the two disorders may be coincidental rather than causal. Only one large population-based study has been carried out to date on dermatomyositis and polymyositis. This study did not report an increased frequency of malignant disease of any type in sufferers, but the study does not subdivide polymyositis and dermatomyositis.[5]

A recent case–control study of 65 patients with biopsy-proven polymyositis and 50 patients with biopsy-proven dermatomyositis reported an incidence of 25 per cent of malignancy in this population.[6] A wide range of solid tumours, including breast, lung, bladder and prostate, were reported, as were two cases of associated Hodgkin's disease. However, 17 per cent of an appropriate age-matched control population also had malignancy and the same range of solid tumours was observed in the control population. The difference in incidence of malignancy between the polymyositis and dermatomyositis population and the control group was not statistically significant, and there was no difference in malignancy incidence between dermatomyositis and polymyositis patients. It should be noted, however, that the power of this study was such that only a fivefold increase in incidence of malignancy in the dermatomyositis group would have been regarded as significant.

Patients suffering from dermatomyositis have been reported to have had a non-cutaneous malignancy apparently completely excised as long as 20 years before the development of their dermatomyositis. At the other end of the spectrum are those patients who have developed polymyositis or dermatomyositis up to 14 years before the detection of their malignancy. These very variable timescales can be difficult to reconcile with a common mechanism in all cases.

In view of the varying frequency with which a malignancy is identified, it can at times be difficult to decide on an appropriate series of investigations for an individual patient with polymyositis or dermatomyositis showing no clinical evidence of malignancy. Personal experience would suggest that the frequency with which an occult malignancy is found after a relatively routine series of investigations at a time shortly after the diagnosis of polymyositis or dermatomyositis is made is high enough to justify investigations at this particular time. In the past a chest X-ray, full barium series, and, in the case of a female, examination of the breasts and gynaecological ultrasound have been considered to be an appropriate battery of investigations. Current clinical practice may be to carry out a CT scan and thus reduce the number of invasive procedures required.

The problem then arises as to whether or not patients should be reinvestigated for malignancies that have not yet declared themselves at the time of presentation with polymyositis and dermatomyositis, and, if this is considered justified, the frequency of these reinvestigations.

There is no agreed protocol of timing of repeat investigations in this situation, and the clinician must be guided by personal experience, by his or her own personal view of the likelihood of an association, and by the patient's clinical condition. The author's personal practice is to carry out a thorough clinical examination and appropriate screening procedures when the patient first presents, and if no malignancy is detected at that stage, to carry out further investigations for malignancy only if a change in the patient's clinical condition warrants repeat investigations.

Autoimmune bullous diseases

Paraneoplastic pemphigus

There are reported cases of coexisting pemphigus and malignancy, particularly thymoma, and, as both are rare diseases, it is considered that this association is more than coincidental. In addition, one patient has been described who developed uncontrollable pemphigus vulgaris and a lymphoma. Tumour homogenate from the lymphoma contained a high titre of pemphigus antibodies.[7]

Recently, Anhalt has described a distinct entity which he has labelled paraneoplastic pemphigus.[8-10] The term describes the coexistence of a pemphigus-like clinical picture with erythema multiforme-type lesions on the palms and soles and also mucosal involvement. The histology shows typical pemphigus suprabasal splits and acantholysis, but also individual dyskeratotic keratinocytes. The immunofluorescence picture shows a combination of both intercellular antibodies and also basement membrane antibodies. Circulating autoantibodies are present directed against desmoglein 1, and also against bullous pemphigoid-like antigens with molecular masses of 230, 210 and 190 kDa. The majority of reported cases to date are associated with leukaemias and lymphomas.

Bullous pemphigoid and malignancy are, from time to time, found coexisting in the same patient, but patients with bullous pemphigoid are usually elderly, and thus there may be no aetiological association.[11] One reported case of bullous pemphigoid in a young male cleared rapidly after identification and removal of a gastrointestinal malignancy, and recurred when the patient developed metastases.[12] Thus, the possibility of malignancy should perhaps be considered in younger patients or in those who do not respond to oral steroid therapy.

Some series suggest that patients with dermatitis herpetiformis have an increased risk of developing gastrointestinal lymphoma,[13] but other workers consider that this is more related to gluten-sensitive enteropathy and coeliac disease than to dermatitis herpetiformis per se.

Migratory erythemas

There are three main types of migratory erythema said to be associated with cutaneous malignancy. These are necrolytic migratory erythema or the glucagonoma syndrome, erythema annulare centrifugum and erythema gyratum repens. All are relatively rare.

Necrolytic migratory erythema (glucagonoma syndrome)

This was first described by Becker et al[14] in 1942 in the American literature and by Church and Crane[15] in 1967 in the British literature.

The clinical features include a cutaneous eruption, frequently involving the genital and suprapubic area, and also the perioral area, with an associated glossitis. The cutaneous lesions present with a slowly expanding erythematous macular rash, which develops a palpable lateral margin of small vesicles. These are rapidly ruptured by the pressure of clothing or bedding, giving rise to a crusted outline.[16,17] If the lesions are marked with an appropriate felt-tip pen it will be seen that they are not constant in site but migrate across the epidermal surface, moving several inches in a few days.

The oral lesions and glossitis may be extremely raw and painful, and may give rise to anorexia. Anaemia and diarrhoea are also associated problems.

A large proportion of, but not all, patients with necrolytic migratory erythema will be found, on investigation, to have a glucagon-producing tumour of the pancreas.[18] This can be diagnosed by demonstrating gross elevation of the plasma glucagon level (normal levels 50–150 pg/l).

Necrolytic migratory erythema is so rare, and the associated pancreatic tumour so common, that investigation for glucagonoma should be carried out routinely in all patients with this condition. The mechanisms for the association of necrolytic migratory erythema and high levels of plasma glucagon are not understood.

Erythema annulare centrifugum and erythema gyratum repens are also rare, and have an association with malignancy not quite as frequent as with migratory necrolytic erythema.

Erythema annulare centrifugum

As the name suggests, this is a characteristic and bizarre pattern of slowly moving polycyclic rings of erythema that are the consequence of central clearance, but with peripheral persistence of large erythematous plaques.[19] The lesions are most frequently seen on the trunk, and as new lesions develop and

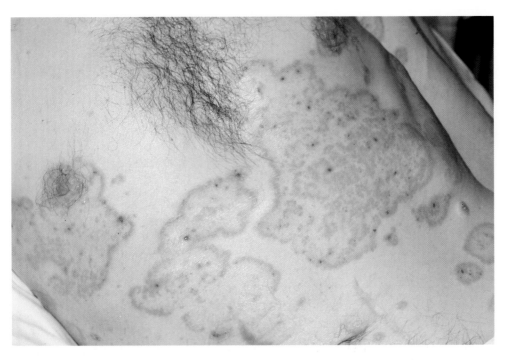

Figure 14.5   Erythema annulare centrifugum with an associated adenocarcinoma of the colon.

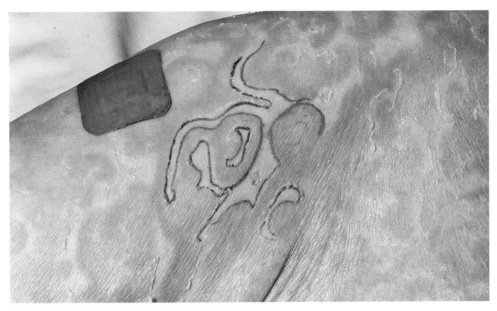

Figure 14.6   Erythema gyratum repens in a female with bladder cancer.

move across the epidermal surface they may join lesions in other sites to give a very striking polycyclic outline (Figure 14.5). The condition is usually asymptomatic, and biopsy will show only a non-specific superficial and deep lymphocytic infiltrate situated around vessels in the dermis.

Erythema gyratum repens

This has an even more bizarre cutaneous presentation with very often the entire skin of the trunk covered with striking mobile polycyclic lesions, resembling woodgrain (Figure 14.6).[20] Once again, the pathological features are non-specific and show only a mild superficial and deep lymphocytic infiltrate.

Malignancies of all types have been reported in association with the two latter variants of migratory erythema. As with dermatomyositis, the more common malignancies are reported most frequently in association with these conditions. Erythema annulare centrifugum is more common than erythema gyratum repens but the association with malignancy is less strong. It is suggested that patients having erythema annulare centrifugum present for more than 3 months should have appropriate screening tests for non-cutaneous malignancies, and that all patients with erythema gyratum repens should have appropriate screening carried out at the time of diagnosis.

Paraneoplastic disorders possibly associated with epidermal growth factor abnormalities

Acanthosis nigricans

Acanthosis nigricans is a rare disease.[21,22] Three main varieties exist. These are a familial inherited type, a type linked with obesity and endocrine disease, and a third, discrete, type, with which malignancy may be associated.

The clinical presentation of acanthosis nigricans is the development of hyperpigmented warty plaques, usually in the groin (Figure 14.7) and axillae.[23] The hands (Figure 14.8) and feet may also be affected, and there is frequently cosmetically distressing perioral involvement (Figure 14.9). Mild pruritus is

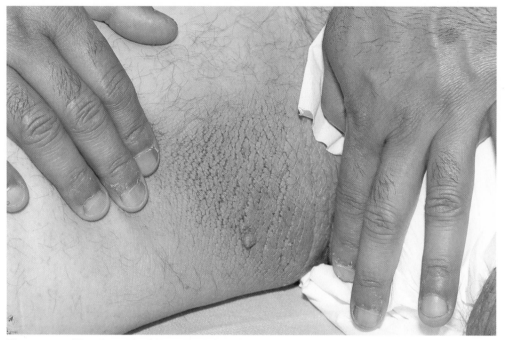

Figure 14.7   Hyperkeratotic pigmented patch in the groin of a patient with acanthosis nigricans.

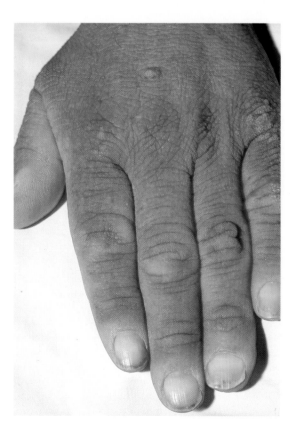

Figure 14.8   Hyperkeratosis and pigmentation on the back of the hand of a patient with acanthosis nigricans and carcinoma of the stomach.

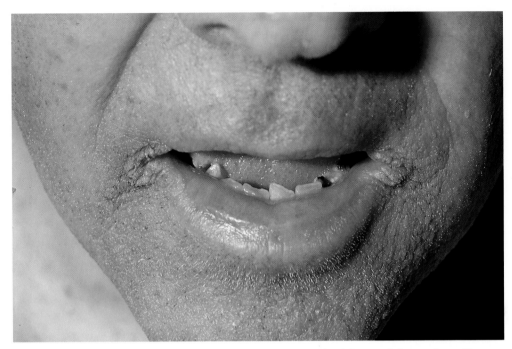

Figure 14.9   Hyperkeratosis and papillomatous lesions at the angle of the mouth in a patient with malignancy-associated acanthosis nigricans.

common, and secondary bacterial colonization may give rise to malodour.

The pathological features of acanthosis nigricans are non-specific. Epidermal acanthosis and hyperkeratosis of the stratum corneum is seen, and there may be horn cysts within the epidermis. The individual features are similar to those seen in the basal cell papillomas described in Chapter 5.

A recent extremely interesting case report of a patient with malignant melanoma and coexistent acanthosis nigricans, the sign of Leser–Trélat, and multiple skin tags, should do much to stimulate research into the relationship between this paraneoplastic group and abnormalities of growth factors or their receptors.[24,25] This patient experienced spontaneous involution of all types of epidermal proliferative lesions after excision of his malignant melanoma. In addition, elevated levels of alpha-transforming growth factor observed circulating in the patient's serum reverted to normal after excision ·of his tumour. Observations of this kind clearly require extension to large series, and it must be stressed that acanthosis nigricans is not a common accompaniment of cutaneous malignant melanoma. Nevertheless, the application of modern molecular biological techniques to this area of dermatology is of great interest.

For patients presenting with clinical evidence of acanthosis nigricans, in whom there is neither a family history nor any history of the associated endocrinological causes and obesity, the likelihood of a malignancy being present is estimated to be approximately 50 per cent. Clearly, this justifies investigation. The majority of reported malignancies are of the gastrointestinal tract, but the lung, the breast and the ovaries are also reported sites.

If the malignancy is removed successfully, the lesions of acanthosis nigricans may remit spontaneously, and, on occasion, recurrence of features of acanthosis nigricans may be the first sign of tumour recurrence.

The sign of Leser–Trélat

The sign of Leser–Trélat is the name given to the sudden appearance of very large numbers of basal cell papillomas (seborrhoeic keratoses) on the skin surface. Aspects of the condition have already been discussed in the section on basal cell papillomas, or seborrhoeic keratoses, in Chapter 5.

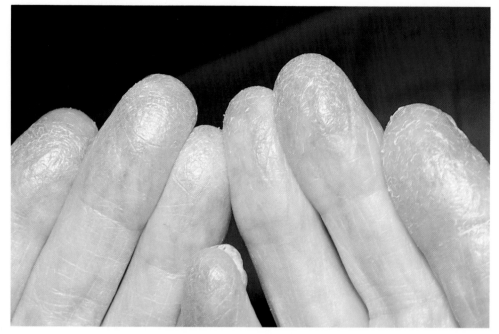

Figure 14.10 Tender, violaceous fingertips in a patient with paraneoplastic acrokeratosis of Bazex (patient of Dr WS Douglas).

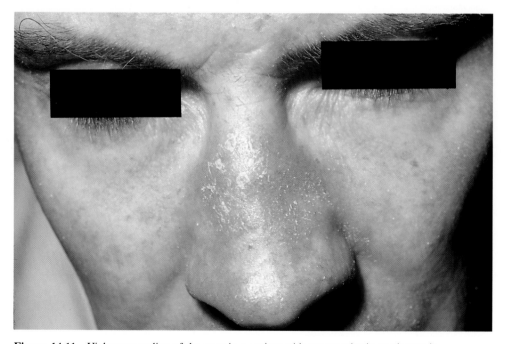

Figure 14.11 Violaceous scaling of the nose in a patient with paraneoplastic acrokeratosis.

For many years it has been suggested that the sudden appearance of very large numbers of basal cell papillomas may be a sign of internal malignancy, and personal observation suggests that on occasion it may be associated with carcinoma of both gastrointestinal tract and bronchus. The mechanism once again is not known, but a role for epidermal growth factor seems likely.[26]

As with acanthosis nigricans, the individual lesions may remit spontaneously following successful removal of the associated tumour.

Multiple acrochordons, or skin tags

The true status of this condition as a marker of internal malignancy is debatable. Multiple acrochordons are a very common feature in middle-aged women around the time of the menopause and later. The great majority of these patients have a purely cosmetic problem, usually with large numbers of small lesions on the neck, and extensive investigations for malignancy would not, in the author's opinion, appear to be justified if acrochordons are the only cutaneous lesion present.

Bazex syndrome (paraneoplastic acrokeratosis)

This condition was first described by Bazex et al in 1965, and a large number of case reports of the condition exist in the French literature.[27] In comparison, there is little written on this topic in the British or North American literature.[28-31]

The condition appears to be associated very frequently with malignancy of the pharynx, larynx, or oesophagus, or secondary tumour in the cervical nodes, and therefore although Bazex syndrome itself appears to be very rare, investigation for malignancy in these sites is not only justified, but essential.

To date the great majority of reported cases are of males aged 40 or older. The clinical features initially are those of a scaling, erythematous, rather psoriasiform eruption involving the distal parts of the fingers and toes (Figure 14.10), and in time also involving the ears and nose (Figure 14.11). In some patients a rather seborrhoeic dermatitis-like picture is seen, and the severity of involvement of the ears may suggest an allergic contact dermatitis or a photosensitivity dermatitis. A violaceous keratoderma may then develop, and the lesions may become widespread. Nail dystrophy and onycholysis are regularly reported (Figure 14.12).

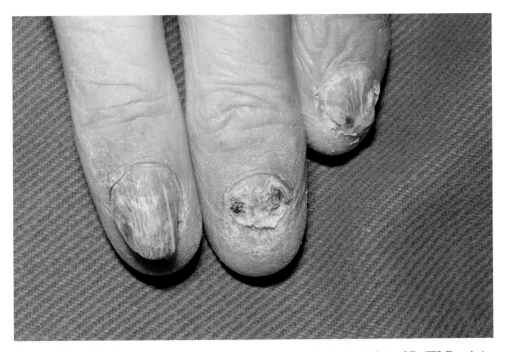

Figure 14.12   Nail changes in a patient with paraneoplastic acrokeratosis (patient of Dr WS Douglas).

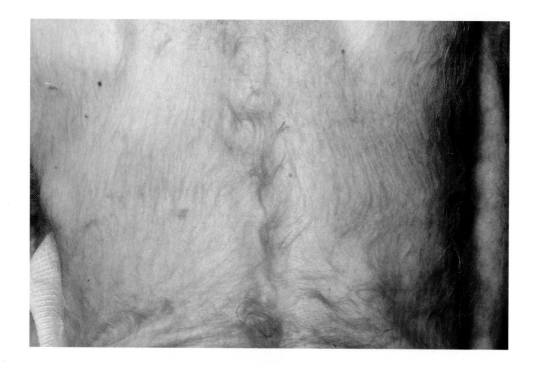

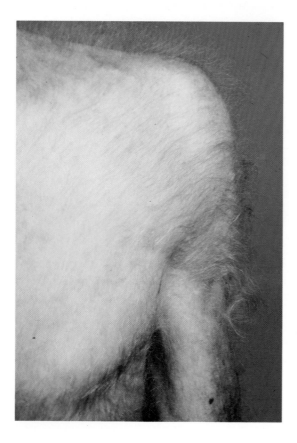

Figures 14.13 and 14.14   A female with ovarian carcinoma and hypertrichosis lanuginosa acquisita.

The dermatopathology is not specific. There is mild epidermal hyperkeratosis and acanthosis overlying a dermis in which there is a focal spongiosis and lymphocytic infiltration.

The malignancies reported to date are predominantly squamous cell carcinomas of the larynx, pharynx and lung, and secondary tumours in the cervical nodes. Cutaneous lesions resolve in most cases after successful identification and removal of the malignant tumour.

Acquired ichthyosis

Acquired ichthyosis appears in many reviews of the cutaneous markers of malignancy but there is no published series which attempts to quantify the frequency of this association. Personal experience would suggest that, although a dry skin is a frequent sequel to chemotherapy in recognized malignant disease, acquired ichthyosis is not a common presenting feature of undetected solid tumours. The published case reports relate mainly to lymphomas and leukaemia, and therefore a full blood examination and sternal marrow puncture would seem a reasonable approach in cases of rapid onset with no obvious aetiological explanation.

Hypertrichosis lanuginosa acquisita[32]

This rare and distressing condition may be associated with malignancy and also occasionally with other serious systemic diseases. The great majority of patients reported on in the literature have an associated malignancy. Two recent case reports indicate that some patients suffering from this condition may have high levels of circulating carcinoembryonic antigen.[33,34] This finding is, of course, non-specific, and the vast majority of patients with high levels of circulating carcinoembryonic antigen do not have hypertrichosis lanuginosa.

The main clinical feature is the sudden appearance of fine, silky hair growth on any body site, commonly the face. The rate of growth may be rapid (Figures 14.13 and 14.14).

Pruritus

In all standard dermatological textbooks, the investigation of pruritus includes a search for an occult malignancy. Pruritus is a relatively common dermatological problem, and the possible causes are numerous. It is more important, therefore, in this situation than in the rarer conditions discussed above to weigh up the relative likelihood of detecting a malignancy, and the real need for extensive and expensive investigations.

A useful study on 125 cases of pruritus followed for up to 6 years puts this in perspective.[35] Two-thirds of this group reported chronic pruritus, and four patients were found to have a malignancy at the time of presenting with pruritus, with a further four developing a malignancy during the follow-up period. This incidence of malignancy is not significantly higher than would be expected in this population, with the exception of lymphomas, which did occur more frequently. Thus, appropriate screening for lymphomas appears clearly justified in cases of persistent pruritus of unidentified cause.

Pruritus is frequently observed in patients who have a recognized lymphoma, but the pruritus may appear up to 2 years before the lymphoma is diagnosed, and may persist, particularly in the case of Hodgkin's disease, after the completion of successful therapy.

15

Approaches to primary and secondary prevention of skin cancer

In the field of cancer prevention and early detection it is important to define clearly the terms commonly used. Prevention of death from a malignancy, in this case malignant melanoma, can be brought about by either primary or secondary prevention. Primary prevention is the prevention of the development of the malignancy itself, and secondary prevention is the prevention of deaths from that malignancy, either by improved therapy or by earlier diagnosis. Thus, in the case of melanoma, primary prevention is usually centred around efforts to avoid excessive sun exposure, while secondary prevention concentrates on public education concerning features of early melanoma, and encouraging self-examination of the skin and attendance for surgical treatment when any possible melanoma is at an early curable stage.

The terms **case finding, screening** and **surveillance** also require definition. Some of the current activities in the field of early detection, while described as screening, are probably more appropriately termed opportunistic or invited case finding rather than screening.

Case finding is the dissemination of information either to the public or to the primary care team of the features of early malignant melanoma and inviting individuals to self-examine their skin and self-refer themselves to an appropriate referral centre if they feel they have a worrying skin lesion. Thus many of the skin cancer fairs held in the past, mainly in North America, are examples of case finding rather than true screening. At these case finding examinations, some

centres offer a free total body skin examination, while others offer free examination of one specific lesion giving rise to concern. A problem with such exercises, discussed below, may be the lack of treatment available or offered and the lack of any regular follow-up to confirm that advice offered has been acted upon.

Screening for melanoma involves the systematic examination of a population. Population screening involves the systematic screening of a selected group coming from one geographic area. The individuals in this population to be screened may be selected on the basis of age, sex or other features. Screening may also be confined to those known to be at increased risk of melanoma, and thus could be confined to those who have a known family history of melanoma, who are known to have multiple naevi, or who have other risk factors.

Surveillance is the ongoing examination at regular intervals of individuals for development of new pigmented lesions which may be early malignant melanoma. The interval at which surveillance examinations take place varies, but is usually between 3 and 6 months. This is clearly a labour-intensive exercise and is currently confined to a small number of centres who have a research interest in this area, examining individuals who are known to be at greatly increased risk of developing primary malignant melanoma. Examples of individuals subjected to surveillance in some centres include those who have already had one primary malignant melanoma and those individuals with both a family history of melanoma and large numbers of benign naevi.

There is as yet no statistically significant proven survival benefit in screening, case finding or surveillance activities other than in females in Scotland. While a number of centres have shown encouraging trends, in reported diagnoses and removal of thinner presumed early melanomas in a population subjected to surveillance, for example, no appropriate control group has been used. Well-constructed controlled trials of the value of these activities are therefore urgently needed, as there is a current trend to introduce screening programmes on the assumption that they must be of benefit. This does require to be proven.

In Europe at the present time activities are ongoing in several countries.[1] These mainly concern early detection and education exercises, but increasingly there is a movement towards primary prevention, with governments, public health departments, national dermatological associations and others mounting campaigns to encourage a cautious approach and advocate sensible sun exposure. In the UK, skin cancer has been targeted in the government's Health of the Nation document, with the stated aim of halting the year-on-year rise in the incidence of skin cancer by the year 2005.

Approaches to early detection of malignant melanoma depend on the hypothesis that if melanoma is detected and removed at an early stage, it will be a thinner tumour, and that this in turn will correlate with increased survival. It is well established from detailed clinicopathological studies correlating features of the primary tumour with prognosis that tumour thickness is in the great majority of such studies the most important determinant of survival. Thus 5-year survival for patients with tumours thinner than 1.5 mm is over 90 per cent, while for those with tumours thicker than 3.5 mm it falls to under 50 per cent. However, studies on patients' history of pigmented lesion growth and tumour thickness suggest that the correlation of the stated duration of a new or growing lesion on the skin and tumour thickness is not absolute. This is clear, for example, in slowly growing melanomas of the lentigo maligna/lentigo maligna melanoma variants, in which the history of slow growth may extend over several years, during which time the tumour has only invaded to 1–2 mm. The other end of this spectrum is the rapidly growing nodular melanoma, where the patient gives a clear history, sometimes supplemented by clinical photographs, of the absence of any lesion in the affected site 4–6 months prior to rapid development of a nodular melanoma which is already 3–4 mm thick at the time of excision.

However, for superficial spreading melanomas a reasonable correlation has been established by Temoshok et al.[2] This shows that for superficial spreading malignant melanomas, which comprise over 70 per cent of all primary cutaneous melanomas, there is a reasonable correlation between the patient's statement of duration of growth of the pigmented lesion in question and tumour thickness. Thus the early-detection approach to malignant melanoma should be successful for superficial spreading lesions, but probably less so for nodular and lentigo maligna melanomas.

A further point to be considered is the question of lead time bias. This has been investigated mainly in the field of breast cancer, and is the suggestion that the time from potential recognition of a tumour to death is constant, and that earlier recognition will not alter that point. Thus early diagnosis could lead to a longer period of follow-up during which time the patient is slowly developing progressive disease, but will not lead to a higher number of survivors at a distant point in time, perhaps 12–18 years after original diagnosis. The problem of lead time bias has not yet been addressed in the field of melanocytic lesions.

Secondary prevention – public education activities

Early-detection campaigns aimed at informing the public at large about the features of possible early malignant melanoma and advising them to seek medical advice require several important features (Table 15.1). The first of these is that there must be general agreement that early malignant melanoma is an entity that can be recognized or at least suspected by relatively untrained eyes. Studies assessing the preoperative diagnostic accuracy of specialist dermatologists have suggested that around 70 per cent of primary cutaneous malignant melanomas may be recognized preoperatively by dermatologists[3] but no similar study has yet been carried out on family doctors and the general public. The accuracy of diagnosis by these groups is likely to be less than 70 per cent, and could be very much less.

Given this fact, it is essential that the features advertised to the public as suggestive of malignant melanoma are relatively broad, and are sensitive but relatively non-specific. In other words every effort must be made to identify all malignant melanomas and include these, although it has to be recognized that this will inevitably include a proportion of benign

Table 15.1 Requirements for public education campaigns in early detection of malignant melanoma.

- Clear, sensitive but relatively non-specific description of early melanoma
- Well publicized
- Access to appropriate media for this
- Primary care medical teams alerted to campaign and ready to handle resultant workload
- Secondary referral facilities (e.g. pigmented lesion clinic available)
- Rapid diagnostic biopsy and pathology facilities
- Rapid access to further definitive surgery as needed

pigmented lesions. These may be either benign lesions arising from the melanocytic series or other pigmented lesions which do not arise from melanocytes, such as angiomas and occasionally pigmented basal cell carcinomas.

Once the clinical features suggestive but not diagnostic of malignant melanoma have been established and appropriately publicized, there must be an appropriate referral or self-referral centre available for members of the public who respond to these campaigns and require medical advice. Thus prior to any public education campaign, it is absolutely essential that the appropriate medical personnel in the area to be subjected to the campaign are primed about the aims and objectives of the campaign and are themselves up-to-date with regard to features of early malignant melanoma and its appropriate initial treatment. In many countries, including the UK, this means preparing the primary care team to deal with pigmented lesions.

As totally accurate preoperative clinical diagnosis is impossible, a proportion of pigmented lesions self-referred by the public may require an excision biopsy to establish a histological diagnosis. This may be carried out either by the primary care physician, or at a specialist referral centre. Whichever is appropriate for the health care system in question, it is essential that members of these groups are acquainted with appropriate techniques and excision margins for excision biopsy of pigmented lesions about which there is any suspicion of early malignant change.

The next requirement is the availability of a rapid and accurate pathology diagnostic service. The

accurate definition of early malignant melanoma and its separation on pathological grounds from reactive but benign melanocytic proliferations can be surprisingly difficult, and centres that plan a large melanoma-recognition campaign do require to be sure that a specialist pathologist who has experience in this area is available. In addition, there must be adequate technical staff involved in pathological processing to provide high-quality specimens relatively rapidly.

A proportion of melanomas diagnosed as a result of increased knowledge and thus self-awareness on the part of the patient and subsequent excision biopsy will require further surgery. Once again, geographic areas planning early-detection activities must be sure that the surgical services in their area have the staff available to carry out any necessary definitive surgery rapidly and effectively.

From the above it will be seen that it is essential that the medical back-up services for early-detection activities are in place. If any part of this necessary chain of medical activity is lacking, the result of an early-detection campaign could be detrimental rather than beneficial, in that the system could become blocked by those alarmed by the publicity, but who do not have melanoma – the worried well – thus preventing appropriate rapid management of those who do have true melanoma.

The public's attention can be drawn to malignant melanoma by a variety of media approaches. These can be transmitted by local or national newspapers, by television or radio, and also by purpose-designed leaflets and posters. Research in many parts of the world has shown that television has the greatest power to reach the greatest number, certainly in those parts of Europe where the number of television channels available is relatively small.[4] However, in the USA, where there are a large number of television channels, local newspapers have been found to be a more effective route. Audits of different approaches to public education have, however, demonstrated that all avenues of publicity do result in some response.

Melanoma early-detection activities

Europe

One of the first early-detection exercises in Europe was that carried out by Cristofolini and colleagues in the province of Trento in Northern Italy.[5] Over the period 1977–85, this group trained dermatologists in the earlier recognition of malignant melanoma, informed general practitioners of these activities, and then explained to the public the necessary aspects of self-examination for early malignant melanoma using leaflets, conferences, television and radio. The control population for this study came from the adjacent neighbouring areas of the Veneto, Alto Adige and Lombardia. Cristofolini and colleagues in their publications do not indicate how they prevented these adjacent areas receiving television, newspaper or radio material.

Analysis of the effect of this campaign has been on the basis of expected and observed deaths in Trentino for the period 1977–85. For men the expected deaths were 40 and the observed 26, while for women the expected deaths were 34 and the observed 26. Thus it has been calculated that 22 lives have been saved as a result of melanoma education. The cost of the campaign was $70 800, and the cost per year of lives saved was calculated at $400.[6] It is of interest to note that this campaign appears to have been more effective in men than women, an observation in contrast to the early findings from the USA and Scotland, where it appears to have been easier to influence women than men.

In Scotland a similar campaign has taken place. In 1985 it was observed that a relatively high proportion of patients in Scotland had melanoma diagnosed when it was thicker than 1.5 mm.[4,7] A campaign was therefore launched, firstly to improve early detection of malignant melanoma by those working in the primary care sector, and thereafter to offer public information on the features of early malignant melanoma and encourage rapid self-referral.

This took place in the spring and early summer of 1985, and the results of these activities have already been published in detail.[8] Five audit measures were built in to the public education campaign (Table 15.2). These were a measure of increasing interest in malignant melanoma, increasing referrals of true malignant melanoma, an increase in the number of thin melanomas excised, an absolute fall in the number of thick melanomas excised, and a fall in melanoma mortality trends. From the early days of the campaign it was apparent that there was an increasing interest in melanoma with a sharp increase in the number of patients referred with histologically proven melanoma. Comparison of the Breslow thickness of melanomas excised in the whole of Scotland in the latter part of 1985–86 and 1987 by comparison with melanomas excised in the years 1980–85 showed a significant increase in the proportion of thin tumours (less than 1.5 mm). This was followed by a fall in the absolute number of thick tumours in

Table 15.2 Appropriate audit measures to evaluate public education activities.

- Is greater interest generated concerning melanoma?
- Are more melanomas diagnosed?
- Initially, are those thinner melanomas than before? (over 2–3 years)
- After 2–3 years does the absolute number of thicker melanomas fall?
- Longer term, does melanoma mortality fall?

women but not in men, and subsequently by a downward mortality trend in women but not in men. This campaign is one of the few which has been carefully audited from the outset, and has provided clear evidence that public education using television, radio, newspapers, leaflets, posters and other measures is an effective method of educating women with early malignant melanoma, but appears to have virtually no effect on men. The reasons for this sex difference are not immediately apparent. One feature, however, may be the extremely useful and informative wave of secondary education published in women's magazines. These may well be an underestimated avenue of health education.

Work carried out by Rampen and colleagues[9,10] in the Netherlands has also been published. This group offered screening in the town of Oss in 1989 and 1990, and 2564 individuals presented themselves for screening. Nine melanomas were suspected in this population, and the cost of the campaign was modest, being estimated at only $6000. It is not clear from the publications whether or not all of the nine suspected melanomas were pathologically confirmed.

In Germany, Hoffman et al[11] have reported on activities in the town of Bochum, where 1467 individuals attended a designated clinic after publicity was generated. Fourteen pathologically-confirmed melanomas were diagnosed in this population, giving a ratio of 1 melanoma diagnosed per 100 individuals examined.

In Austria, campaigns carried out in 1988 and 1989 showed a sharp rise in the number of melanomas diagnosed from 169 in 1988 to 213 in 1989.[12] The average thickness of these melanomas fell from 1.4 to 1.1 mm. However, after 1989 the number of diagnoses fell again, suggesting that regular reminder campaigns are necessary if the impetus begun by early-detection activities is to be maintained.

Work carried out in Switzerland, in the Canton of Basle, has been reported by Bulliard et al.[13] Initial work was carried out in 1986, with an augmentation campaign in 1989. There was a doubling in the number of newly diagnosed cases of cutaneous melanoma immediately after the 1986 campaign, with a statistically significant drop in the age at diagnosis and a non-significant drop in tumour thickness. However, the recall campaign in 1989 did not appear to produce any significant changes.

The USA

Over the past decade similar exercises have been carried out in the USA, mainly under the guidance of the American Academy of Dermatology. These efforts have mainly related to offers of free skin cancer screening clinics, held at outdoor and social events such as county fairs, or at easily accessible sites such as shopping malls.[14–16] A major problem in the US studies to date is that, for ethical reasons, individuals thought to have melanoma have not been followed up or offered treatment, but only advised to seek medical help. Attempts to review these individuals have indicated that by no means all took this advice, and the published results suggest that these activities are labour-intensive and expensive for the number of melanomas found, although a reasonable number of non-melanoma skin cancers are detected incidentally.

Australia

In Australia, early-detection activities have been carried out for many years, mainly in Queensland.[17] Concomitant with this activity, there has been a fall in mean melanoma thickness at the time of excision, and it has been assumed that this is attributable to public education, although no specific review programme of the results of the educational activities has been published.

Conclusion

In summary, therefore, a large number of countries are currently carrying out early-detection exercises. It is highly desirable that such activities are carefully audited to determine their true worth and to identify those areas of public education which are of greatest value. It is necessary, therefore, to know the number of melanomas and the distribution of tumour thickness in the population to be offered education for 3 or 4 years preceding any educational activity, and to follow these figures after the educational activity takes place. Over time it is also necessary to continue to observe tumour thickness. A fall in the absolute number of thick tumours would be an excellent marker of an effective campaign, but a fall only in the **proportion** of these tumours would not be adequate, as it is possible that the campaign has resulted in increased referral of only very early and possibly non-progressor lesions. Mortality figures must, of course, be available. These activities are best carried out on a population basis, so the figures for the above measures must be available for the whole population, not just for one referral centre. This can give rise to problems in areas where there is an increasing trend for office-based surgeons, dermatologists or plastic surgeons to excise thin melanomas in an office setting, as not all may be sent for adequate pathological reporting, leading to incomplete cancer registration. Nevertheless, the overall impression is that early detection and melanoma publicity campaigns do lead to presentation of thinner melanomas. If all thin melanomas are lesions that would in time have become thicker tumours, then these activities should lead to a fall in melanoma-associated mortality. As yet this has only been demonstrated in Scotland.[8]

Primary prevention of malignant melanoma

Primary prevention of malignant melanoma is a longer-term exercise. From what is known about the growth kinetics of malignant melanoma, it is likely that trends in falling melanoma mortality and falling tumour thickness might be seen within 3–5 years of mounting a public education campaign aimed at secondary melanoma, but the latent interval between initiation of a tumour and development of melanoma may be longer than 20 years. Thus primary prevention activities need to be carried out on a very long-term basis. At the present time a large number of European countries are offering advice to their public on safe sun exposure,[1] on the assumption that excessive exposure to natural UV radiation is the most important aetiological agent in developing malignant melanoma. Epidemiological studies strongly support this hypothesis, and furthermore there is increasing evidence that sunlight exposure in early childhood is a significant risk factor for subsequent development of malignant melanoma as an adult some 20–30 years later. However, the exact wavelength and action spectrum for the development of malignant melanoma is not yet established.

Activities currently in progress in the UK, Sweden and other European countries are aimed at encouraging a safe sun approach to exposure to natural UV radiation. Specific items in these safe sun approaches include avoidance of noonday sun, the use of shade such as trees or sun umbrellas, the use of protective clothing such as hats and T-shirts, and the use of a high-SPF sunscreen at all times. These activities are inherently more difficult to monitor and audit than early-detection activities, but there does appear, on the basis of large surveys carried out by national magazines, to be greater awareness of the hazards of sun exposure with regard to both early aging and the development of cutaneous malignancy. However, there is still considerable room for improvement and enhancement of knowledge on the part of the public. For example, in a survey of 22 000 individuals carried out in the UK in 1993 by a popular women's magazine, it was found that the most popular sunscreen had an SPF of only 4. In 1993 the UK Cancer Research Campaign mounted a 'Play Safe In The Sun' activity campaign, similar to those promoted in Australia. The emphasis has been that it is possible to enjoy activities in the sunlight in Europe while taking appropriate precautions to prevent excessive sun exposure which could lead initially to sunburn and possibly later to cutaneous malignancy. The main points to be emphasized in the safe sun approach are avoidance of noonday sun, the use of natural shade (such as trees), the use of appropriate, comfortable clothing (such as wide-brimmed hats and cotton T-shirts), and only then the sensible use of high-SPF sunscreens (Table 15.3).

The importance of avoiding excessive sun exposure in early life has been recognized recently, and so emphasis has switched to the education of young mothers and school-age children. A wealth of educational material is now available for primary school children in a variety of languages.

The field of assessment of primary melanoma prevention is a new one for many clinicians. This has been pioneered for many years in Australia,[18] and it is important to recognize that knowledge and attitude changes precede behavioural change. It is also essential to deliver primary prevention educational material in a way in which it is easily assimilated by the appropriate age range, and does not cause aversion due to

Table 15.3 Safe sun education points.

- Avoid direct exposure to noonday sun
- Seek natural shade (trees) or create it yourself (sun umbrellas)
- Use wide-brimmed hats and T-shirts as comfortable protective clothing
- Use high-SPF (>15) broad-spectrum sunscreens sensibly to reduce risk of damage
- Apply thickly and reapply every 2–3 hours
- Protect the skin of children at all times

alarm or fear. A recent publication by Boldeman and colleagues[19] from Sweden has illustrated that health education designed to encourage sensible sun exposure has been disseminated through Swedish pharmacies, schools, colleges of nursing science and pre-school teachers. Information diffusion has been good, and it remains to be seen whether or not there will be an associated change in behaviour.

Assessment of the efficacy of primary prevention campaigns is necessarily a long-term goal. Clearly the desired end result is a fall in the incidence of malignant melanoma. With increasing availability of leisure time, and reports of a fall in ozone levels in the northern hemisphere, it would be expected that without any primary prevention activities the incidence of malignant melanoma would continue to rise as it has done in Europe for the past 20 years, and furthermore that this rise might be rather steeper than has been observed to date. Thus it may be more realistic to expect some flattening of the increase in incidence curve following primary prevention campaigns rather than an absolute fall. There is not as yet any evidence of any reversing trend in the steadily rising incidence of malignant melanoma in all European countries for which data are available.

Primary prevention activities also refer to the avoidance of excessive exposure to artificial UV radiation as well as to natural sunlight. In northern European countries sunbeds and sun lamps have been popular mainly during the winter months, to promote the year-round tan. There are now four case–control studies, from Canada, from the UK and from other European countries,[20–22] all of which show that excessive use of UV sunbeds is an additional risk factor for malignant melanoma. Primary prevention activities also therefore advise against excessive exposure to artificial UV radiation.

One approach to primary prevention of melanoma is to target the section of the population at greatest risk of melanoma. In Europe this may be an appropriate strategy, as the incidence of melanoma, although rising rapidly, is still relatively low. In contrast, in high-incidence countries, such as Australia, the policy is to target the whole population.

An approach to defining the high-risk sector of the population in the UK has been made by ourselves in carrying out a case–control study to determine the most important risk factors for melanoma. It was observed by appropriate statistical analysis that the four most important independent and statistically significant risk factors were total number of banal naevi, presence of freckling, presence of three or more clinically atypical or dysplastic naevi and a history of three or more episodes of severe sunburn. From this material a melanoma risk factor chart has been devised which is in regular use in a number of clinics. This categorizes the population into four main groups, with the fourth group containing those at significantly increased risk of developing melanoma who merit additional advice against excessive sun exposure, and possibly in some cases surveillance (Table 15.4). The work carried out and published in 1989 in the UK[23] has recently been extended and confirmed in a population in Germany.[24,25]

Sun avoidance and sensible sun exposure is the mainstay of advice on primary prevention. At the present time a number of manufacturers are encouraging the use of devices which give an indication when a certain measured level of UV has reached the device, which is placed on the skin. These monitors, which have a variety of trade names, are suggested as

Table 15.4 Groups possibly meriting melanoma surveillance.

Past history of primary melanoma	Second primary risk × 90
Multiple (more than 3) clinically atypical naevi No family history	Relative risk × 90
Multiple atypical naevi Positive family history	Relative risk × 100–400

being an appropriate way of offering 'safe' sun exposure.[26] However, it must be remembered that sun exposure has cumulative deleterious effects on the skin, and at the present time it is not possible to define any safe level of sun exposure. For this reason these sun exposure devices cannot be given any medical recommendation.

In conclusion, melanoma early detection and prevention in Europe is currently at a relatively early stage compared with that in Australia but appropriate educational activities for limiting the incidence of melanoma and for improving the knowledge of the public are being identified.

It is essential that ongoing audit of the efficacy of these systems is carried out so that the more effective approaches can be widely disseminated and those which are less effective can be brought to an appropriate conclusion.

References

Chapter 1

1 Potten CS, Location of clonogenic cells in the epidermis and the structural arrangement of the epidermal proliferative unit. In: Cairnie AB, Lach PK, Osmond S, eds, *Stem cells of renewing cell populations.* (Academic Press: New York 1976) 91–102.

2 Costarelis G, Sun TT, Lavker RM, Label retaining cells reside in the bulge area of pilosebaceous unit, *Cell* (1990) **61**:1329–37.

3 Marks R, Measurement of biological ageing in human epidermis, *Br J Dermatol* (1981) **104**:627–33.

4 Montagna W, Morphology of the aging skin. In: Montagna W, ed, *Advances in biology of skin,* vol 6, *Aging.* (Pergamon Press: Oxford 1965):1–16.

5 Fenske NA, Lober CW, Structural and functional changes of normal aging skin, *J Am Acad Dermatol* (1986) **15**:571–85.

6 Morison WL, What is the function of melanin? *Arch Dermatol* (1985) **121**:1160–2.

7 Calanchini-Postizzi E, Frenk E, Long-term actinic damage in sun-exposed vitiligo and normally pigmented skin, *Dermatologica* (1987) **174**:266–72.

8 Okoro AN, Albinism in Nigeria: a clinical and social study, *Br J Dermatol* (1975) **92**:485–92.

9 Gilchrest BA, Blog FB, Szabo G, Effects of aging and chronic sun exposure on melanocytes in human skin, *J Invest Dermatol* (1979) **73**:141–3.

10 Rowden G, The Langerhans cell, *CRC Crit Rev Immunol* (1981) **5**:95–180.

11 Tamaki K, Katz SI, Ontogeny of Langerhans cells, *J Invest Dermatol* (1980) **75**:12–13.

12 Silberberg I, Apposition of mononuclear cells to Langerhans cells in contact allergic reactions, *Acta Derm Venereol (Stockholm)* (1973) **53**:1–12.

13 Merkel F, Tastzellen und Taskörperchen bei den Hausthieren und beim Menschen, *Arch Mikrosk Anat* (1876) **11**:636–52.

14 Camisa C, Weissmann A, The Merkel cell, *Am J Dermatopathol* (1982) **6**:527–35.

15 Serafino WE, Austin KF, Mediators of immediate hypersensitivity reactions, *N Engl J Med* (1987) **317**:30–4.

16 Hawkins RA, Claman HN, Clerk RAF et al, Increased dermal mast cell populations in progressive systemic sclerosis: a link in chronic fibrosis? *Ann Intern Med* (1985) **102**:182–6.

Chapter 2

1 Yuspa SH, Cutaneous chemical carcinogenesis, *J Am Acad Dermatol* (1986) **15**:1031–44.

2 Iannaccone PM, Gardner RL, Harris H, The cellular origin of chemically induced tumors, *J Cell Sci* (1978) **29**:249–69.

3 Brookes P, Lawley PD, Evidence for binding of polynuclear aromatic hydrocarbons to the nucleic acids of mouse skin: relation between carcinogenic hydrocarbons and their binding to DNA, *Nature* (1964) **202**:781–4.

4 Blumberg PM, In vitro studies on the mode of action of the phorbol esters, potent tumor promotors, *CRC Crit Rev Toxicol* (1980) **8**:153–234.

5 Blumberg PM, Jaken S, Konig B et al, Mechanism of action of the phorbol ester tumor promoters: specific receptors for lipophilic ligands, *Biochem Pharmacol* (1984) **33**:933–40.

6 Berridge MJ, Inositol triphosphate and diacylglycerol as second messengers, *Biochem J* (1984) **220**:345–60.

7 Burgoyne RD, Control of exocytosis, *Nature* (1987) **328**:112–13.

8 Klein-Szanto AJP, Slaga TJ, Effects of peroxides on rodent skin: epidermal hyperplasia and tumor promotion, *J Invest Dermatol* (1982) **79**:30–4.

9   Kurokawa Y, Takamura N, Matsushima Y et al, Studies on the promoting and complete carcinogenic activities of some oxidizing chemicals in skin carcinogenesis, *Cancer Lett* (1984) **24**:299–304.

10 Elwood JM, Gallagher RP, Stapleton PJ, No association between malignant melanoma and acne or psoriasis, *Br J Dermatol* (1986) **115**:573–6.

11 Jones SK, MacKie RM, Hole DJ et al, Further evidence for the safety of tar in psoriasis, *Br J Dermatol* (1985) **113**:97–101.

12 Pawlowski A, Lea PJ, Nevi and melanoma induced by chemical carcinogens in laboratory animals: similarities and differences with human lesions, *J Cutan Pathol* (1983) **10**:81–110.

13 Kripke ML, Sass ER, eds, *International conference on ultraviolet carcinogenesis 1978*, National Cancer Institute Monograph 50. DHEW Publication no. (NIH) 78 1532. (US Department of Health, Education and Welfare: Bethesda 1978).

14 MacKie RM, Elwood JM, Hawk JLM, Links between exposure to ultraviolet radiation and skin cancer, *J R Coll Physicians Lond* (1987) **21**:91–6.

15 Holman CDJ, Armstrong BK, Heenan PJ, Relationship of cutaneous melanoma to individual sunlight exposure habits, *J Natl Cancer Inst* (1986) **76**:403–14.

16 Elwood JM, Gallagher RP, Davison J et al, Sunburn, sun tan and the risk of cutaneous melanoma – the Western Canada melanoma study, *Br J Cancer* (1985) **51**:543–9.

17 Okoro AN, Albinism in Nigeria: a clinical and social study, *Br J Dermatol* (1975) **92**:485–92.

18 Titus JG, ed, *Effects of changes in stratospheric ozone and global climate*, vol. 1, *Overview*; vol 2, *Stratospheric ozone* (US Environmental Protection Agency: Washington DC 1986).

19 Kerr RA, The ozone hole reaches a new low, *Science* (1993) **262**:501.

20 Manney GL, Froidevaux L, Waters JW et al, Chemical depletion of ozone in the Arctic lower stratosphere during winter (1993), *Nature* (1994) **370**:429–33.

21 Moan J, Dahlback A, The relationship between skin cancers, solar radiation and ozone depletion, *Br J Cancer* (1992) **65**:916–21.

22 Stern RS, Long-term use of psoralens and ultraviolet A for psoriasis: evidence for efficacy and cost savings, *J Am Acad Dermatol* (1986) **14**:520–6.

23 Stern RS, Thibodeau LA, Kleinerman RA et al, Risk of cutaneous carcinoma in patients treated with oral methoxsalen photochemotherapy for psoriasis, *N Engl J Med* (1979) **300**:809–13.

24 Stern RS, Laird N, Melski J et al, Cutaneous squamous-cell carcinoma in patients treated with PUVA, *N Engl J Med* (1984) **310**:1156–61.

25 Stern RS, Lange R, The carcinogenic risk of treatments for severe psoriasis. Photochemotherapy follow up study, *Cancer* (1994) **73**:2759–64.

26 Tanew A, Honigsmann H, Ortel B et al, Non-melanoma skin tumors in long-term photochemotherapy treatment of psoriasis, *J Am Acad Dermatol* (1986) **15**:960–5.

27 Henseler T, Christophers E, Honigsmann H et al, Skin tumors in the European PUVA study, *J Am Acad Dermatol* (1987) **16**:108–16.

28 Gibbs NK, Honigsmann H, Young AR, PUVA treatment strategies and cancer risk, *Lancet* (1986) **i**:150–1.

29 Lever L, Farr P, PUVA induced skin cancer. Malignant or premalignant lesions occur in half of high dose patients, *Br J Dermatol* (1993) **129**(supp 42):21.

30 Rhodes AR, Stern RS, Melski JW, The PUVA lentigo: an analysis of predisposing factors, *J Invest Dermatol* (1983) **81**:459–63.

31 Strickland PT, Photocarcinogenesis by near-ultraviolet (UVA) radiation in Sencar mice, *J Invest Dermatol* (1986) **87**:272–5.

32 Sterenborg HJCM, van der Leuen JC, Tumorigenesis by long wave UVA radiation. In: Sterenborg HJCM, ed, *Investigations on the action spectrum of tumorigenesis by ultraviolet radiation* (MD thesis: Utrecht 1987):79–82.

33 Sverdlow A, English JSC, MacKie RM et al, Fluorescent lights, ultraviolet lamps and risk of cutaneous melanoma, *BMJ* (1988) **297**:647–50.

34 Walter SD, Marrott ID, From L et al, The association of cutaneous malignant melanoma with the use of sunbeds and sunlamps, *Am J Epidemiol* (1990) **131**:232–43.

35 Westerdahl J, Olsson H, Masback A et al, Use of sunbeds or sunlamps and malignant melanoma in southern Sweden, *Am J Epidemiol* (1994) **140**:691–9.

36 Traenkle HL, *X-ray induced cancer in man*, National Cancer Institute Monograph (1963) **10**:423–40.

37 Lindelof B, Incidence of malignant skin tumors in 14 140 patients after Grenz-ray treatment for benign skin disorders, *Arch Dermatol* (1986) **122**:1391–5.

38 Abel EA, Sendagorta E, Hoppe RT, Cutaneous malignancies and metastatic squamous cell carcinoma following topical therapies for mycosis fungoides, *J Am Acad Dermatol* (1986) **14**:1029–38.

39 Evered D, Clark S, eds, *Papilloma viruses*. Ciba Foundation Symposium 120 (John Wiley: Chichester (1986).

40 Bernard HU, Apt D, Transcriptional control and cell type specificity of HPV gene expression, *Arch Dermatol* (1994) **130**:210–15.

41 Durst M, Kleinheinz A, Holz M et al, The physical state of human papillomavirus type 16 DNA in benign and malignant genital tumours, *J Gen Virol* (1985) **66**:1515–22.

42 Meanswell CA, Cox MF, Blackledge G et al, HPV 16 DNA in normal and malignant cervical epithelium: implications for the aetiology and behaviour of cervical neoplasia, *Lancet* (1987) **i**:703–7.

43 Leading article, Human papilloma viruses and cervical cancer. A fresh look at the evidence, *Lancet* (1987) **i**:725–6.

44 Lutzner M, Croissant O, Ducasse MF et al, A potentially oncogenic human papillomavirus HPV 5 found in

2 renal allograft patients, *J Invest Dermatol* (1980) **75**:353–6.

45 Quan MB, Moy RL, The role of human papilloma virus in carcinoma, *J Am Acad Dermatol* (1991) **25**:698–705.

46 Gupta AK, Cardella CJ, Haberman HF, Cutaneous malignant neoplasms in patients with renal transplants, *Arch Dermatol* (1986) **122**:1288–93.

47 Boyle J, MacKie RM, Briggs JD et al, Cancer, warts and sunshine in renal transplant patients, *Lancet* (1984) **i**:702–5.

48 Bunney MH, Barr BB, McLaren K et al, Human papilloma virus type 5 and skin cancer in renal allograft patients, *Lancet* (1987) **ii**:151–2.

49 Kaplan MH, Sadick N, McNutt NS et al, Dermatologic findings and manifestations of acquired immunodeficiency syndrome (AIDS), *J Am Acad Dermatol* (1987) **16**:485–506.

50 Gottlieb G, Ragaz A, Friedman-Kien AE et al, A preliminary communication on extensively disseminated Kaposi's sarcoma in homosexual men, *Am J Dermatopathol* (1981) **3**:111–14.

51 Chang Y, Cesarmen E, Pessin M et al, Identification of herpes virus like DNA sequences in AIDS associated Kaposi's sarcoma, *Science* (1994) **266**:1865–69.

52 Lisby G, Reitz MS, Vejlsgaard GL, No detection of HTLV-1 DNA in punch skinbiopsies from patients with cutaneous T cell lymphoma by polymerase chain reaction, *J Invest Dermatol* (1992) **98**:417–20.

53 Yuspa S, Dugosz AA, Cheng CK et al, Role of oncogenes and tumour suppressor genes in multistage carcinogenesis, *J Invest Dermatol* (1994) **103**:90S–95S.

54 Balmain A, Pragnell IB, Mouse skin carcinomas induced in vivo by chemical carcinogens have a transforming Harvey-ras oncogene, *Nature* (1983) **303**:72–4.

55 Piercall WE, Goldberg LH, Tainsky MA et al, Ras gene mutation and amplification in human non melanoma skin cancers, *Mol Carcinogen* (1991) **4**:196–202.

56 Carr J, MacKie RM, Point mutations in the N ras oncogene in malignant melanoma and congenital naevi, *Br J Dermatol* (1994) **131**:72–7.

57 Albino AP, Nanus DM, Mentle IR et al, Analysis of ras oncogenes in malignant melanoma and precursor lesions: correlation of point mutations with differentiation phenotype, *Oncogene* (1989) **4**:1363–74.

58 Ball NJ, Yohn JJ, Morelli JG et al, Ras mutations in human melanoma. A marker of malignant progression, *J Invest Dermatol* (1994) **102**:285–90.

59 Basset Seguin N, Moles JP, Mils V et al, TP53 tumour suppressor gene and skin carcinogenesis, *J Invest Dermatol* (1994) **103**:102S–6S.

60 Ziegler A, Leffell DJ, Kunala S et al, Mutation hotspots due to sunlight in the p53 gene of non melanoma skin cancers, *Proc Natl Acad Sci USA* (1993) **90**:4216–20.

61 Ziegler A, Jonason AS, Leffell DJ et al, Sunburn and p53 in the onset of skin cancer, *Nature* (1994) **372**:773–6.

62 MacFarlane-Burnett F, *Self and not-self* (Cambridge University Press: Cambridge 1969).

63 Houghton AN, Real FX, Davis LJ et al, Phenotypic heterogeneity of melanoma, *J Exp Med* (1987) **164**:812–29.

64 Holzmann B, Brocker EB, Lehmann JM et al, Tumor progression in human malignant melanoma: five stages defined by their antigenic phenotypes, *Int J Cancer* (1987) **39**:466–71.

65 Elliot A, MacKie RM, Docherty V et al, A comparative study of sensitivity and specificity of radio labelled monoclonal antibody and computerised tomography in the detection of sites of disease in human malignant melanoma, *Br J Cancer* (1989) **59**:600–4.

66 Kripke ML, Immunology and photocarcinogenesis, *J Am Acad Dermatol* (1986) **14**:149–55.

Chapter 3

1 Presser SE, Taylor JR, Clinical diagnostic accuracy of basal cell carcinoma, *J Am Acad Dermatol* (1987) **16**:988–90.

2 Kopf AW, Mintzis M, Bart RS, Diagnostic accuracy in malignant melanoma, *Arch Dermatol* (1975) **111**:1291–2.

3 MacKie, RM, An aid to preoperative assessment of pigmented lesions of the skin, *Br J Dermatol* (1971) **85**:232–8.

4 Pehamberger H, Steiner A, Wolff K, In vivo epiluminescence microscopy. Improvement of early diagnosis of melanoma, *J Am Acad Dermatol* (1987) **17**:571–83.

5 Steiner A, Pehamberger H, Wolff K, In vivo epiluminescence of pigmented lesions. II Diagnosis of small pigmented lesions and early detection of melanoma, *J Am Acad Dermatol* (1987) **17**:584–91.

6 Bahmer FA, Fritsch P, Kreusch J et al, Terminology in surface microscopy, *J Am Acad Dermatol* (1990) **23**:1159–62.

7 Soyer HP, Smolle J, Leitinger G et al, Diagnostic reliability of dermoscopic criteria for detecting malignant melanoma, *Dermatology* (1995) **190**:25–30.

8 Swanson NA, *Atlas of cutaneous surgery* (Little, Brown: Boston 1986).

9 Robinson J, *Fundamentals of skin biopsy* (Year Book Medical Publishers: Chicago 1986).

10 Burge S, Rayment R, *Simple skin surgery* (Blackwell: Oxford 1986).

11 Henderson DW, Papadimitriou JM, Coleman M, *Ultrastructural appearance of tumours* (Churchill Livingstone: Edinburgh 1986).

12 Polak JM, Van Noorden S, eds, *Immunocytochemistry. Modern methods and applications*, 2nd edn. (John Wright: Bristol 1986).

13 Weiss LM, Hu E, Woods GS et al, Clonal rearrangement of T cell receptor genes in mycosis fungoides and dermatopathic lymphadenopathy, *N Engl J Med* (1985) **313**:539–44.

14 Le Boit PE, Parslow TG, Gene rearrangements in dermatopathology, *Am J Dermatopathol* (1987) **9**:212–18.

15 Headington JT, Roth MS, Ginsburg D et al, T-cell receptor gene rearrangement in regressing atypical histiocytosis, *Arch Dermatol* (1987) **123**:1183–7.

16 Zacarian SA, *Cryosurgery* (Mosby: St Louis 1985).

17 Kuflik EG, Cryosurgery updated, *J Am Acad Dermatol* (1994) **31**:925–44.

18 Mohs FE, *Chemosurgery. Microscopically controlled surgery for skin cancer* (Charles C Thomas: Springfield, Illinois 1978).

19 Rapini RP, On the definition of Mohs surgery, *Arch Dermatol* (1992) **128**:673–7.

20 Swanson NA, Mohs surgery, *Arch Dermatol* (1983) **119**:761–73.

21 Spittle M, Radiotherapy in dermatology. In: Champion RH, Burton J, Ebling FJG, eds, *Textbook of Dermatology* 4th edn (Blackwell: Oxford 1992).

22 Van Scott EJ, Kalmanson JD, Complete remission of mycosis fungoides lymphoma induced by topical nitrogen mustard (HN2). Control of delayed hypersensitivity to HN2 by desensitization and by induction of specific immunologic tolerance, *Cancer* (1973) **32**:18–30.

23 Zackheim HS, Epstein EH, Crain WR, Topical BCNU for cutaneous T cell lymphoma, *J Am Acad Dermatol* (1990) **22**:802–10.

24 Price NM, Deneau DG, Hoppe RT, The treatment of mycosis fungoides with ointment-based mechlorethamine, *Arch Dermatol* (1982) **118**:234–7.

25 Wolf G, Multiple functions of vitamin A, *Physiol Rev* (1984) **64**:873–937.

26 Lippman SM, Kessler JF, Meyskens FL, Retinoids as preventive and therapeutic anti-cancer agents, *Cancer Treat Rep* (1987) **71**:391–405.

27 Grupper CH, Beretti B, Cutaneous neoplasia and etretinate. In: Spitzy KH, Karrer R, eds, *Proceedings of 13th international congress of chemotherapy* (VH Egermann: Vienna 1983): 24–7.

28 Peck GL, Therapy and prevention of skin cancer. In: Saurat JH, ed, *Retinoids. New trends in research and therapy* (S Karger: Basel 1985): 345–54.

29 Meyskens FL, Gilmartin E, Alberts DS et al, Activity of isotretinoin against squamous cell cancers and preneoplastic lesions, *Cancer Treat Rep* (1982) **66**:1315–19.

30 Meyskens FL, Booth AE, Goff P et al, Randomized trial of BCG and vitamin A for stages I & II cutaneous melanoma. In: Jones SE, Salmon SE, eds, *Adjuvant therapy of cancer 5* (Grune & Stratton: Orlando 1987).

31 Neely SM, Mehlmauer M, Feinstein DI, The effect of isotretinoin in 6 patients with CTCL, *Arch Intern Med* (1987) **147**:529–31.

32 Moriarty M, Dunn J, Darragh A et al, Etretinate in treatment of actinic keratoses. A double blind crossover study, *Lancet* (1982) **i**:364–5.

33 Legha SS, Interferons in the treatment of malignant melanoma, *Cancer* (1986) **57**:1675–7.

34 Cascinelli N, Bufalino R, Morabito R, MacKie RM, Results of the adjuvant interferon study in the World Health Organisation melanoma programme, *Lancet* (1994) **343**:913–14.

35 Parry EJ and MacKie RM, Management of cutaneous lymphoma, *BMJ* (1994) **308**:858–9.

36 Trattner A, Reizis Z, David M et al, Therapeutic effect of intralesional interferon in classical Kaposi's sarcoma, *Br J Dermatol* (1993) **129**:590–3.

37 Tur E, Brenner S, Michalevicz R, Low dose recombinant interferon alpha treatment for classical Kaposi's sarcoma, *Arch Dermatol* (1993) **129**:1297–300.

38 Dupuy J, Price M, Lynch G et al, Intralesional interferon alpha and zidovudine in epidemic Kaposi's sarcoma, *J Am Acad Dermatol* (1993) **28**:966–72.

39 Rosenberg SA, Yang JC, Topalian JC et al, Treatment of 283 consecutive patients with metastatic melanoma or renal cell carcinoma using high dose bolus interleukin 2, *JAMA* (1994) **271**:907–13.

40 Hart IR, Vile RG, Targeted therapy for melanoma, *Current Opinion Onco* (1994) **6**:221–2.

41 Irie RF, Morton DL, Regression of cutaneous malignant melanoma by intradermal injection with human monoclonal to ganglioside GD2, *Proc Natl Acad Sci USA* (1986) **83**:8694–8.

42 Spitler LE, del Rio M, Khentigan A et al, Therapy of patients with malignant melanoma using a monoclonal antimelanoma antibody ricin A chain immunotoxin, *Cancer Res* (1987) **47**:1717–23.

43 Edelson R, Berger C, Gaspara F, Treatment of cutaneous T cell lymphoma by extracorporeal photochemotherapy. Preliminary results, *N Engl J Med* (1987) **316**:297–303.

44 Armus S, Keyes B, Cahill C et al, Successful treatment of cutaneous T-cell lymphoma with photopheresis, *J Am Acad Dermatol* (1990) **23**:898–902.

45 Zic J, Arzubiaga C, Salhany KE et al, Extracorporeal photopheresis for treatment of cutaneous T-cell lymphoma, *J Am Acad Dermatol* (1992) **27**:729–36.

46 Dougherty TJ, Henderson PW, Schwartz S et al, *Photodynamic therapy* (Marcel Dekker: New York 1992) 1–15.

47 Lin CW, Selective localisation of photosensitisers in tumours: a review of the phenomenon and possible associated mechanisms. In: Kessel D et al, eds, *Photodynamic therapy of neoplastic disease* (CRC Press: Boca Raton 1990) 79–101.

48 Wilson BD, Mang TS, Stoll H et al, Photodynamic therapy for the treatment of basal cell carcinoma, *Arch Dermatol* (1992) **128**:1597–601.

49 Lui H, Anderson RR, Photodynamic therapy in dermatology, *Arch Dermatol* (1992) **128**:1631–6.

50 Hersey P, Melanoma vaccines. Current status and future prospects, *Drugs* (1994) **47**:373–82.

51 Livingston PO, Wong GYC, Adluris S et al, Improved survival in stage 3 melanoma patients treated with GM2 antibodies, *J Clin Oncol* (1994) **12**:1036–44.

52 Black HS, Herd JA, Goldberg LH et al, Effect of a low fat diet on the incidence of actinic keratosis, *N Engl J Med* (1994) **330**:1272–5.

53 Thompson SC, Jolley D, Marks R, Reduction of solar keratoses by regular sunscreen use, *N Engl J Med* (1993) **329**:1147–51.

54 Weiss JS, Ellis CN, Headington JT et al, Topical tretinoin improves photoaged skin, *JAMA* (1988) **259**:527–32.

55 Ellis CN, Weiss JS, Hamilton TA et al, Sustained improvement with prolonged topical tretinoin for photoaged skin, *J Am Acad Dermatol* (1990) **23**:629–37.

Chapter 4

1 Kaposi M, In: Hebra F, Kaposi M, eds, *On disease of the skin including the exanthemata*, vol. 3 (New Sydenham Society: London 1874) 252.

2 Robbins JH, Xeroderma pigmentosum. An inherited disease with sun sensitivity, multiple cutaneous neoplasms and abnormal DNA repair, *Ann Intern Med* (1974) **80**:221–30.

3 Hashem N, Brosma D, Keijzer W et al, Clinical characteristics, DNA repair and complemental groups in xeroderma pigmentosum patients from Egypt, *Cancer Res* (1980) **40**:13–18.

4 Cleaver JE, Zelle B, Hashem N et al, Xeroderma pigmentosum patients from Egypt. II. Preliminary correlations of epidemiology, clinical symptoms and molecular biology, *J Invest Dermatol* (1981) **77**:96–119.

5 Kraemer KH, Slov H, Xeroderma pigmentosum, *Clin Dermatol* (1985) **2**:33–58.

6 Kraemer KH, Lee MM, Scotto J, Xeroderma pigmentosum. Cutaneous, ocular and neurologic abnormalities in 830 published cases, *Arch Dermatol* (1987) **123**:241–50.

7 Scully RE, Mark EJ, McNeely WF et al, Case records of the Massachussetts General Hospital, *N Engl J Med* (1987) **317**:1008–20.

8 de Sanctis C, Cacchione A, L'idiozica xerodermica, *Riv Sper Fremiat Med Leg Alienazioni Merit* (1932) **56**:269–74.

9 English JSC, Swerdlow A, The risk of malignant melanoma, internal malignancy and mortality in xeroderma pigmentosum patients, *Br J Dermatol* (1987) **117**:463–70.

10 Cole J, Arlett CF, Green MHL, 6-Thioguanine resistant mutant frequency is elevated in the circulating T lymphocytes of xeroderma pigmentosum (abstract), *Br J Dermatol* (1988) **118**:285.

11 Cleaver JE, Defective replication repair of DNA in xeroderma pigmentosum, *Nature* (1968) **218**:652–4.

12 Cleaver JE, DNA damage and repair in light sensitive human skin disease (review), *J Invest Dermatol* (1970) **54**:181–95.

13 Pawsey SA, Magnus IA, Ramsay CA et al, Clinical, genetic and DNA repair studies on a consecutive series of patients with xeroderma pigmentosum, *Q J Med* (1979) **190**:179–210.

14 Tanaka K, Miura N, Satokata I et al, Analysis of a human DNA excision repair gene involved in group A xeroderma pigmentosum and containing a zinc finger domain, *Nature* (1990) **348**:73–6.

15 van Oostrom C, de Vries A, Verbeek SJ et al, Cloning and characteristics of the mouse X pac gene, *Nucleic Acids Research* (1994) **22**:11–14.

16 Gozukara EM, Parris CN, Weber CA et al, The human DNA repair gene ERCC2 corrects UV hypersensitivity and UV hypermutability of a shuttle vector replicated in xeroderma pigmentosum group D cells, *Cancer Res* (1994) **54**:3837–44.

17 Jung E, A new form of molecular defect in xeroderma pigmentosum, *Nature* (1970) **228**:361–2.

18 Burk PG, Lutzner MA, Clark DD, UV-stimulated thymidine incorporation in xeroderma pigmentosum lymphocytes, *J Lab Clin Med* (1971) **77**:759–67.

19 Cleary JE, Greave AE, Coriell LL et al, Xeroderma pigmentosum variants, *Cytogenet Cell Genet* (1981) **31**:188–92.

20 Lehmann A, Kirk Bell S, Arlett C et al, Xeroderma pigmentosum cells with normal levels of excision repair have a defect in DNA synthesis after UV irradiation, *Proc Natl Acad Sci USA* (1975) **72**:219–23.

21 Gorlin RJ, The naevoid basal cell carcinoma syndrome, *Medicine* (1987) **66**:98–113.

22 Gorlin RJ, Goltz RW, Multiple naevoid basal cell epitheliomas, jaw cysts and bifid ribs. A syndrome, *N Engl J Med* (1960) **262**:908–12.

23 Howell JB, Caro MR, The basal cell naevus, *Arch Dermatol* (1959) **79**:67–80.

24 Howell JB, Naevoid basal cell carcinoma syndrome. Profile of genetic and environmental features in oncogenesis, *J Am Acad Dermatol* (1984) **11**:98–104.

25 Binkley GW, Johnson HH, Epithelioma adenoides cysticum: basal cell nevi, agenesis of the corpus callosum and dental cysts, *Arch Dermatol* (1951) **63**:73–84.

26 Farndon PA, Del Mastro RG, Evans D et al, Location of gene for Gorlin's Syndrome, *Lancet* (1992) **339**:581–2.

27 Reis A, Kuster W, Linss G et al, Localisation of the gene for the naevoid basal cell carcinoma syndrome, *Lancet* (1992) **339**:300–3.

28 Bale AE, Gailani MR, Leffell DJ et al, Naevoid basal cell carcinoma syndrome, *J Invest Dermatol* (1994) **103**:126s–130s.

29 Compton JG, Goldstein AM, Turner M et al, Fine mapping of the locus for naevoid basal cell carcinoma syndrome on chromosome 9q, *J Invest Dermatol* (1994) **103**:178–81.

30 Howell JB, Freeman RG, Structure and significance of the pits and their tumors in the nevoid basal cell carcinoma syndrome, *J Am Acad Dermatol* (1980) **2**:224–38.

31 Ringborg U, Lambert B, Landegren J et al, Decreased UV-induced DNA repair synthesis in peripheral leukocytes from patients with the nevoid basal cell carcinoma syndrome, *J Invest Dermatol* (1981) **76**:268–70.

32 Goldstein AM, Bale SJ, Peck G et al, Sun exposure and basal cell carcinomas in the naevoid basal cell carcinoma syndrome, *J Am Acad Dermatol* (1993) **29**:34–41.

33 Martin N, Strong L, Spiro RH, Radiation-induced skin cancer of head and neck, *Cancer* (1970) **25**:61–71.

34 Clark WH, Reimer RR, Greene M et al, Origins of familial malignant melanomas from heritable melanocytic lesions, *Arch Dermatol* (1978) **114**:732–5.

35 Lynch HT, Frichot BC, Lynch JF et al, Familial atypical mole malignant melanoma syndrome, *J Med Genet* (1978) **15**:352–60.

36 NIH consensus conference report, *JAMA* (1992) **268**:1314–19.

37 Bale S, Dracopoli NC, Tucker MA et al, Mapping the gene for hereditary malignant melanoma–dysplastic naevus syndrome to chromosome 1p, *N Engl J Med* (1989) **320**:1367–72.

38 Canon Albright LA, Goldgar DE, Meyer LJ et al, Assignment of a locus for familial melanoma MLM to chomosome 9p13–22, *Science* (1992) **258**:1148–52.

39 Goldstein AM, Dracopoli NC, Ho EC et al, Further evidence for a locus for cutaneous melanoma–dysplastic naevus on chromosome 1p and evidence for genetic heterogeneity, *Am J Hum Genet* (1993) **52**:537–50.

40 Goldstein AM, Dracopoli NC, Engelstein M et al, Linkage of cutaneous malignant melanoma–dysplastic naevi to chromosome 9p and evidence for genetic heterogeneity, *Am J Hum Genet* (1994) **54**:489–96.

41 Walker GJ, Palmer JM, Walters MK et al, Refined localisation of the melanoma MLM gene on chromosome 9p by analysis of allelic deletions, *Oncogene* (1994) **9**:819–24.

42 Kamb A, Gruis A, Weaver Feldhaus J et al, A cell cycle regulator potentially involved in genesis of many tumour types, *Science* (1994) **264**:436–9.

43 Lynch HT, Fusaro RM, eds, *Hereditary malignant melanoma* (CRC Press: Boca Raton 1991).

44 Seywright M, Doherty VR, MacKie RM, Proposed alternative terminology and subclassification of so called dysplastic naevi, *J Clin Pathol* (1986) **39**:189–94.

45 Greene MH, Clark WH, Tucker MA et al, High risk of melanoma in melanoma-prone families with dysplastic naevi, *Arch Intern Med* (1985) **102**:458–65.

46 MacKie RM, Multiple melanoma and atypical melanocytic naevi. Evidence of an activated and expanded melanocytic system, *Br J Dermatol* (1982) **107**:621–9.

47 Kopf AW, Lindsay AC, Rogers GS et al, Relationship of nevocytic nevi to sun exposure in dysplastic nevus syndrome, *J Am Acad Dermatol* (1985) **12**:656–62.

48 Currie AR, Ferguson-Smith J, Multiple primary spontaneous-healing squamous cell carcinomata of the skin, *J Pathol Bacteriol* (1952) **64**:827–31.

49 Goudie DR, Yuille MAR, Leversha MA et al, Multiple self-healing squamous epitheliomata (ESS 1) mapped to chromosome 9q 22–q31 in families with common ancestry, *Nat Gene* (1993) **3**:165–9.

50 Ferguson-Smith MA, Wallace D, James Z et al, Multiple self-healing squamous epitheliomata, *Birth Defects* (1971) **7**:157–63.

51 Muir EG, Bell AJY, Barlow KA, Multiple primary carcinomata of the colon, duodenum and larynx associated with keratoacanthoma of the face, *Br J Surg* (1967) **54**:191–6.

52 Torre D, Multiple sebaceous tumours, *Arch Dermatol* (1968) **98**:549.

53 Bakker PM, Tjon A, Joe SS, Multiple sebaceous gland tumours with multiple tumours of internal organs. A new syndrome? *Dermatologica* (1971) **142**:50–4.

54 Lynch HT, Lynch PM, Pester J et al, The cancer family syndrome. Rare cutaneous phenotypic linkage or Torre's syndrome, *Arch Intern Med* (1981) **141**:607.

55 Finian MC, Connolly SM, Sebaceous gland tumours and systemic disease. A clinico-pathological analysis, *Medicine* (1984) **63**:232–42.

56 Starink TM, van der Veen JPW, Arwert F et al, The Cowden syndrome. A clinical and genetic study in 21 patients, *Clin Genet* (1986) **29**:222–33.

57 Lloyd KM, Dennis M, Cowden's disease. A possible new symptom complex with multiple system involvement, *Ann Intern Med* (1963) **58**:136–42.

58 Brownstein MH, Mehregan AH, Bikowski JB et al, The dermatopathology of Cowden's syndrome, *Br J Dermatol* (1979) **100**:667–73.

59 Brownstein MH, Wolf M, Bkowski JB et al, Cowden's disease. A cutaneous marker of breast cancer, *Cancer* (1978) **41**:2393–8.

60 Starink TM, Cowden's disease. Analysis of 14 new cases, *J Am Acad Dermatol* (1984) **11**:1127–41.

61 Nuss D, Aeling JL, Clemons DE et al, Multiple hamartoma syndrome, *Arch Dermatol* (1978) **114**:743–6.

62 Gardner EJ, A genetic and clinical study of intestinal polyposis, a predisposing factor for carcinoma of the skin and rectum, *Am J Hum Genet* (1951) **3**:167–76.

63 Gardner EJ, Richards RC, Multiple cutaneous and subcutaneous lesions occurring simultaneously with hereditary polyposis and osteomatosis, *Am J Hum Genet* (1953) **5**:139–47.

64 Weary PE, Linthicum A, Cawley EP et al, Gardner's syndrome. A family group study and review, *Arch Dermatol* (1964) **90**:20–30.

65 Leppard BJ, Bussey HJR, Gardner's syndrome with epidermoid cysts showing features of pilomatrixomas, *Clin Exp Dermatol* (1976) **1**:75–82.

66 Cooper PH, Fechner RE, Pilomatricoma-like changes in the epidermal cysts of Gardner's syndrome, *J Am Acad Dermatol* (1985) **8**:639–44.

67 Peutz JLA, On a very remarkable case of familial polyposis of the mucous membrane of the intestinal tract and nasopharynx accompanied by peculiar pigmentation of the skin and mucous membrane, *Ned Tijdschr Geneeskd* (1921) **10**:134–46.

68 Jeghers H, McKusick VA, Katz KH, Generalized intestinal polyposis and melanin spots of the oral mucosa, lip and digits. A syndrome of diagnostic significance, *N Engl J Med* (1949) **241**:1031–6.

69 Burdiek D, Prior JT, Scanlon GT, Peutz–Jeghers syndrome. A clinico-pathological study of a large family with a ten year follow-up, *Cancer* (1963) **16**:854–67.

70   Dozois RR, Judd ES, Dahlin DC et al, The Peutz–Jeghers syndrome. Is there a predisposition to the development of intestinal malignancy? *Arch Surg* (1969) **98**:509–17.

71   Trau H, Schewach-Millet M, Fisher BK et al, Peutz–Jeghers syndrome and bilateral breast carcinoma, *Cancer* (1982) **50**:788–92.

72   Linos DA, Dozois RR, Dahlin DC et al, Does Peutz–Jeghers syndrome predispose to gastrointestinal malignancy? A later look, *Arch Surg* (1981) **116**:1182–4.

73   Giardiello RM, Welsh SB, Hamilton SR et al, Increased risk of cancer in the Peutz–Jeghers syndrome, *N Engl J Med* (1987) **316**:1511–14.

74   Zinsser F, Atrophia cutis reticularis cum pigmentatione, dystrophia unguium et leukoplakia oris, *Ikonographia Dermatol (Hyoto)* (1910) **5**:219–23.

75   Cole HN, Rauschkolb JE, Toomey J, Dyskeratosis congenita with pigmentation, dystrophia unguis and leukokeratosis oris, *Arch Dermatol Syph* (1930) **21**:71–95.

76   Sirinavin C, Trowbridge AA, Dyskeratosis congenita. Clinical features and genetic aspects, *J Med Genet* (1975) **12**:339–47.

77   Costello MJ, Buncke CM, Dyskeratosis congenita, *Arch Dermatol* (1956) **73**:123–32.

78   Fudenberg HH, Active and suppressor T cells. Diminution in a patient with dyskeratosis congenita and first degree relatives, *Gerontology* (1979) **25**:231–4.

79   Carter DM, Pan M, Gaynor A et al, Psoralen DNA cross-linking photoadducts in dyskeratosis congenita: delay in excision and promotion of sister chromatid exchange, *J Invest Dermatol* (1979) **73**:97–101.

80   Carney JA, Gordon H, Carpenter PC et al, The complex of myxomas, spotty pigmentation and endocrine overactivity, *Medicine* (1985) **64**:270–83.

81   Shenoy BV, Carpenter PC, Carney JA, Bilateral primary pigmented nodular adrenocortical disease. Rare cause of the Cushing syndrome, *Am J Surg Pathol* (1984) **8**:335–40.

82   Schweizer-Cagiamet M, Froesh ER, Hedinger C, Primary adrenocortical nodular dysplasia with Cushing's syndrome and cardiac myxomas. A peculiar familial disease, *Virchow's Archiv Pathol Anat* (1980) **397**:183–90.

83   Atherton DJ, Pitcher DW, Wells RS et al, A syndrome of various cutaneous pigmented lesions, myxoid neurofibromata and atrial myxoma: the NAME syndrome, *Br J Dermatol* (1980) **103**:421–9.

84   Rhodes AR, Silverman RA, Harrist TJ et al, Mucocutaneous lentigines, cardiomucocutaneous myxomas, and multiple blue nevi: the 'LAMB' syndrome, *J Am Acad Dermatol* (1984) **10**:72–82.

Chapter 5

1   Su WPD, Histopathologic varieties of epidermal nevus, *Am J Dermatopathol* (1982) **4**:161–70.

2   Cramer SF, Mandel MA, Hauler R et al, Squamous cell carcinoma arising in a linear epidermal nevus, *Arch Dermatol* (1981) **117**:222–4.

3   Altman J, Mehregan AH, Inflammatory linear verrucous epidermal nevus, *Arch Dermatol* (1971) **104**:385–9.

4   Kaidbey KH, Kurban AK, Dermatitic epidermal nevus, *Arch Dermatol* (1971) **104**:166–71.

5   Dupré A, Christol B, Inflammatory linear verrucous epidermal nevus. A pathological study, *Arch Dermatol* (1977) **113**:767–9.

6   Solomon LM, Fretzin DF, Dewald RL, The epidermal nevus syndrome, *Arch Dermatol* (1968) **97**:273–85.

7   Becker SW, Concurrent melanosis and hypertrichosis in distribution of nevus unius lateris, *Arch Dermatol Syph* (1949) **60**:155–60.

8   Copeman PWM, Wilson Jones E, Pigmented hairy epidermal naevus (Becker), *Arch Dermatol* (1965) **92**:249–51.

9   Urbanek RW, Johnson WC, Smooth muscle hamartoma associated with Becker's nevus, *Arch Dermatol* (1978) **114**:104–6.

10   Sanderson KV, The structure of seborrhoeic keratoses, *Br J Dermatol* (1968) **80**:588–93.

11   Mevorah B, Mishima Y, Cellular response of seborrhoeic keratoses following croton oil irritation and surgical trauma, *Dermatologica* (1965) **131**:452–62.

12   Becker SW, Seborrhoeic keratosis and verruca with special reference to the melanotic variety, *Arch Dermatol* (1951) **63**:358–72.

13   Connors RC, Ackerman AB, Histologic pseudomalignancies of the skin, *Arch Dermatol* (1976) **112**:1767–80.

14   Ronchese F, Keratoses, cancer and the sign of Leser and Trélat, *Cancer* (1965) **18**:1003–6.

15   Dantzig P, Sign of Leser–Trélat, *Arch Dermatol* (1973) **108**:700–1.

16   Liddell K, Seborrhoeic keratoses and cancer of the large bowel, *Br J Dermatol* (1975) **92**:449–52.

17   Helwig EB, Inverted follicular keratosis. In: *Seminar on the skin: neoplasms and dermatoses*. American Society of Clinical Pathologists, International Congress of Clinical Pathology, Washington, DC, 1954 (American Society of Clinical Pathologists 1955).

18   Mehregan A, Follicular keratosis, *Arch Dermatol* (1964) **89**:229–35.

19   Spielvogel RL, Austin C, Ackerman AB, Inverted follicular keratosis is not a specific keratosis but a verruca vulgaris (or seborrhoeic keratosis) with squamous eddies, *Am J Dermatopathol* (1983) **5**:427–42, and following articles.

20   Sim-Davis D, Marks R, Wilson Jones E, The inverted follicular keratosis, *Acta Derm-Venereol (Stockholm)* (1976) **56**:337–44.

21   Birt AR, Hogg GR, Dubé WJ, Hereditary multiple fibrofolliculomas with trichodiscomas and acrochordons, *Arch Dermatol* (1977) **113**:1674–7.

22   Fujita WH, Barr RJ, Headley JL, Multiple fibrofolliculomas with trichodiscomas and acrochordons, *Arch Dermatol* (1981) **117**:32–5.

23   Ubogy-Rainey Z, James WD, Lupton GP et al, Fibrofolliculomas, trichodiscomas, and acrochordons: the

Birt–Hogg–Dubé syndrome, *J Am Acad Dermatol* (1987) **16**:452–7.

24 Pinkus H, Coskey R, Burgess GH, Trichodiscoma. A benign tumor related to haarscheibe (hair disk), *J Invest Dermatol* (1974) **63**:212–18.

25 Degos R, Civatte J, Clear cell acanthoma. Experience of 8 years, *Br J Dermatol* (1970) **83**:248–54.

26 Fine RM, Chernosky ME, Clinical recognition of clear-cell acanthoma (Degos'), *Arch Dermatol* (1969) **100**:559–63.

27 Trau H, Fisher BK, Schewach-Millet M, Multiple clear cell acanthomas, *Arch Dermatol* (1980) **116**:433–4.

28 Wells GC, Wilson Jones E, Degos' acanthoma, *Br J Dermatol* (1967) **79**:249–58.

29 Kyrle J, Hyperkeratosis follicularis et parafollicularis in cutem penetrans, *Arch Dermatol Syph (Berlin)* (1916) **123**:466–93.

30 Hood AF, Hardegen GL, Zarate AR et al, Kyrle's disease in patients with chronic renal failure, *Arch Dermatol* (1982) **118**:85–8.

31 Carter VH, Constantine VS, Kyrle's disease. I. Clinical findings in five cases and review of literature, *Arch Dermatol* (1968) **97**:624–32.

32 Constantine VS, Carter VH, Kyrle's disease. II. Histopathologic findings in five cases and review of the literature, *Arch Dermatol* (1968) **97**:633–9.

33 Flegel H, Hyperkeratosis lenticularis perstans, *Hautarzt* (1958) **9**:362–4.

34 Bean SF, The genetics of hyperkeratosis lenticularis perstans, *Arch Dermatol* (1972) **106**:72.

35 Beveridge GW, Langlands AO, Familial hyperkeratosis lenticularis perstans associated with tumours of the skin, *Br J Dermatol* (1973) **88**:453–8.

36 Raffle EJ, Rogers J, Hyperkeratosis lenticularis perstans, *Arch Dermatol* (1969) **100**:423–8.

37 Squier CA, Eady RAJ, Hopps RM, The permeability of epidermis lacking normal membrane-coating granules: an ultrastructural tracer study of Kyrle–Flegel disease, *J Invest Dermatol* (1978) **70**:361–4.

38 Lindemayr H, Jurecka W, Retinoic acid in the treatment of hyperkeratosis lenticularis perstans Flegel. *Acta Derm-Venereol (Stockholm)* (1982) **62**:89–91.

39 McGavran MH, Binnington B, Keratinous cysts of the skin, *Arch Dermatol* (1966) **94**:499–508.

40 Leppard BJ, Sanderson KV, The natural history of trichilemmal cysts, *Br J Dermatol* (1976) **94**:379–90.

41 Leppard BJ, Sanderson KV, Wells RS, Hereditary trichilemmal cysts, *Clin Exp Dermatol* (1977) **2**:23–32.

42 Pinkus H, 'Sebaceous cysts' are trichilemmal cysts, *Arch Dermatol* (1969) **99**:544–55.

Chapter 6

1 Marks R, Ponsford MW, Selwood TS et al, Non-melanotic skin cancer and solar keratoses in Victoria, *Med J Aust* (1983) **2**:619–22.

2 Marks R, Jolley D, Lectas S, Foley P, The role of childhood exposure to sunlight in the development of solar keratoses and non melanocytic skin cancer, *Med J Aust* (1990) **152**:62–6.

3 Marks R, Non-melanoma skin cancer and solar keratoses in Australia, *Eur J Epidemiol* (1985) **1**:319–22.

4 Marks R, Selwood TS, Solar keratoses. The association with erythemal ultraviolet radiation in Australia, *Cancer* (1985) **56**:2332–6.

5 Marks R, Foley P, Goodman G et al, Spontaneous remission of solar keratoses. The case for conservative management, *Br J Dermatol* (1986) **115**:649–55.

6 Dodson JM, Despain J, Hewett J, Clark P, Malignant potential of actinic keratoses and the controversy over treatment, *Arch Dermatol* (1991) **127**:1029–31.

7 Bercovitch L, Topical chemotherapy of actinic keratoses of the upper extremity with tretinoin and 5-fluorouracil: a double-blind controlled study, *Br J Dermatol* (1987) **116**:549–52.

8 Rahbari H, Pinkus H, Large cell acanthoma, *Arch Dermatol* (1978) **114**:49–52.

9 Winkler M, Knoetchen erkrankung am helix, *Arch Dermatol Syph (Berlin)* (1915) **121**:278–85.

10 Santa Cruz DJ, Chondrodermatitis nodularis helicis. A transepidermal perforating disorder, *J Cutan Pathol* (1980) **7**:70–5.

11 Goette DK, Chondrodermatitis nodularis chronica helicis: a perforating necrotic granuloma, *J Am Acad Dermatol* (1980) **2**:148–54.

12 Goldschmidt H, Sherwin WK, Reactions to ionizing radiation, *J Am Acad Dermatol* (1980) **3**:551–79.

13 Bowen JT, Precancerous dermatosis, *J Cutan Dis* (1912) **30**:241–55.

14 Bowen JT, Precancerous dermatosis. The further course of two cases previously reported, *Arch Dermatol* (1920) **1**:23–4.

15 Brownstein MH, Rabinowitz AD, The precursors of squamous cell carcinoma, *Int J Dermatol* (1979) **18**:1–16.

16 Kao GF, Graham JH, Premalignant and malignant cutaneous disorders of the head and neck. In: *Otolaryngology*, vol. 5, ch. 58 (Harper & Row: New York 1986).

17 Kao GF, Carcinoma arising in Bowen's disease, *Arch Dermatol* (1986) **122**:1124–6.

18 Graham JH, Helwig EB, Bowen's disease and its relationship to systemic cancer, *Arch Dermatol* (1959) **80**:133–59.

19 Callen JP, Headington J, Bowen's and non-Bowen's squamous intraepidermal neoplasia of the skin, *Arch Dermatol* (1980) **116**:422–6.

20 Arbesmann H, Ranshoff DF, Is Bowen's disease a predictor for the development of internal malignancy? A methodological critique of the literature, *JAMA* (1987) **257**:516–18.

21 Peterka ES, Lynch FW, Goltz RW, An association between Bowen's disease and internal cancer, *Arch Dermatol* (1961) **84**:623–9.

22 Moller R, Nielsen A, Reymann F et al, Squamous cell carcinoma of the skin and internal malignant neoplasms, *Arch Dermatol* (1979) **115**:304–5.

23 Chute CG, Chuang TY, Bergstralh EJ, Su WPD, The subsequent risk of internal cancer with Bowen's disease, *JAMA* (1991) **266**:816–19.

24 Epstein E, Association of Bowen's disease with visceral cancer, *Arch Dermatol* (1960) **82**:349–51.

25 Queyrat L, Erythroplasie du gland, *Bull Fr Soc Dermatol Syph* (1911) **22**:378–82.

26 Goette DK, Erythroplasia of Queyrat, *Arch Dermatol* (1974) **110**:271–3.

27 Wade TR, Kopf AW, Ackerman AB, Bowenoid papulosis of the genitalia, *Arch Dermatol* (1979) **115**:306–8.

28 Bhawan J, Multicentric pigmented Bowen's disease. A clinically benign squamous cell carcinoma in situ, *Gynaecol Oncol* (1980) **10**:201–5.

29 Kaufman RH, Dressmann GR, Burek J et al, Herpes virus-induced antigens in squamous cell carcinoma in situ of the vulva, *N Engl J Med* (1987) **305**:483–8.

30 Berger BW, Hori Y, Multicentric Bowen's disease of the genitalia, *Arch Dermatol* (1978) **114**:1698–9.

31 Paget J, A disease of the mammary areola preceding cancer of the mammary gland, *St Bartholomew's Hosp Rep* (1874) **10**:87–91.

32 Ashikari H, Park K, Huvos AG, Paget's disease of the breast, *Cancer* (1970) **26**:680–5.

33 Culberson JD, Horn RC, Paget's disease of the nipple, *Arch Surg* (1959) **72**:224–31.

34 Gunn RA, Gallagher HS, Vulvar Paget's disease, *Cancer* (1980) **46**:590–4.

35 Helwig EB, Graham JH, Anogenital Paget's disease. A clinicopathological study, *Cancer* (1963) **16**:387–403.

36 Fisher ER, Beyer F, Differentiation of neoplastic lesions characterised by large vacuolated intraepidermal (Pagetoid) cells, *Arch Pathol* (1959) **67**:140–5.

37 Penneys NS, Nadji M, Morales A, Carcinoembryonic antigen in benign sweat gland tumors, *Arch Dermatol* (1982) **118**:225–7.

38 Jadassohn J, Bemerkungen zur Histologie der systematisierten Naevi und uber 'Talgdrusen-Naevi', *Arch Dermatol Syph (Berlin)* (1895) **33**:355–94.

39 Mehregan AH, Pinkus H, Life history of organoid naevi, *Arch Dermatol* (1965) **91**:574–88.

40 Wilson Jones E, Heyl T, Naevus sebaceus, *Br J Dermatol* (1970) **82**:99–117.

41 Domingo J, Helwig EB, Malignant neoplasms associated with the naevus sebaceus of Jadassohn, *J Am Acad Dermatol* (1979) **1**:545–56.

42 MacCormack H, Scarff RW, Molluscum sebaceum, *Br J Dermatol* (1936) **48**:624–9.

43 Musso L, Spontaneous resolution of molluscum sebaceum, *Proc R Soc Med* (1950) **43**:838–9.

44 Ghadially FN, Barton BW, Kerridge DF, The etiology of keratoacanthoma, *Cancer* (1963) **16**:603–11.

45 Rook A, Whimster I, Le keratoacanthome, *Arch Belges Dermatol* (1950) **6**:1–12.

46 Rook A, Whimster I, Keratoacanthoma. A 30 year retrospect, *Br J Dermatol* (1979) **100**:41–7.

47 Silberberg I, Kopf AW, Baer RL, Recurrent keratoacanthoma of the lip, *Arch Dermatol* (1962) **86**:44–53.

48 Calnan CD, Haber H, Molluscum sebaceum, *J Path Bact* (1955) **69**:61–6.

49 Mibelli V, Porokeratosis. In: Morris MA, ed, *International atlas of rare skin diseases*, 27th edn (Leopold Voss: Hamburg 1899) 8–10.

50 Bloom D, Abramowitz EW, Porokeratosis Mibelli, *Arch Dermatol* (1943) **47**:1–15.

51 Eyre WG, Carson WE, Linear porokeratosis of Mibelli, *Arch Dermatol* (1972) **105**:426–9.

52 Chernosky ME, Freeman RG, Disseminated superficial actinic porokeratosis, *Arch Dermatol* (1967) **96**:611–24.

53 Chernosky ME, Anderson DE, Disseminated superficial actinic porokeratosis, *Arch Dermatol* (1969) **99**:401–7.

54 Chernosky ME, Anderson DE, Disseminated superficial actinic porokeratosis. Genetic aspects, *Arch Dermatol* (1969) **99**:408–12.

55 Guss SB, Osbourn RA, Lutzner MA, Porokeratosis plantaris, palmaris et disseminata, *Arch Dermatol* (1971) **104**:366–73.

56 MacMillan AL, Roberts SOB, Porokeratosis of Mibelli after renal transplantation, *Br J Dermatol* (1974) **90**:45–54.

57 Bencini PL, Tarantino A, Grimalt R, Ponticelli C, Caputo R, Porokeratosis and immunosuppression, *Br J Dermatol* (1995) **132**:74–8.

58 Lederman JS, Sober AJ, Lederman GS, Immunosuppression: a cause of porokeratosis? *J Am Acad Dermatol* (1985) **13**:75–9.

59 Reed RJ, Leone P, Porokeratosis a mutant clonal keratosis of the epidermis. I. Histogenesis, *Arch Dermatol* (1970) **101**:340–7.

60 Taylor AMR, Harnden DG, Fairburn EA, Chromosomal instability associated with susceptibility to malignant disease in patients with porokeratosis of Mibelli, *J Natl Cancer Inst* (1973) **51**:371–8.

61 Goerttler EA, Jung EG, Porokeratosis Mibelli and skin carcinoma. A critical review, *Humangenetik* (1975) **26**:291–6.

62 Pinkus H, Premalignant fibroepithelial tumors of the skin, *Arch Dermatol* (1953) **67**:598–615.

Chapter 7

1 Jacob A, An ulcer of peculiar character which attacks the eyelid and other parts of the face, *Dublin Hosp Rep Commun* (1827) 232–9.

2 Gellin GA, Kopf AW, Garfinkel L, Basal cell epithelioma, *Arch Dermatol* (1965) **91**:38–45.

3 Giles G, Marks R, Foley P, The incidence of non-melanocytic skin cancer in Australia, *BMJ* (1988) **296**:13–17.

4 Miller DL, Weinstock M, Nonmelanoma skin cancer in the United States: incidence, *J Am Acad Dermatol* (1994) **30**:774–8.

5 Reizner GT, Chuang TY, Elpern DJ, Stone JL, Farmer ER, Basal cell carcinoma in Kauai, Hawaii: the highest documented incidence in the United States, *J Am Acad Dermatol* (1993) **29**:184–9.

6 Marks R, Staples M, Giles GG, Trends in non-melanocytic skin cancer treated in Australia: the second national survey, *Int J Cancer* (1993) **53**:585–90.

7 Levi F, Franceschi S, Te VC et al, Trends of skin cancer in the Canton of Vaud, 1976–1992, *Br J Cancer* (1995) in press.

8 Kricker A, Armstrong BK, English DR, Heenan PJ, Pigmentary and cutaneous risk factors for non-melanocytic skin cancer – a case–control study, *Int J Cancer* (1991) **48**:650–62.

9 Kricker A, Armstrong BK, English DR, Sun exposure and non-melanocytic skin cancer, *Cancer Causes and Control* (1994) **5**:367–92.

10 Emmett AJJ, Broadbent G, Basal cell carcinoma in Queensland, *Aust NZ J Surg* (1981) **51**:576–90.

11 Marshall DR, The clinical and pathological effects of prolonged solar exposure. Part II. The association with basal cell carcinoma, *Aust NZ J Surg* (1968) **38**:89–97.

12 Panje WR, Ceilly RI, The influence of embryology of the mid face in the spread of epithelial malignancies, *Laryngoscope* (1979) **89**:1914–20.

13 Ewing MR, The significance of a single injury in the causation of basal cell carcinoma of the skin, *Aust NZ J Surg* (1971) **41**:140–7.

14 Rich JD, Shesol BF, Horne DW, Basal cell carcinoma arising in a smallpox vaccination site, *J Clin Pathol* (1980) **33**:134–5.

15 Connolly JG, Basal cell carcinoma occurring in burn scars, *Can Med Assoc J* (1960) **83**:1433–4.

16 Emmett AJJ, Basal cell carcinoma. In: Emmett AJJ, O'Rourke NGE, eds, *Malignant skin tumours* (Churchill-Livingstone:Edinburgh 1982) 32.

17 Darier J, Ferand M, L'epitheliome pavimenteux mixte et intermedaire, *Ann Dermatol Syph (Paris)* (1955) **82**:124–39.

18 Borel DM, Cutaneous basosquamous carcinoma. A review of the literature and report of 35 cases, *Arch Pathol* (1973) **95**:293–7.

19 Presser SE, Taylor JR, Clinical diagnostic accuracy of basal cell carcinoma, *J Am Acad Dermatol* (1987) **16**:988–90.

20 Lang PG, McKelvey AC, Nicholson JH, Three dimensional reconstruction of the superficial multicentric basal cell carcinoma using serial sections and a computer, *Am J Dermatopathol* (1987) **9**:198–203.

21 Scanlon EF, Volkmer DD, Oviedo MA, Metastatic basal cell carcinoma, *J Surg Oncol* (1980) **15**:171–80.

22 Gormley DE, Hirsch P, Aggressive basal cell carcinoma of the scalp, *Arch Dermatol* (1978) **114**:782–3.

23 Pollack SW, Goslen JB, Sherertz EF et al, The biology of basal cell carcinoma. A review, *J Am Acad Dermatol* (1982) **7**:569–77.

24 Krompecher E, *Der basalzellenkrebs* (Gustav Fischer: Jena 1903) 241–56.

25 Van Scott EJ, Reinertson RP, The modulating influence of stromal environment on epithelial cells studied in human autotransplants, *J Invest Dermatol* (1961) **36**:109–17.

26 Cooper M, Pinkus H, Intrauterine transplantation of rat basal cell carcinoma as a model for reconversion of malignant to benign growth, *Cancer Res* (1977) **73**:2544–52.

27 Brownstein MH, Shapiro L, Desmoplastic trichoepithelioma, *Cancer* (1977) **40**:2979–86.

28 MacDonald DM, Wilson Jones E, Marks R, Sclerosing epithelial hamartoma, *Clin Exp Dermatol* (1977) **2**:153–60.

29 Weinstein GD, Frost P, Cell proliferation in human basal cell carcinoma, *Cancer Res* (1970) **30**:724–8.

30 Kerr JFR, Searle J, A suggested explanation for the paradoxically slow growth rate of basal cell carcinomas that contain mitotic figures, *J Pathol* (1972) **107**:41–4.

31 Weedon D, Searle J, Kerr JFR, Apoptosis. Its nature and implications for dermatopathology, *Am J Dermatopathol* (1979) **1**:133–44.

32 Hashimoto K, Brownstein MH, Localised amyloidosis in basal cell epitheliomas, *Acta Derm-Venereol (Stockholm)* (1973) **53**:331–9.

33 McNutt NS, Ultrastructural comparison of the interface between epithelium and stroma in basal cell carcinoma and control human skin, *Lab Invest* (1976) **35**:132–42.

34 Montandon D, Kocher O, Gabbiani G, Cancer invasiveness: immunofluorescent and ultrastructural methods of assessment, *Plast Reconstr Surg* (1982) **69**:365–71.

35 Yamanishi Y, Dubbous MK, Hashimoto K, Effect of collagenolytic activity in basal cell epithelioma of the skin on reconstituted collagen and physical properties and kinetics of the crude enzyme, *Cancer Res* (1972) **32**:2551–60.

36 Sloane JP, The value of typing basal cell carcinomas in predicting recurrence after surgical excision, *Br J Dermatol* (1977) **96**:127–32.

37 Domerus H, Stevens PJ, Metastatic basal cell carcinoma, *J Am Acad Dermatol* (1984) **10**:1043–60.

38 Weedon D, Wall D, Metastatic basal cell carcinoma, *Med J Aust* (1975) **2**:177–9.

39 Mikhail GR, Nims LP, Kelly AP et al, Metastatic basal cell carcinoma, *Arch Dermatol* (1977) **113**:1261–9.

40 Robinson JK, What are adequate treatment and follow up care for nonmelanoma cutaneous cancer? *Arch Dermatol* (1987) **123**:331–2.

41 McGrouther DAM, Treatment of basal cell carcinoma. A plastic surgeon's view, *Br J Dermatol* (1987) **117**:399.

Chapter 8

1 Beadle PC, Bullock D, Bedford G et al, Accuracy of skin cancer incidence data in the United Kingdom, *Clin Exp Dermatol* (1982) **7**:255–60.

2   Giles GG, Marks R, Foley P, The incidence of non-melanocytic skin cancer in Australia, *BMJ* (1988) **296**:13–17.

3   Marks R, Staples M, Giles GG, Trends in non-melanocytic skin cancer treated in Australia: the second national survey, *Int J Cancer* (1993) **53**:585–90.

4   Miller DL, Weinstock A, Nonmelanoma skin cancer in the United States: incidence, *J Am Acad Dermatol* (1994) **30**:774–77.

5   Levi F, Franceschi S, Te VC, et al, Trends of skin cancer in the Canton of Vaud, 1976–1992, *Br J Cancer* (1995) in press.

6   Weinstock MA, Bogaars A, Ashley M et al, Nonmelanoma skin cancer mortality, *Arch Dermatol* (1991) **127**:1194–7.

7   Kricker A, Armstrong BK, English DR et al, Pigmentary and cutaneous risk factors for non-melanocytic skin cancer – a case–control study, *Int J Cancer* (1991) **48**:650–62.

8   Kricker A, Armstrong BK, English DR, Sun exposure and non-melanocytic skin cancer, *Cancer Causes and Control* (1994) **5**:367–92.

9   Ramani ML, Bennett RG, High prevalence of skin cancer in World War II servicemen stationed in the Pacific theater, *J Am Acad Dermatol* (1993) **28**:733–7.

10 Vitasa BC, Taylor HR, Strickland PT et al, Association of nonmelanoma skin cancer and actinic keratosis with cumulative solar ultraviolet exposure in Maryland watermen, *Cancer* (1990) **65**:2811–17.

11 Potter M, *Percival Potts' contribution to cancer research*, National Cancer Institute Monograph 10 (US Department of Health, Education and Welfare: Bethesda 1963) 1–6.

12 Paris JA, *Pharmacologica*, 3rd edn (London 1822).

13 Neubauer O, Arsenical cancers: a review, *Br J Cancer* (1947) **1**:192–251.

14 Henry SA, Occupational cutaneous cancer attributable to certain chemicals in industry, *Br Med Bull* (1947) **4**:389–98.

15 Southam AH, Wilson SR, Cancer of the scrotum: the aetiology and clinical features, and treatment of the disease, *BMJ* (1922) **2**:971–3.

16 Woodhouse DL, Environmental carcinogenesis with special reference to mineral oil carcinogenesis. In: Rook A, ed, *Progress in the biological sciences in relation to dermatology* (Cambridge University Press: Cambridge 1960) 356–69.

17 Unna PG, *The histopathology of diseases of the skin* (Churchill: Edinburgh 1896) 7–19.

18 Dubreuilh W, Epitheliomas of primary origin, *Ann Dermatol Syph* (1907) **8**:387–95.

19 Hyde JN, On the influence of light in the production of cancer of the skin, *Am J Med Sci* (1906) **131**:1–9.

20 Findlay GM, Ultra-violet light and skin cancer, *Lancet* (1928) **ii**:1070–3.

21 Blum HF, Sunlight and cancer of the skin, *J Natl Cancer Inst* (1940) **1**:397–421.

22 Rusch HP, Kline BE, Baumann CA, Carcinogenesis by ultraviolet rays with reference to wavelength and therapy, *Arch Pathol* (1941) **31**:135–47.

23 MacDonald EJ, The epidemiology of skin cancer, *J Invest Dermatol* (1959) **32**:379–82.

24 Brash DE, Rudolph JA, Simon JA et al, A role for sunlight in skin cancer: UV-induced p53 mutations in squamous cell carcinoma, *Proc Natl Acad Sci USA* (1991) **88**:10124–28.

25 Ziegler A, Jonason AS, Leffel DJ et al, Sunburn and p53 in the onset of skin cancer, *Nature* (1994) **372**:773–6.

26 Oettle AG, Skin cancer in Africa. In: Potter M, ed, National Cancer Institute Monograph 10 (US Department of Health, Education and Welfare: Bethesda 1963) 197–205.

27 Vitaliano PP, Urbach F, The relative importance of risk factors in non-melanoma carcinoma, *Arch Dermatol* (1980) **116**:454–6.

28 Aubry F, McGibbon B, Risk factors of squamous cell carcinoma of the skin. A case control study in the Montreal region, *Cancer* (1985) **55**:907–11.

29 Jones SK, MacKie RM, Hole DJ et al, Further evidence for the safety of tar in psoriasis, *Br J Dermatol* (1985) **113**:97–107.

30 Larko O, Swanbeck G, Is UVB treatment of psoriasis safe? *Acta Derm Venereol (Stockholm)* (1982) **62**:507–12.

31 Cartwright RA, Hughes BR, Cunliffe WJ, Malignant melanoma, benzoyl peroxide and acne. A pilot epidemiological case control investigation, *Br J Dermatol* (1988) **118**:239–43.

32 Warin AP, Davies M, Frost T, More than 1000 J/cm² of UVA for PUVA treatment of psoriasis, *Br J Dermatol* (1995) **132**:151–2.

33 Stern RS, Laird N, The carcinogenic risk of treatments for severe psoriasis. Photochemotherapy follow-up study, *Cancer* (1994) **73**:2759–64.

34 Lewis FM, Shah M, Messenger AG et al, Metastatic squamous-cell carcinoma in patient receiving PUVA, *Lancet* (1994) **344**:1157.

35 Sedlin ED, Fleming JL, Epidermoid carcinoma arising in chronic osteomyelitic foci, *J Bone Surg Am* (1963) **45**:827–30.

36 Glucksman A, A comparison of the histogenesis of radiation and chemically-induced skin cancer. In: Rook AJ, ed, *Progress in the biological sciences in relation to dermatology* (Cambridge University Press: Cambridge 1960) 343–55.

37 Cade S, Radiation-induced cancer in man, *Br J Radiol* (1957) **30**:393–402.

38 Benton EC, Bunney MH, Barr BB et al, Skin cancers and their relationship to human papilloma virus infection in a group of renal allograft recipients (abstract), *Br J Dermatol* (1988) **118**:270.

39 Elliott JA, Welton DG, Epithelioma. A report of 1742 treated patients, *Arch Dermatol* (1946) **53**:307–32.

40 Kligman LH, Kligman AM, Reflections on heat, *Br J Dermatol* (1984) **110**:369–75.

41 Ackermann LV, Verrucous carcinoma of the oral cavity, *Surgery* (1948) **23**:670–9.

42 Headington JT, Verrucous carcinoma, *Cutis* (1978) **21**:207–11.

43 Foye G, Marshall MR, Minkowitz S, Verrucous carcinoma of the vulva, *Obstet Gynecol* (1969) **34**:384–90.

44 Okagaki T, Clark BA, Zachow KR et al, Presence of human papillomavirus in verrucous carcinoma (Ackerman) of the vagina. Immunocytochemical, ultrastructural and DNA hybridization studies, *Arch Pathol Lab Med* (1984) **108**:567–70.

45 Aird I, Daintree Johnson H, Lennox B, Epithelioma cuniculatum. A variety of squamous carcinoma peculiar to the foot, *Br J Surg* (1954) **42**:245–50.

46 Kao G, Graham JH, Helwig EB, Carcinoma cuniculatum, *Cancer* (1982) **49**:2395–403.

47 Johnson WC, Helwig EB, Adenoid squamous carcinoma, *Cancer* (1966) **19**:1639–50.

48 Broders S, Practical points in the microsurgic grading of carcinoma, *NY State J Med* (1932) **32**:667–80.

49 Mohs FE, *Chemosurgery* (Charles C. Thomas: Springfield, Ill. 1978).

50 Tromovitch TA, Stegman SJ, Microscopically controlled excision of cutaneous tumour, *Cancer* (1977) **41**:653–8.

51 Moller R, Reymann F, Hou-Jensen K, Metastases in dermatological patients with squamous cell carcinoma, *Arch Dermatol* (1979) **115**:703–5.

Chapter 9

1 Bolognia J, Reticulated black solar lentigo, *Arch Dermatol* (1992) **128**:934–40.

2 Nicholls EM, Development and elimination of pigmented moles and anatomical distribution of malignant melanoma, *Cancer* (1973) **32**:192–201.

3 MacKie RM, English J, Aitchison TC et al, The number and distribution of benign melanocytic naevi in a healthy British population, *Br J Dermatol* (1985) **113**:167–74.

4 Lund HZ, Stobbe GD, The natural history of the pigmented naevus: factors of age and anatomic location, *Am J Pathol* (1949) **25**:1117–45.

5 Stegmaier OC, Natural regression of the melanocytic naevus, *J Invest Dermatol* (1959) **32**:413–21.

6 Maize JC, Foster G, Age-related changes in melanocytic naevi, *Clin Exp Dermatol* (1979) **4**:49–58.

7 Weedon D, Unusual features of naevocellular naevi, *J Cutan Pathol* (1982) **9**:284–92.

8 Schrader WA, Helwig EB, Balloon cell naevi, *Cancer* (1967) **20**:1502–14.

9 Spitz S, Malignant melanoma of childhood, *Am J Pathol* (1948) **24**:591–601.

10 Brownstein WE, Multiple agminated juvenile melanoma, *Arch Dermatol* (1972) **106**:89–91.

11 Gould DJ, Bleehen SS, Multiple agminate juvenile melanoma, *Clin Exp Dermatol* (1980) **5**:63–5.

12 Smith SA, Day CL Jr, Vander Ploeg DE, Eruptive widespread Spitz naevi, *J Am Acad Dermatol* (1986) **15**:1155–9.

13 Weedon D, Little JH, Spindle and epithelioid cell naevi in children and adults, *Cancer* (1977) **40**:217–25.

14 Peters MS, Goellner JR, Spitz naevi and malignant melanomas of childhood and adolescence, *Histopathology* (1986) **10**:1289–1302.

15 Casso E, Grin Jorgensen C, Grant Kels J, Spitz naevi, *J Am Acad Dermatol* (1992) **27**:901–13.

16 Barr RJ, Morales RV, Graham JH, Desmoplastic naevus, *Cancer* (1980) **46**:557–64.

17 MacKie RM, Doherty VR, The desmoplastic naevus, *Histopathology* (1992) **20**:207–11.

18 Sutton RL, An unusual variety of vitiligo (Leukoderma acquisitum centrifugum), *J Cutan Dis* (1916) **34**:797–801.

19 Frank SB, Cohen HJ, The halo naevus, *Arch Dermatol* (1964) **89**:367–73.

20 Copeman PWM, Lewis MG, Phillips TM et al, Immunological associations of the halo naevus with cutaneous malignant melanoma, *Br J Dermatol* (1973) **88**:127–37.

21 Reed RJ, Ichinose H, Clark WH Jr et al, Common and uncommon melanocytic naevi and borderline melanomas, *Semin Oncol* (1975) **2**:119–47.

22 Sagebiel RW, Chinn EK, Egbert BM, Pigmented spindle cell naevus: clinical and histologic review of 90 cases, *Am J Surg Pathol* (1984) **8**:645–53.

23 Mehregan AH, King JR, Multiple target-like pigmented naevi, *Arch Dermatol* (1972) **105**:129–30.

24 Happle R, Kokarden naevus, *Hautarzt* (1974) **25**:594–6.

25 Elder DE, Goldman LI, Goldman SC et al, Dysplastic naevus syndrome: a phenotypic association of sporadic cutaneous melanoma, *Cancer* (1980) **46**:1787–94.

26 Nordlund JJ, Kirkwood J, Forget BM et al, Demographic study of clinically atypical (dysplastic) naevi in patients with melanoma and comparison subjects, *Cancer Res* (1985) **45**:1855–6.

27 Kelly JW, Crutcher WA, Sagebiel RW, Clinical diagnosis of dysplastic melanocytic naevi, *J Am Acad Dermatol* (1986) **14**:1044–52.

28 Roush GC, Barnhill RL, Duray PH et al, Diagnosis of the dysplastic naevus in different populations, *J Am Acad Dermatol* (1986) **14**:419–25.

29 English DR, Menz J, Heenan PJ et al, The dysplastic naevus syndrome in patients with cutaneous malignant melanoma in Western Australia, *Med J Aust* (1986) **145**:194–8.

30 NIH consensus conference, Diagnosis and treatment of early melanoma (leading article), *JAMA* (1992) **268**:1314–20

31 Elder DE, The dysplastic naevus, *Pathology* (1985) **17**:291–7.

32 Sagebiel RW, Banda PW, Schneider JS et al, Age distribution and histologic patterns of dysplastic naevi, *J Am Acad Dermatol* (1985) **13**:975–82.

33 Seywright M, Doherty VR, MacKie RM, Proposed alternative terminology of the so-called dysplastic naevus syndrome, *J Clin Pathol* (1986) **39**:189–94.

34 Dorsey CS, Montgomery H, Blue naevus and its distinction from Mongolian spot and the naevus of Ota, *J Invest Dermatol* (1954) **22**:225–36.

35 Rodriguez HA, Ackerman LV, Cellular blue naevus, *Cancer* (1968) **21**:393–405.

36 Ota M, Tanino H, The naevus fusco-caeruleus ophthalmomaxillaris and its relationship to pigmentary changes in the eye, *Tokyo Med J* (1939) **63**:1243–4.

37 Mishima Y, Mevorah B, Naevus Ota and Naevus Ito in American Negroes, *J Invest Dermatol* (1961) **36**:133–54.

38 Ito M, Studies on melanin: XXII. Naevus fusco-caeruleus acromiodeltoideus, *Tohoku J Exp Med* (1954) **60**:10–20.

39 Schoenfeld RJ, Pinkus H, The recurrence of naevi after incomplete removal, *Arch Dermatol* (1958) **78**:30–5.

40 Watanabe S, Takahashi H, Treatment of the naevus of Ota with the Q switched ruby laser, *N Engl J Med* (1994) **331**:1745–51.

41 Spann CR, Owen LG, Hodge SJ, The labial melanotic macule, *Arch Dermatol* (1987) **123**:1029–31.

42 Kopf AW, Bart RS, Hennessey P, Congenital naevocytic naevi and malignant melanomas, *J Am Acad Dermatol* (1979) **1**:123–30.

43 Walton RG, Jacobs AH, Cox AJ, Pigmented lesions in newborn infants, *Br J Dermatol* (1976) **95**:389–96.

44 Kroon S, Clemmensen OJ, Hastrup N, Incidence of congenital melanocytic naevi in newborn babies in Denmark, *J Am Acad Dermatol* (1987) **17**:422–6.

45 Osburn K, Schosser RH, Everett MA, Congenital pigmented and vascular lesions in newborn infants, *J Am Acad Dermatol* (1987) **16**:788–92.

46 Reed WB, Becker SW, Becker SW Jr et al, Giant pigmented naevi, melanoma and leptomeningeal melanocytosis, *Arch Dermatol* (1965) **91**:100–19.

47 Mark GJ, Mihm MC, Liteplo MG et al, Congenital melanocytic naevi of the small and garment type: clinical, histologic and ultrastructural studies, *Hum Pathol* (1973) **4**:395–418.

48 Silvers DN, Helwig EB, Melanocytic naevi in neonates, *J Am Acad Dermatol* (1981) **4**:166–75.

49 Rhodes AR, Wood WC, Sober AJ et al, Non-epidermal origin of malignant melanoma associated with giant congenital cellular naevus, *Plast Reconstr Surg* (1981) **67**:782–4.

50 Stewart DM, Altman J, Mehregan AH, Speckled lentiginous naevus, *Arch Dermatol* (1978) **114**:895–6.

51 Stern JB, Haupt HM, Aaronson CM, Malignant melanoma in a speckled lentiginous naevus, *Int J Dermatol* (1990) **29**:583–4.

52 Rhodes AR, Mihm M, Origin of cutaneous melanoma in a congenital dysplastic naevus spilus, *Arch Dermatol* (1990) **126**:500–5.

53 Bolognia JL, Fatal melanoma arising in a zosteriform speckled lentiginous naevus, *Arch Dermatol* (1991) **127**:1240–1.

54 Lorentzen M, Pers M, Brettville Jensen G, The incidence of malignant transformation in giant pigmented naevi, *Scand J Plast Reconstr Surg* (1977) **11**:163–7.

55 Rhodes AR, Sober AJ, Day CL et al, The malignant potential of small congenital naevocellular naevi, *J Am Acad Dermatol* (1982) **6**:230–41.

56 Illig L, Weidner F, Hundeiker M et al, Congenital naevi less than 10 cm as precursors to melanoma, *Arch Dermatol* (1985) **121**:1274–81.

57 Kopf AW, MacKie RM, Rhodes AR et al, Summary of workshop on congenital naevi as precursors to melanoma. In: Veronesi U, Cascinelli N, Santinami M, eds, *Cutaneous melanoma* (Academic Press: London 1987) 261–79.

Chapter 10

1 Franceschi S, La Vecchia C, Lucchini F et al, The epidemiology of cutaneous malignant melanoma: aetiology and European data, *Eur J Cancer Prevention* (1991) **1**:9–22.

2 MacKie R, Hunter JAA, Aitchison TC et al, Cutaneous malignant melanoma, Scotland, 1979–89, *Lancet* (1992) **339**:971–5.

3 McHenry PM, Hole DJ, MacKie R, Melanoma in people aged 65 and over in Scotland, 1979–89, *BMJ* (1992) **304**:746–9.

4 Maclennan R, Green AC, McLeod GRC et al, Increasing incidence of cutaneous melanoma in Queensland Australia, *J Natl Cancer Inst* (1992) **84**:1427–31.

5 Elwood JM, Recent developments in melanoma epidemiology, *Mel Res* (1993) **3**:149–56.

6 Van der Esch EP, Muir CS, Nectoux J et al, Temporal change in diagnostic criteria as a cause of the increase of malignant melanoma over time is unlikely, *Int J Cancer* (1991) **47**:483–90.

7 Lee JAH, Scott J, Melanoma: linked temporal and latitude changes in the United States, *Cancer Causes and Control* (1993) **4**:413–18.

8 Thorn M, Ponten F, Bergstom R et al, Trends in tumour characteristics and survival of malignant melanoma 1960–84: a population-based study in Sweden, *Br J Cancer* (1994) **70**:743–48.

9 Khlat M, Vail A, Parkin M et al, Mortality from melanoma in migrants to Australia: variation by age at arrival and duration of stay, *Am J Epidemiol* (1992) **135**:1103–13.

10 MacKie RM, Hole D, Audit of public education to encourage earlier detection of malignant melanoma, *BMJ* (1992) **304**:1012–15.

11 MacKie RM, Freudenberger TC, Aitchison T, Personal risk factor chart for malignant melanoma, *Lancet* (1989) **ii** 487–9.

12 Garbe C, Buttner P, Weiss J et al, Risk factors for developing malignant melanoma, *J Invest Dermatol* (1994) **102**:695–9.

13 NIH Consensus conference report, Diagnosis and treatment of early malignant melanoma, *JAMA* (1992) **268**:1314–20.

14 MacKie RM, McHenry P, Hole D, Accelerated detection with prospective surveillance for cutaneous melanoma in high risk groups, *Lancet* (1993) **341**:1618–20.

15 Carey W, Thompson CJ, Synnestvedt M et al, Dysplastic naevi as a melanoma risk factor in patients with familial melanoma, *Cancer* (1994) **74**:3118–25.

16 Elwood JM, Gallagher RP, Hill GB et al, Cutaneous melanoma in relation to intermittent and constant sun exposure – the Western Canada Melanoma Study, *Int J Cancer* (1985) **35**:427–33.

17 Osterlind A, Tucker MA, Stone BJ et al, The Danish case-control study of cutaneous malignant melanoma. II. Importance of UV-light exposure, *Int J Cancer* (1988) **42**: 319–24.

18 Green A, MacLennan R, Youl P et al, Site distribution of cutaneous melanoma in Queensland, *Int J Cancer* (1993) **53**:232–6.

19 White E, Kirkpatrick CS, Lee JAH, Case-control study of malignant melanoma in Washington State 1. Constitutional factors and sun exposure, *Am J Epidemiol* (1994) **139**:857–68.

20 Armstrong BK, Kricker A, How much melanoma is caused by sun exposure? *Mel Res* (1993) **3**:395–401.

21 Kirkpatrick CS, White E, Lee JAH, Case-control study of malignant melanoma in Washington State. II. Diet, alcohol and obesity, *Am J Epidemiol* (1994) **139**:869–80.

22 Nelemans PJ, Verbeek ALM, Rampen F, Non solar factors in melanoma risk, *Clin Dermatol* (1992) **10**:51–63.

23 Walter SD, Marrett LD, From L et al, The association of cutaneous melanoma with the use of sunlamps and sunbeds, *Am J Epidemiol* (1990) **131**:232–43.

24 Sverdlow AJ, English J, MacKie R et al, Fluorescent lights ultraviolet lamps and the risk of melanoma, *Br Med J* (1988) **297**:647–50.

25 Westerdahl J, Olsson H, Masback A et al, Use of sunbeds or sunlamps and malignant melanoma in southern Sweden, *Am J Epidemiol* (1994) **140**:691–9.

26 Elwood JM, Could melanoma be caused by fluorescent light? In: Gallagher RP et al, eds, *Epidemiology of malignant melanoma* (Springer Verlag: Berlin 1986) 127–36.

27 Beral V, Evans S, Shaw H et al, Oral contraceptive use and malignant melanoma in Australia, *Br J Cancer* (1984) **50**:681–5.

28 Lee JAH, Merrill JM, Sunlight and the aetiology of malignant melanoma. A synthesis, *Med J Aust* (1970) **2**:846–51.

29 Klein-Szanto AJP, Silvers WK, Mintz B, Ultraviolet radiation-induced malignant skin melanoma in melanoma-susceptible transgenic mice, *Cancer Res* (1994) **54**:4560.

30 Clark WH, From L, Bernardino EA et al, The histogenesis and biologic behaviour of primary human malignant melanomas of the skin, *Cancer Res* (1969) **29**:705–26.

31 Cox NH, Jones SK, MacKie RM, Malignant melanoma of the head and neck in Scotland: an eight-year analysis of trends in prevalence, distribution and prognosis, *Q J Med* (1987) **64**:661–70.

32 Conley J, Latter R, Orr W, Desmoplastic malignant melanoma. A rare variant of spindle cell melanoma, *Cancer* (1971) **28**:914–36.

33 Reed RJ, Leonard DD, Neurotropic melanoma. A variant of desmoplastic melanoma, *Am J Surg Pathol* (1979) **3**:301–11.

34 Burden AD, Vestey JP, MacKie RM, Multiple primary melanomas, *BMJ* (1994) **309**:375.

35 MacKie RM, An aid to preoperative assessment of pigmented lesions of the skin, *Br J Dermatol* 1971 **85**:232–8.

36 Pehamberger H, Binder M, Steiner A et al, In vivo epiluminescence microscopy, *J Invest Dermatol* (1993) **100**:356s–62s.

37 Kenet R, Kang S, Kenet BJ et al, Clinical diagnosis of pigmented lesions using epiluminescence microscopy, *Arch Dermatol* (1993) **129**:157–74.

38 Breslow A, Tumour thickness level of invasion and node dissection in stage 1 cutaneous melanoma, *Ann Surg* (1975) **182**:572–5.

39 Keefe M, MacKie RM, The relationship between risk of death from clinical stage 1 cutaneous melanoma and thickness of primary tumour; no evidence for steps in risk, *Br J Cancer* (1991) **64**:598–602.

40 Clark WH, Elder D, Guerry D et al, A study of tumour progression. The precursor lesions of superficial spreading and nodular melanoma, *Hum Pathol* (1984) **15**:1147–65.

41 Guerry D, Synnestvedt M, Elder D et al, Lessons from tumour progression. The invasive radial growth phase of melanoma is commonly incapable of metastasis and is indolent, *J Invest Dermatol* (1993) **100**:342s–45s.

42 Gromet MA, Epstein WL, Blois MS, The regressing thin melanoma. A distinctive lesion with metastatic potential, *Cancer* (1978) **42**:2282–92.

43 McGovern VJ, Shaw HM, Milton GW, Prognosis in patients with thin melanoma: influence of regression, *Histopathology* (1983) **7**:673–80.

44 Kelly JW, Sagebiel RW, Blois MS, Regression in malignant melanoma. A histologic feature without independent prognostic significance, *Cancer* (1985) **56**:2287–91.

45 Soong SJ, Formula expressing a relationship among thickness and time after diagnosis and survival probability in patients with malignant melanoma, *Int J Biomed Computing* (1994) **37**:171–80.

46 MacKie RM, Aitchison T, Sirel JM et al, Prognostic models for subgroups of melanoma patients from the Scottish Melanoma Group database 1979–86 and their subsequent validation, *Br J Cancer* (1995) **71**:173–6.

47 Taylor BA, Hughes LE, Policy of selective excision for primary cutaneous malignant melanoma, *Eur J Surg Oncol* (1985) **11**:7–13.

48 Morton DL, Wen DR, Wong JH et al, Technical details of intraoperative mapping for early stage melanoma, *Arch Surg* (1992) **127**:1392–9.

49 Klaase JM, Kroon BBR, van Geel AN et al, Limb recurrence free interval and survival in patients with recurrent melanoma of the limbs treated with normothermic isolated limb perfusion, *J Am Coll Surg* (1994) **178**:564–72.

50 MacKie RM, Bufalino R, Morabito A et al, Lack of effect of pregnancy on outcome of melanoma, *Lancet* (1991) **337**:653–5.

51 Stables G, Doherty V, MacKie RM, Nine years experience of BELD chemotherapy for metastatic melanoma, *Br J Dermatol* (1992) **127**:505–9.

52 Peschel RE, Fischer JJ, Radiation therapy. In: Nathanson L, ed, *Management of advanced melanoma* (Churchill Livingstone: New York 1986) 113–43.

53 Harwood AR, Conventional radiotherapy in the treatment of lentigo maligna and lentigo maligna melanoma, *J Am Acad Dermatol* (1982) **6**:310–16.

54 Hartmann H, Lischka G, Maligner blauer Naevus, *Hautarzt* (1972) **23**:175–8.

Chapter 11

1 Alibert JLM, *Tableau du plan fongoide* (Barrois l'Aine: Paris 1806).

2 Bazin PAE, *Leçons sur le traitement des maladies chroniques en general affections de la peau* (Delahaye: Paris 1870).

3 Sézary A, Bouvrain Y, Erythrodermie avec présence de cellules monstreuses dans le derme et le sang circulant, *Bull Soc Fr Dermatol Syph* (1938) **45**:245–60.

4 Lutzner MA, Hobbs JW, Horvath P, Ultrastructure of abnormal cells in Sézary syndrome, mycosis fungoides and parapsoriasis en plaque, *Arch Dermatol* (1971) **103**:375–86.

5 Edelson RL, Kirkpatrick CH, Shevach EN et al, Preferential cutaneous infiltration by neoplastic thymus-derived lymphocytes, *Ann Intern Med* (1974) **80**:685–92.

6 Thomas JA, Janossy G, Graham-Brown RAC et al, The relationship between T lymphocyte subsets and Ia-like antigen positive non-lymphoid cells in early stages of cutaneous T cell lymphoma, *J Invest Dermatol* (1982) **78**:169–76.

7 MacKie RM, Turbitt ML, The use of a double-label immunoperoxidase monoclonal antibody technique in the investigation of patients with mycosis fungoides, *Br J Dermatol* (1982) **106**:379–84.

8 Weiss LM, Hu E, Wood GS et al, Clonal rearrangements of T-cell receptor genes in mycosis fungoides and

dermatopathic lymphadenopathy, *N Engl J Med* (1985) **313**:539–44.

9 Fivenson DP, Hanson CA, Nickoloff BJ, Localisation of clonal T cells to the epidermis in cutaneous T cell lymphoma, *J Am Acad Dermatol* (1994) **31**:717–23.

10 Fischmann AB, Bunn PA Jr, Guccion JG et al, Exposure to chemicals, physical agents, and biologic agents in mycosis fungoides and the Sézary syndrome, *Cancer Treat Rep* (1979) **63**:591–6.

11 Greene MH, Dalager NA, Lamberg SI et al, Mycosis fungoides: epidemiologic observations, *Cancer Treat Rep* (1979) **63**:597–606.

12 Cohen SR, Stenn KS, Braverman IM et al, Mycosis fungoides: clinicopathologic relationships, survival and therapy in 59 patients with observations on occupation as a new prognostic factor, *Cancer* (1980) **46**:2654–66.

13 Tuyp E, Burgoyne A, Aitchison T et al, A case control study of possible causative factors in mycosis fungoides, *Arch Dermatol* (1987) **123**:196–200.

14 Tan RS-H, Butterworth CM, McLaughlin H et al, Mycosis fungoides – a disease of antigen persistence, *Br J Dermatol* (1974) **91**:607–16.

15 MacKie RM, Hypothesis. The initial event in mycosis fungoides is a viral infection of the epidermal Langerhans cell, *Lancet* (1981) **ii**:283–5.

16 Thiers BH, Controversies in mycosis fungoides, *J Am Acad Dermatol* (1982) **7**:1–16.

17 Lisby G, Reitz MS, Veiljsgaard GL, No detection of HTLV 1 DNA in punch skin biopsies from patients with cutaneous T cell lymphoma by polymerase chain reaction, *J Invest Dermatol* (1992) **98**:417–20.

18 Lamberg SI, Green SB, Byar DP et al, Clinical staging for cutaneous T cell lymphoma, *Ann Intern Med* (1984) **100**:187–92.

19 Koch SE, Zackheim HS, Williams ML et al, Mycosis fungoides beginning in childhood and adolescence, *J Am Acad Dermatol* (1987) **17**:563–70.

20 Edelson RL, T cell lymphoma: mycosis fungoides, Sézary syndrome and other variants, *J Am Acad Dermatol* (1980) **2**:89–106.

21 Burke JS, Colby TV, Dermatopathic lymphadenopathy. Comparison of cases associated and unassociated with mycosis fungoides, *Am J Surg Pathol* (1981) 5:343–52.

22 Block JB, Edgcomb J, Eisen A et al, Mycosis fungoides. Natural history and aspects of its relationship to other malignant lymphomas, *Am J Med* (1963) **34**:228–35.

23 Epstein EH Jr, Levin DL, Schein P et al, Mycosis fungoides. Survival, prognostic features, response to therapy and autopsy findings, *Medicine* (1972) **51**:61–72.

24 Rosen ST, Gore R, Brennan J et al, Evaluation of computed tomography and radionuclide scanning in the staging of cutaneous T cell lymphoma, *Arch Dermatol* (1986) **22**:884–6.

25 Keenan AM, Weinstein JN, Mulshine JL et al, Immunolymphoscintigraphy in patients with lymphoma after subcutaneous injection of indium-111-labeled T101 monoclonal antibody, *J Nucl Med* (1987) **28**:42–6.

26 Wantzin GL, Larsen JK, Christensen IJ et al, Early diagnosis of cutaneous T cell lymphoma by DNA flow cytometry on skin biopsies, *Cancer* (1984) **54**:1348–52.

27 Holloway KB, Flowers FP, Ramos Caro FA, Therapeutic alternatives in cutaneous T cell lymphoma, *J Am Acad Dermatol* (1992) **27**:367–78.

28 Gilchrest BA, Parrish JA, Tannenbaum L et al, Oral methoxsalen photochemotherapy of mycosis fungoides, *Cancer* (1976) **38**:683–9.

29 Vella Briffa D, Warin AP, Photochemotherapy in mycosis fungoides. A study of 73 patients, *Lancet* (1980) **ii**:49–53.

30 Molin L, Thomsen K, Volden G et al, Photochemotherapy (PUVA) in the pre-tumour stage of mycosis fungoides, *Acta Derm-Venereol (Stockholm)* (1980) **61**:47–51.

31 Abel EA, Sendagorta E, Hoppe RT et al, PUVA treatment of erythrodermic and plaque-type mycosis fungoides, *Arch Dermatol* (1987) **123**:897–901.

32 MacKie RM, Foulds IS, McMillan EM et al, The histological changes observed in the skin of patients with mycosis fungoides receiving photochemotherapy, *Clin Exp Dermatol* (1980) **5**:405–13.

33 Cox NH, Jones SK, Downey DJ et al, Cutaneous and ocular side-effects of oral photochemotherapy: results of an 8-year follow-up study, *Br J Dermatol* (1987) **116**:145–52.

34 Van Scott EJ, Kalmanson JD, Complete remission of mycosis fungoides lymphoma induced by topical nitrogen mustard, *Cancer* (1973) **32**:18–30.

35 Price NM, Hoppe RT, Deneau DG, Ointment-based mechlorethamine treatment for mycosis fungoides, *Cancer* (1983) **52**:2214–19.

36 Abel EA, Sendagorta E, Hoppe RT, Cutaneous malignancies and metastatic squamous cell carcinoma following topical therapies for mycosis fungoides, *J Am Acad Dermatol* (1986) **14**:1029–38.

37 Zackheim HS, Epstein E, Crain WR, Topical BCNU for cutaneous T cell lymphoma. A 15 year experience in 143 patients, *J Am Acad Dermatol* (1990) **22**:802–10.

38 Hoppe RT, Fuks Z, Bagshaw MA, The rationale for curative radiotherapy in mycosis fungoides, *Int J Radiat Oncol Biol Phys* (1977) **2**:843–51.

39 Spittle M, Electron beam therapy, *Bull Cancer (Paris)* (1977) **64**:305–11.

40 Braverman IM, Yager NB, Chen M et al, Combined total body electron beam irradiation and chemotherapy for mycosis fungoides, *J Am Acad Dermatol* (1987) **16**:45–60.

41 Kessler JF, Jones SE, Levine N et al, Isotretinoin and cutaneous helper T-cell lymphoma (mycosis fungoides), *Arch Dermatol* (1987) **123**:201–4.

42 Tousignant J, Raymond GP, Light MJ, Treatment of cutaneous T cell lymphoma with the arotinoid Ro 13 6298, *J Am Acad Dermatol* (1987) **16**:167–71.

43 Molin L, Thomsen K, Volden G et al, Oral retinoids in mycosis fungoides and Sézary syndrome: a comparison of isotretinoin and etretinate, *Acta Derm-Venereol (Stockholm)* (1987) **67**:232–6.

44 Mahrle G, Thiele B, Retinoids in cutaneous T cell lymphomas, *Dermatologica* (1987) **175**(suppl 1): 145–50.

45 Bunn PA Jr, Foon KA, Ihde DC et al, Recombinant leukocyte A interferon: an active agent in advanced cutaneous T cell lymphomas, *Ann Intern Med* (1984) **101**:484–7.

46 Bunn PA Jr, Ihde DC, Foon KA, The role of recombinant interferon alfa-2a in the therapy of cutaneous T cell lymphomas, *Cancer* (1986) **57**:1689–95.

47 Vonderheid EC, Thompson R, Smiles KA et al, Recombinant interferon alfa-2b in plaque-phase mycosis fungoides, *Arch Dermatol* (1987) **123**:757–63.

48 Thestrup-Pedersen K, Hammer R, Kaltoft K et al, Treatment of mycosis fungoides with recombinant interferon a-2a (Roferon-A) alone and in combination with etretinate (Tigason), *Br J Dermatol* (1988) **118**:811–18.

49 Parry EJ, MacKie RM, Management of cutaneous T cell lymphoma with PUVA and interferon, *BMJ* (1994) **308**:858–9.

50 Edelson R, Berger C, Gasparro F et al, Treatment of cutaneous T cell lymphoma by extracorporeal photochemotherapy, *N Engl J Med* (1987) **316**:297–303.

51 Zic J, Arsubiaga C, Salhany KE et al, Extracorporeal photopheresis for cutaneous T cell lymphoma, *J Am Acad Dermatol* (1992) **27**:729–36.

52 Heald P, Rook A, Perez M et al, Treatment of erythrodermic cutaneous T cell lymphoma with extracorporeal photochemotherapy, *J Am Acad Dermatol* (1992) **27**:427–33.

53 Burrows NP, Humanised monoclonal antibody therapy for psoriasis with radiolabeled monoclonal antibodies, *Radiology* (1987) **165**:297–304.

54 Willemze R, Diagnostic criteria in Sézary's syndrome, *J Invest Dermatol* (1983) **81**:392–7.

55 Weiselthier J, Koh H, Sézary syndrome. Diagnosis prognosis and critical review of treatment options, *J Am Acad Dermatol* (1990) **22**:381–401.

56 Buechner SA, Winkelmann RK, Sézary syndrome. A clinicopathologic study of 39 cases, *Arch Dermatol* (1983) **119**:979–86.

57 Winkelmann RK, Perry HO, Muller SA et al, Treatment of Sézary syndrome, *Mayo Clin Proc* (1974) **49**:590–2.

58 Woringer F, Kolopp P, Lésion érythematosquameuse polycyclique de l'avant bras évoluant depuis 6 ans chez un garconnet de 13 ans. Histologiquement infiltrat intraépidermique d'apparence tumorale, *Ann Derm-Venereol* (1939) **10**:945–58.

59 Mandojana RM, Helwig EB, Localized epidermotropic reticulosis (Woringer–Kolopp disease), *J Am Acad Dermatol* (1983) **8**:813–29.

60 MacKie RM, Turbitt ML, A case of Pagetoid reticulosis bearing the T cytotoxic suppressor surface marker on the lymphoid infiltrate: further evidence that Pagetoid reticulosis is not a variant of mycosis fungoides, *Br J Dermatol* (1984) **110**:89–94.

61 Geerts MI, Kaiserling E, Kint A, Microenvironment of Woringer–Kolopp disease, *Dermatologica* (1982) **164**:15–29.

62 Willemze R, Beljaards RC, Spectrum of primary cutaneous CD 30 Ki 1 positive lymphoproliferative disorders, *J Am Acad Dermatol* (1993) **28**:973–80.

63 Macaulay WL, Lymphomatoid papulosis, *Arch Dermatol* (1968) **97**:23–30.

64 Thomsen K, Wantzin GL, Lymphomatoid papulosis. A follow-up study of 30 patients, *J Am Acad Dermatol* (1987) **17**:632–6.

65 Willemze R, Meyer CJLM, Van Vloten WA et al, The clinical and histological spectrum of lymphomatoid papulosis, *Br J Dermatol* (1982) **107**:131–44.

66 Lederman JS, Sober AJ, Harrist TJ et al, Lymphomatoid papulosis following Hodgkin's disease, *J Am Acad Dermatol* (1987) **16**:331–5.

67 Wantzin GL, Thomsen K, Methotrexate in lymphomatoid papulosis, *Br J Dermatol* (1984) **111**:93–5.

68 Ive FA, Magnus IA, Warin RP et al, 'Actinic reticuloid': a chronic dermatosis associated with severe photosensitivity and the histological resemblance to lymphoma, *Br J Dermatol* (1969) **81**:469–85.

69 Kingston TP, Lowe NJ, Sofen HL et al, Actinic reticuloid in a black man: successful therapy with azathioprine, *J Am Acad Dermatol* (1987) **16**:1079–83.

70 Black MM, Wilson Jones E, 'Lymphomatoid' pityriasis lichenoides: a variant with histological features simulating a lymphoma, *Br J Dermatol* (1972) **86**:329–47.

71 Liebow AA, Carrington CRB, Friedmann PJ, Lymphomatoid granulomatosis, *Hum Pathol* (1972) **3**:457–8.

72 Katzenstein A-LA, Carrington CB, Liebow AA, Lymphomatoid granulomatosis. A clinicopathologic study of 152 cases, *Cancer* (1979) **43**:360–73.

73 Kessler S, Lund HZ, Leonard DD, Cutaneous lesions of lymphomatoid granulomatosis. Comparison with lymphomatoid papulosis, *Am J Dermatopathol* (1981) **3**:115–27.

74 Jambrosic J, From L, Assaad DA et al, Lymphomatoid granulomatosis, *J Am Acad Dermatol* (1987) **17**:621–31.

75 Willemze R, Meijer CJLM, Sentis HJ et al, Primary cutaneous large cell lymphomas of follicular center cell origin. A clinical follow-up study of 19 patients, *J Am Acad Dermatol* (1987) **16**:518–26.

76 Wick MR, Mills SE, Scheithauer BW et al, Reassessment of malignant 'angioendotheliomatosis'. Evidence in favour of its reclassification as 'intravascular lymphomatosis', *Am J Surg Pathol* (1986) **10**:112–23.

77 Willemze R, Kruyswijk MRJ, De Bruin CD et al, Angiotropic (intravascular) large cell lymphoma of the skin previously classified as malignant angioendotheliomatosis, *Br J Dermatol* (1987) **116**:393–9.

78 White RM, Patterson JW, Cutaneous involvement in Hodgkin's disease, *Cancer* (1985) **55**:1136–45.

79 Toonstra J, Van Der Putte SCJ, Kalsbeek GL, Multilobulated cutaneous T cell lymphoma, *Dermatologica* (1983) **166**:128–35.

80 Rowland Payne CME, Meyrick Thomas RH, Black MM, Crosti's indolent lymphoma and persistent superficial dermatitis, *Clin Exp Dermatol* (1984) **9**:303–8.

81 Pinkus GS, Said GW, Hargreaves H, Malignant lymphoma, T cell type. A distinct morphological variety with large multilobulated nuclei, *Am J Clin Pathol* (1979) **72**:540–50.

82 Wells GC, Whimster IW, Subcutaneous angiolymphoid hyperplasia with eosinophilia, *Br J Dermatol* (1969) **81**:1–15.

83 Wilson Jones E, Bleehen SS, Pseudo or atypical pyogenic granuloma, *Br J Dermatol* (1969) **81**:804–16.

84 Pinkus H, Alopecia mucinosa, *Arch Dermatol* (1957) **76**:419–26.

85 Emmerson RW, Follicular mucinosis, *Br J Dermatol* (1969) **81**:395–413.

86 Lichtenstein L, Histiocytosis X integration of eosinophilic granuloma of bone, Letterer–Siwe disease, and Schuller Christian disease as related manifestations of a single nosologic entity, *Arch Pathol* (1953) **56**:84–102.

87 Writing Group of the Histiocyte Society, Histiocytic syndromes in children, *Lancet* (1987) **i**:208–9.

88 Esterly NB, Maurer HS, Gonzalez-Crussi F, Histiocytosis X: a seven-year experience at a children's hospital, *J Am Acad Dermatol* (1985) **13**:481–96.

89 Vollum DI, Letterer–Siwe disease in the adult, *Clin Exp Dermatol* (1979) **4**:395–406.

90 Helm KF, Lookingbill DP, Marks J Jr, A clinical and pathological study of histiocytosis X in adults, *J Am Acad Dermatol* (1993) **29**:166–70.

91 Pritchard J, Histiocytosis X: natural history and management in childhood, *Clin Exp Dermatol* (1979) **4**:421–33.

92 Longaker MA, Frieden IJ, Leboit P, Sherertz EF, Congenital self healing Langerhans cell histiocytosis. The need for long term follow up, *J Am Acad Dermatol* (1994) **31**:910–16.

Chapter 12

1 Hashimoto K, Lever WF, *Appendage tumours of the skin* (Charles C Thomas: Springfield, Ill. 1968).

2 Headington JT, Tumours of the hair follicle. A review, *Am J Clin Pathol* (1976) **85**:480–514.

3 Azzopardi JG, Laurini R, Inverted follicular keratosis, *J Clin Pathol* (1975) **28**:465–71.

4 Pinkus H, Cosket R, Burgess GH, Trichodiscoma, *J Invest Dermatol* (1974) **63**:212–18.

5 Balus L, Crovato F, Breathnach AS, Familial multiple trichodiscomas, *J Am Acad Dermatol* (1986) **15**:603–7.

6 Mehregan AH, Butler JD, A tumour of the follicular infundibulum, *Arch Dermatol* (1961) **83**:924–7.

7 Headington JT, French AJ, Primary neoplasms of the hair follicle, *Arch Dermatol* (1962) **86**:430–41.

8 Wong Ty, Suster S, Tricholemmal carcinoma, *Am J Dermatopathol* (1994) **16**:463–73.

9 Malherbe A, Chenantais J, Note sur l'épithéliome calcifié des glandes sebacées, *Prog Med* (1880) **8**:826–8.

10 Schlechter MD, Hartsough NA, Guttman FM, Multiple pilomatricomas, *Pediatr Dermatol* (1984) **2**:23–5.

11 Forbis R, Helwig EB, Pilomatrixoma, *Arch Dermatol* (1961) **83**:606–18.

12 Harper PS, Calcifying epithelioma of Malherbe, *Arch Dermatol* (1972) **106**:76–8.

13 Rothman D, Kendall AB, Baldi A, Giant pilomatricoma, *Arch Surg* (1976) **111**:86–7.

14 Lopansri S, Mihm MC, Pilomatrixoma carcinoma, *Cancer* (1980) **45**:2368–73.

15 Giudicci AA, Hyman AB, Ectopic sebaceous glands, *Dermatologica* (1962) **125**:44–63.

16 Prioleau PG, Santa Cruz DJ, Sebaceous gland neoplasms, *J Cutan Pathol* (1984) **11**:396–414.

17 Rulon DB, Helwig EB, Cutaneous sebaceous neoplasms, *Cancer* (1974) **33**:82–102.

18 Rao NA, Hidayat AA, McLean IW et al, Sebaceous carcinoma of the ocular adnexa, *Hum Pathol* (1982) **13**:113–22.

19 Doxanas MT, Green WR, Sebaceous gland carcinoma. A review of 40 cases, *Arch Ophthalmol* (1984) **102**:245–9.

20 Mehregan AH, Supernumerary nipple. A histologic study, *J Cutan Pathol* (1981) **8**:96–104.

21 Smith JD, Chernovsky ME, Apocrine hidrocystoma, *Arch Dermatol* (1974) **109**:700–2.

22 Pinkus H, Life history of naevus syringadenomatosus papilliferus, *Arch Dermatol* (1954) **69**:305–22.

23 Mecker JH, Neubecker RD, Helwig EB, Hidradenoma papilliferum, *Am J Clin Pathol* (1962) **37**:182–95.

24 Warkel RL, Selected apocrine neoplasms, *J Cutan Pathol* (1984) **11**:437–49.

25 Paties C, Taccagni GL, Papotti M, Valente G, Zangrandi A, Aloi F, Apocrine carcinoma of the skin, *Cancer* (1993) **71**:375–81.

26 Urbach F, Graham JH, Goldstein J, Dermal eccrine cylindroma, *Arch Dermatol* (1963) **88**:888–94.

27 Crain RC, Helwig EB, Dermal eccrine cylindroma, *Am J Clin Pathol* (1961) **35**:504–15.

28 Brownstein MH, The genodermopathology of adnexal tumours, *J Cutan Pathol* (1984) **11**:457–65.

29 Luger A, Das Cylindrom der Haut und seine maligne Degeneration, *Arch Dermatol Syph (Berlin)* (1949) **188**:155–80.

30 Weedon D, Eccrine tumours. A selective review, *J Cutan Pathol* (1984) **11**:421–36.

31 Smith JLS, Coburn JG, Hidroacanthoma simplex, *Br J Dermatol* (1956) **68**:400–18.

32 Pinkus H, Rogin JR, Goldman P, Eccrine poroma, *Arch Dermatol* (1956) **74**:511–21.

33 Bottles K, Sagebiel RW, McNutt NS et al, Malignant eccrine poroma, *Cancer* (1984) **53**:1579–85.

34 Mehregan AH, Hashimoto K, Rahbari H, Eccrine adenocarcinoma, *Arch Dermatol* (1983) **119**:104–16.

35 Winkelmann RK, McLeod WA, The dermal duct tumour, *Arch Dermatol* (1966) **94**:50–5.

36 Smith JD, Chernovsky ME, Hidrocystomas, *Arch Dermatol* (1973) **108**:676–9.

37 Sperling LC, Sakas EL, Eccrine hidrocystomas, *J Am Acad Dermatol* (1982) **7**:763–70.

38 Kersting DW, Helwig EB, Eccrine spiradenomas, *Arch Dermatol* (1956) **73**:199–227.

39 Keasbey LE, Hadley GC, Clear cell hidradenoma. Three cases with widespread metastases, *Cancer* (1954) **7**:934–52.

40 Johnson BL, Helwig EB, Eccrine acrospiroma, *Cancer* (1969) **23**:641–57.

41 Hirsch P, Helwig EB, Chondroid syringoma, *Arch Dermatol* (1961) **84**: 835–47.

42 Harrist TJ, Aretz TH, Mihm MC et al, Cutaneous malignant mixed tumour, *Arch Dermatol* (1981) **117**:719–24.

43 Hashimoto K, Gross BG, Lever WF, Syringoma, *J Invest Dermatol* (1966) **46**:150–66.

44 Yung CW, Soltani K, Bernstein JE et al, Unilateral naevoid syringoma, *J Am Acad Dermatol* (1981) **4**:412–16.

45 Urban CD, Cannon JR, Cole RD, Eruptive syringomas in Down's syndrome, *Arch Dermatol* (1981) **117**:374–9.

46 Mendoza S, Helwig EB, Mucinous carcinoma of the skin, *Arch Dermatol* (1971) **103**:69–78.

47 Cooper PH, Adelson G, Holthaus W, Primary cutaneous adenoid cystic carcinoma, *Arch Dermatol* (1984) **120**:774–77.

48 Seab JA, Graham JH, Primary cutaneous adenoid cystic carcinoma, *J Am Acad Dermatol* (1987) **17**:113–18.

49 Goldstein DJ, Barr RJ, Santa Cruz D, Microcystic adnexal carcinoma. A distinct clinicopathological entity, *Cancer* (1982) **50**:566–72.

50 Lupton GP, McMarlin SL, Microcystic adnexal carcinoma, *Arch Dermatol* (1986) **122**:286–9.

51 Cooper PH, Microcystic adnexal carcinoma, *Arch Dermatol* (1986) **122**:261–4.

Chapter 13

1 Enzinger FM, Weiss SW, *Soft tissue tumours* 2nd edn (CV Mosby: St Louis 1988).

2 Argenyi ZB, Recent developments in cutaneous neural neoplasms, *J Cutan Pathol* (1993) **20**:97–108.

3 Das Gupta TK, Brasfield RD, Strong EW et al, Benign solitary schwannomas (Neurilemmomas), *Cancer* (1969) **24**:355–66.

4 Megahed M, Plexiform schwannoma, *Am J Dermatopathol* (1994) **16**:288–93.

5 Megahed M, Ruzicka T, Cellular schwannoma, *Am J Dermatopathol* (1994) **16**:418–21.

6 Reed RJ, Fine RM, Meltzer HD, Palisaded, encapsulated neuromas of the skin, *Arch Dermatol* (1972) **106**:865–70.

7 Megahed M, Palisaded encapsulated neuroma, *Am J Dermatopathol* (1994) **16**:120–5.

8 Megahed M, Histopathological variants of neurofibroma, *Am J Dermatopathol* (1994) **16**:486–95.

9 Cawthon RM, A major sequence of the NF type 1 gene, *Cell* (1990) **62**:193–200.

10 D'Agostino AN, Soule EH, Miller RH, Sarcomas of the peripheral nerves and somatic soft tissues associated with multiple neurofibromatosis (von Recklinghausen's disease), *Cancer* (1963) **16**:1015–27.

11 Giordillo PP, Helson L, Hajdu SI et al, Malignant schwannoma. Clinical characterizing and response to therapy, *Cancer* (1981) **47**:2503–9.

12 Frigerio B, Capella C, Eusebi V et al, Merkel cell carcinoma of the skin: the structure and origin of normal Merkel cells, *Histopathology* (1983) 7:229–49.

13 Merkel F, Tastzellen und Tastkörperchen bei den Hausthieren und beim Menschen, *Arch Mikrosk Anat* (1876) **11**:636–52.

14 Warner TFCS, Uno H, Reza Hafez G et al, Merkel cells and Merkel cell tumours, *Cancer* (1983) **52**:238–45.

15 Toker C, Trabecular carcinoma of the skin, *Arch Dermatol* (1972) **105**:107–10.

16 Tang C-K, Toker C, Trabecular carcinoma of the skin. An ultrastructural study, *Cancer* (1978) **42**:2311–21.

17 Leong AS-Y, Phillips GE, Pieterse AS et al, Criteria for the diagnosis of primary endocrine carcinoma of the skin (Merkel cell carcinoma). A histological, immuno-histochemical and ultrastructural study of 13 cases, *Pathology* (1986) **18**:393–9.

18 Hall PA, D'Ardenne AJ, Butler MG et al, Cytokeratin and laminin immunostaining in the diagnosis of neuroendocrine tumours, *Histopathology* (1986) **10**:1179–91.

19 Murray JC, Pollack SV, Pinnell SR, Keloids: a review, *J Am Acad Dermatol* (1981) **4**:461–70.

20 Linares HA, Larson DC, Early differential diagnosis between hypertrophic and non-hypertrophic healing, *J Invest Dermatol* (1974) **62**:514–16.

21 Cerio R, Spaull J, Jones EW, Dermatofibroma: a tumor of dermal dendrocytes? *J Cutan Pathol* (1987) **14**:351.

22 Arnold HL, Tildon IL, Histiocytoma cutis, *Arch Dermatol* (1943) **47**:498–516.

23 Caron GA, Clink HM, Clinical association of basal cell epithelioma with histiocytoma, *Arch Dermatol* (1964) **90**:271–3.

24 Schoenfeld RJ, Epidermal proliferations overlying histiocytomas, *Arch Dermatol* (1964) **90**:266–70.

25 Nickel WR, Reed WB, Tuberous sclerosis, *Arch Dermatol* (1962) **85**:209–26.

26 Darier J, Ferrand M, Dermatofibromas progressifs et récidivants ou fibrosarcomes de la peau, *Ann Dermatol Syph* (1924) **5**:545–62.

27 Taylor HB, Helwig EG, Dermatofibrosarcoma protuberans. A study of 115 cases, *Cancer* (1962) **15**:717–25.

28 Bednar B, Storiform neurofibromas of the skin, pigmented and non-pigmented, *Cancer* (1957) **10**:368–75.

29 Dahl L, Atypical fibroxanthoma of the skin. A clinico-pathological study of 57 cases, *Acta Pathol Microbiol Scand* (1976) **84**:183–201.

30 Fretzin DF, Helwig EB, Atypical fibroxanthoma of the skin. A clinicopathological study of 140 cases, *Cancer* (1973) **31**:1541–52.

31 Worrell JT, Ansari MQ, Ansari SJ, Cockerell CJ, Atypical fibroxanthoma. DNA ploidy analysis of 14 cases with possible histogenetic implications, *J Cutan Pathol* (1993) **20**:211–15.

32 Michie BA, Reid RP, Fallowfield ME, Aneuploidy in atypical fibroxanthoma DNA content: quantitation of 10 cases by image analysis, *J Cutan Pathol* (1994) **20**:404–7.

33 O'Brien JE, Stout AP, Malignant fibrous xanthomas, *Cancer* (1964) **17**:1445–58.

34 Weiss SW, Enzinger FM, Malignant fibrous histiocytoma. An analysis of 200 cases, *Cancer* (1978) **41**:2250–66.

35 Fletcher CDM, McKee PH, Sarcomas – a clinico-pathological guide with particular reference to cutaneous manifestation. I. Dermatofibrosarcoma protuberans, malignant fibrous histiocytoma and the epithelioid sarcoma of Enzinger, *Clin Exp Dermatol* (1984) **9**:451–65.

36 Enzinger FM, Angiomatoid malignant fibrous histiocytoma, *Cancer* (1979) **44**:2147–57.

37 Warner J, Wilson Jones E, Pyogenic granuloma recurring with multiple satellites. A report of 11 cases, *Br J Dermatol* (1968) **80**:218–27.

38 Johnson WC, The pathology of cutaneous vascular tumours. A review, *Int J Dermatol* (1976) **15**:239–70.

39 Imperial R, Helwig EB, Angiokeratoma, *Arch Dermatol* (1967) **95**:166–75.

40 Masson P, Le glomus neuromyo-artériel des regions tactiles et ses tumeurs, *Lyon Chir* (1924) **21**:257–80.

41 Goodman TF, Abele DC, Multiple glomus tumours, *Arch Dermatol* (1971) **103**:11–23.

42 Rycroft RJG, Menter MA, Sharvill DE et al, Hereditary multiple glomus tumours, *Trans St John's Hosp Dermatol Soc* (1975) **61**:70–81.

43 Tsuneyoshi M, Enjoji M, Glomus tumour, *Cancer* (1982) **50**:1601–7.

44 Whimster IW, The pathology of lymphangioma circumscriptum, *Br J Dermatol* (1976) **94**:473–86.

45 Wilson Jones E, Malignant vascular tumours, *Clin Exp Dermatol* (1976) **1**:287–312.

46 Maddox JC, Evans HL, Angiosarcoma of skin and soft tissue. A study of 44 cases, *Cancer* (1981) **48**:1907–21.

47 Leader M, Collins M, Petel J et al, Staining for Factor VIII-related antigen and Ulex europaeus agglutinin 1 in 230 tumours. An assessment of their specificity for angiosarcoma and Kaposi's sarcoma, *Histopathology* (1986) **10**:1153–63.

48 Holden CA, Spittle MF, Wilson Jones E, Angiosarcoma of the face and scalp. Prognosis and treatment, *Cancer* (1987) **48**:1907–21.

49 Reynolds WA, Winkelman RK, Soule EH, Kaposi's sarcoma. A review, *Medicine (Baltimore)* (1965) **44**:419–43.

50 Lemlich G, Schwam L, Lebwohl M, Kaposi's sarcoma and acquired immunodeficiency syndrome, *J Am Acad Dermatol* (1987) **16**:319–25.

51 Friedman Kien AE, Kaposi's sarcoma in HIV infected homosexual men, *Lancet* (1990) **335**:168–70.

52 Chang Y, Cesarman E, Pessin MS et al, Identification of herpes like DNA sequences in Aids associated Kaposi's sarcoma, *Science* (1994) **266**:1865–9.

53 Cox FH, Helwig EG, Kaposi's sarcoma. A review, *Cancer* (1959) **12**:289–98.

54 Blumenfeld W, Egbert BM, Sagebiel RW, Differential diagnosis of Kaposi's sarcoma, *Arch Pathol Lab Med* (1985) **109**:123–7.

55 Piette WW, The incidence of second malignancies in subsets of Kaposi's sarcoma, *J Am Acad Dermatol* (1987) **16**:855–61.

56 Headington JT, Beals TF, Niederhuber JE, Primary leiomyosarcoma of skin, *J Cutan Pathol* (1977) **4**:308–17.

57 Stout AP, Liposarcoma – the malignant tumour of lipoblasts, *Ann Surg* (1944) **119**:86–107.

58 Enzinger FM, Clear cell sarcoma of tendons and aponeuroses. An analysis of 21 cases, *Cancer* (1968) **18**:1163–72.

59 Bearman RM, Noe J, Kempson R, Clear cell sarcoma with melanin pigment, *Cancer* (1975) **36**:977–90.

60 Boudreaux D, Waisman J, Clear cell sarcoma with melanogenesis, *Cancer* (1978) **41**:1387–92.

61 Brady LW, O'Neill EA, Farber SH, Unusual sites of metastases, *Semin Oncol* (1972) **4**:59–64.

62 Mehregan AH, Metastatic carcinoma to the skin, *Dermatologica* (1961) **123**:311–25.

63 Brownstein MH, Helwig EB, Patterns of cutaneous metastases, *Arch Dermatol* (1972) **105**:862–8.

Chapter 14

1 Bohan A, Peter JB, Polymyositis and dermatomyositis, *N Engl J Med* (1975) **292**:344–7.

2 Christianson HB, Brunsting LA, Perry HO, Dermatomyositis. Unusual features, complications and treatment, *Arch Dermatol* (1956) **74**:581–9.

3 Arundell FD, Wilkinson RD, Haserick JR, Dermatomyositis and malignant neoplasms in adults, *Arch Dermatol* (1960) **82**:772–5.

4 Callen JP, Hyla JF, Bole GG Jr et al, The relationship of dermatomyositis and polymyositis to internal malignancy, *Arch Dermatol* (1980) **116**:295–8.

5 Medsger TA Jr, Dawson WN, Masi AT, The epidemiology of polymyositis, *Am J Med* (1970) **48**:715–23.

6 Lakhanpal S, Bunch TW, Ilstrup DM et al, Polymyositis dermatomyositis and malignant lesions: does an association exist? *Mayo Clin Proc* (1986) **61**:645–53.

7 Saikia NK, Extraction of pemphigus antibodies from a lymphoid neoplasm and its possible relationship to pemphigus vulgaris, *Br J Dermatol* (1972) **86**:411–14.

8 Anhalt GJ, Kim SC, Stanley JR, Paraneoplastic pemphigus, *N Engl J Med* (1990) **323**:1729–35.

9 Camisa C, Helm TN, Liu YC et al, Paraneoplastic pemphigus, *J Am Acad Dermatol* (1992) **27**:547–53.

10 Horn TD, Anhalt GJ, Histologic features of paraneoplastic pemphigus, *Arch Dermatol* (1992) **128**:1091–95.

11 Stone SP, Schroeter AL, Bullous pemphigoid and associated malignant neoplasms, *Arch Dermatol* (1975) **111**:991–4.

12 Saikia NK, MacKie RM, McQueen A, A case of bullous pemphigoid and figurate erythema in association with metastatic spread of carcinoma, *Br J Dermatol* (1973) **88**:331–4.

13 Mansson T, Malignant disease in dermatitis herpetiformis, *Acta Derm-Venereol (Stockholm)* (1971) **51**:379–82.

14 Becker SW, Khan D, Rothman S, Cutaneous manifestations of internal malignant tumours, *Arch Dermatol* (1942) **45**:1069–81.

15 Church RE, Crane WAJ, A cutaneous syndrome associated with islet-cell carcinoma of the pancreas, *Br J Dermatol* (1967) **79**:284–6.

16 Mallinson CN, Bloom SR, Warin AP et al, A glucagonoma syndrome, *Lancet* (1974) **ii**:15–17.

17 Binnick AN, Spencer SK, Dennison WL Jr et al, Glucagonoma syndrome, *Arch Dermatol* (1977) **113**:749–54.

18 Goodenberger DM, Lawley TJ, Strober W et al, Necrolytic migratory erythema without glucagonoma, *Arch Dermatol* (1979) **115**:1429–32.

19 Lazar P, Cancer, erythema annulare centrifugum, autoimmunity, *Arch Dermatol* (1963), **87**:246–51.

20 Gammel JA, Erythema gyratum repens, *Arch Dermatol* (1952) **66**:494–505.

21 Curth HO, Significance of acanthosis nigricans, *Arch Dermatol* (1952) **66**:80–100.

22 Curth HO, Aschner BM, Genetic studies on acanthosis nigricans, *Arch Dermatol* (1959) **79**:55–66.

23 Rigel DS, Jacobs MI, Malignant acanthosis nigricans: a review, *J Dermatol Surg Oncol* (1980) **6**:923–7.

24 Ellis DL, Kafka SP, Chow JC et al, Melanoma, growth factors, acanthosis nigricans, the sign of Leser Trélat, and multiple acrochordons, *N Engl J Med* (1987) **317**:1582–7.

25 Abeloff MD, Paraneoplastic syndromes. A window on the biology of cancer, *N Engl J Med* (1987) **317**:1598–1600.

26 Curry SS, King LE, The sign of Leser Trélat, *Arch Dermatol* (1980) **116**:1059–60.

27 Bazex A, Salvador R, Dupre A et al, Syndrome paranéoplastique a type d'hyperkeratose des extremités, *Bull Soc Fr Dermatol Syph* (1965) **72**:182–7.

28 Bazex A, Griffiths A, Acrokeratosis paraneoplastica - a new cutaneous marker of malignancy, *Br J Dermatol* (1980) **102**:301–6.

29 Jacobsen FK, Abildtrup N, Laursen SO et al, Acrokeratosis paraneoplastica (Bazex' syndrome), *Arch Dermatol* (1984) **120**:502–4.

30 Pecora AL, Landsman L, Imgrund SP et al, Acrokeratosis paraneoplastica (Bazex' syndrome), *Arch Dermatol* (1983) **119**:820–6.

31 Richard M, Giroux J-M, Acrokeratosis paraneoplastica (Bazex' syndrome), *J Am Acad Dermatol* (1987) **16**:178–83.

32 Ikeya T, Izumi A, Suzuki M, Acquired hypertrichosis lanuginosa, *Dermatologica* (1978) **156**:274–82.

33 Price ML, Hall Smith SP, Hypertrichosis lanuginosa, *Clin Exp Dermatol* (1985) **10**:255–7.

34 Jemec GBE, Hypertrichosis lanuginosa acquisita, *Arch Dermatol* (1986) **122**:805–8.

35 Paul R, Paul R, Jansen CT, Itch and malignancy prognosis in generalized pruritus: a 6-year follow-up of 125 patients, *J Am Acad Dermatol* (1987) **16**:1179–82.

Chapter 15

1 MacKie RM, Osterlind A, Ruiter D et al, Report on consensus meeting of the EORTC Melanoma Group on educational needs for primary and secondary prevention of melanoma in Europe, *Eur J Cancer* (1991) **27**:1317–23.

2 Temoshok L, Di Clement RJ, Sweet DM et al, Factors relating to patient delay in seeking attention for cutaneous malignant melanoma, *Cancer* (1984) **54**:3048–53.

3 Grin CM, Kopf AW, Welkovich B et al, Accuracy in the clinical diagnosis of malignant melanoma, *Arch Dermatol* (1990) **126**:763–6.

4 Doherty VR, MacKie RM, Experience of a public education programme on early detection of cutaneous malignant melanoma, *BMJ* (1988) **287**:388–91.

5 Cristofolini M, Zumiani M, Boi S et al, Community detection of early melanoma, *Lancet* (1986) **i**:18.

6 Cristofolini M, Bianchi R, Sebastiana B et al, Analysis of the cost effectiveness ratio of the health campaign for the early diagnosis of cutaneous melanoma in Trentino, Italy, *Cancer* (1993) **71**:370–4.

7 Doherty VR, MacKie RM, Reasons for poor prognosis in British patients with cutaneous malignant melanoma, *BMJ* (1986) **292**:987–9.

8 MacKie RM, Hole D, Audit of public education campaign to encourage earlier detection of malignant melanoma, *BMJ* (1992) **304**:1012–15.

9 Rampen FHJ, van Huystee BEWL, Kiemeney LALM, Melanoma/skin cancer screening clinics: experiences in the Netherlands, *J Am Acad Dermatol* (1991) **25**:776–7.

10 Rampen FHJ, Berretty PJM, van Huystee BEWL et al, Lack of selective attendance of participants at skin cancer/melanoma screening clinics, *J Am Acad Dermatol* (1993) **29**:423–7.

11 Hoffmann K, Dirschka Th, Schatz H et al, A local education campaign on early diagnosis of malignant melanoma, *Eur J Epidemiol* (1993) **9**:591–8.

12 Pehamberger H, Binder M, Knollmayer S et al, Immediate effects of a public education campaign on prognostic feature of melanoma, *J Am Acad Dermatol* (1993) **29**:106–9.

13 Bulliard JL, Raymond L, Levi F et al, Prevention of cutaneous melanoma: an epidemiological evaluation of the Swiss campaign, *Rev Epiderm Santé Publ* (1992) **40**:431–8.

14 Koh HK, Lew RA, Prout MN, Screening for melanoma/skin cancer: theoretic and practical considerations, *J Am Acad Dermatol* (1989) **20**:159–72.

15 Koh HK, Geller AC, Miller DR et al, Who is being screened for melanoma/skin cancer? *J Am Acad Dermatol* (1991) **24**:271–7.

16 Goldenhersh MA, Melanoma screening: critique and proposal, *J Am Acad Dermatol* (1993) **28**:642–4.

17 Mcleod GR, Control of melanoma in a high risk population, *Pigment Cell* (1988) **9**:131–40.

18 Marks R, Hill D, *The public health approach to melanoma control: prevention and early detection* (Australian Cancer Society: Melbourne 1992) 23–4.

19 Boldeman C, Ullen H, Mansson-Brahme E et al, Primary prevention of malignant melanoma in the Stockholm Cancer Prevention Programme, *Eur J Cancer Prevention* (1993) **2**:441–6.

20 Walter SD, Marrett LD, From L et al, Association of cutaneous malignant melanoma with the use of sunbeds and sunlamps, *Am J Epidemiol* (1990) **131**:232–4.

21 Sverdlow AJ, English JSC, MacKie RM et al, Fluorescent lamps, ultraviolet lamps and the risk of cutaneous melanoma, *BMJ* (1987) **297**:647–50.

22 Autier P, Dore J-F, Lejeune F et al, Cutaneous malignant melanoma and exposure to sunlamps or sunbeds: an EORTC multicenter case-control study in Belgium, France and Germany, *Int J Cancer* (1994) **58**:809–13.

23 MacKie RM, Freudenberger T, Aitchison TC, Personal risk factor chart for melanoma, *Lancet* (1989) **ii**:487–90.

24 Garbe C, Buttner P, Weiss J et al, Risk factors for developing cutaneous melanoma and criteria for identifying persons at risk: multicenter case-control study of the central malignant melanoma, *J Invest Dermatol* (1994) **102**:695–9.

25 Garbe C, Buttner P, Weiss J et al, Associated factors in the prevalence of more than 50 common melanocytic nevi, atypical melanocytic nevi, and actinic lentigines: multicenter case-control study of the central malignant melanoma registry of the German Dermatological Society, *J Invest Dermatol* (1994) **102**:700–5.

26 Moseley H, MacKie RM, Ferguson J, The suitability of SunCheck patches and Tanscan cards for monitoring the sunburning effectiveness of sunlight, *Br J Dermatol* (1993) **128**:75–8.

Index